COVID-19 and Gastrointestinal Disease: Current Insights and Future Management

COVID-19 and Gastrointestinal Disease: Current Insights and Future Management

Editor

Hemant Goyal

MDPI • Basel • Beijing • Wuhan • Barcelona • Belgrade • Manchester • Tokyo • Cluj • Tianjin

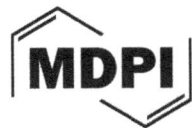

Editor
Hemant Goyal
The Wright Center for
Graduate Medical Education
USA

Editorial Office
MDPI
St. Alban-Anlage 66
4052 Basel, Switzerland

This is a reprint of articles from the Special Issue published online in the open access journal *Journal of Clinical Medicine* (ISSN 2077-0383) (available at: https://www.mdpi.com/journal/jcm/special_issues/COVID_GD).

For citation purposes, cite each article independently as indicated on the article page online and as indicated below:

LastName, A.A.; LastName, B.B.; LastName, C.C. Article Title. *Journal Name* **Year**, *Volume Number*, Page Range.

ISBN 978-3-0365-6089-2 (Hbk)
ISBN 978-3-0365-6090-8 (PDF)

© 2022 by the authors. Articles in this book are Open Access and distributed under the Creative Commons Attribution (CC BY) license, which allows users to download, copy and build upon published articles, as long as the author and publisher are properly credited, which ensures maximum dissemination and a wider impact of our publications.
The book as a whole is distributed by MDPI under the terms and conditions of the Creative Commons license CC BY-NC-ND.

Contents

Marko Zelenika, Marko Lucijanic, Tomislav Bokun, Tonci Bozin, Mislav Barisic Jaman, Ida Tjesic Drinkovic, Frane Pastrovic, Anita Madir, Ivica Luksic, Nevenka Piskac Zivkovic, et al.
FibroScan-AST Score Predicts 30-Day Mortality or Need for Mechanical Ventilation among Patients Hospitalized with COVID-19
Reprinted from: *J. Clin. Med.* **2021**, *10*, 4355, doi:10.3390/jcm10194355 1

Liliana Łykowska-Szuber, Karolina Wołodźko, Anna Maria Rychter, Aleksandra Szymczak-Tomczak, Iwona Krela-Kaźmierczak and Agnieszka Dobrowolska
Liver Injury in Patients with Coronavirus Disease 2019 (COVID-19)—A Narrative Review
Reprinted from: *J. Clin. Med.* **2021**, *10*, 5048, doi:10.3390/jcm10215048 13

Gian Eugenio Tontini, Giovanni Aldinio, Nicoletta Nandi, Alessandro Rimondi, Dario Consonni, Massimo Iavarone, Paolo Cantù, Angelo Sangiovanni, Pietro Lampertico and Maurizio Vecchi
An Unprecedented Challenge: The North Italian Gastroenterologist Response to COVID-19
Reprinted from: *J. Clin. Med.* **2022**, *11*, 109, doi:10.3390/jcm11010109 25

Dragos Serban, Laura Carina Tribus, Geta Vancea, Anca Pantea Stoian, Ana Maria Dascalu, Andra Iulia Suceveanu, Ciprian Tanasescu, Andreea Cristina Costea, Mihail Silviu Tudosie, Corneliu Tudor, et al.
Acute Mesenteric Ischemia in COVID-19 Patients
Reprinted from: *J. Clin. Med.* **2022**, *11*, 200, doi:10.3390/jcm11010200 33

Yamile Zabana, Ignacio Marín-Jiménez, Iago Rodríguez-Lago, Isabel Vera, María Dolores Martín-Arranz, Iván Guerra, Javier P. Gisbert, Francisco Mesonero, Olga Benítez, Carlos Taxonera, et al.
Nationwide COVID-19-EII Study: Incidence, Environmental Risk Factors and Long-Term Follow-Up of Patients with Inflammatory Bowel Disease and COVID-19 of the ENEIDA Registry
Reprinted from: *J. Clin. Med.* **2022**, *11*, 421, doi:10.3390/jcm11020421 55

Krzysztof Kaliszewski, Dorota Diakowska, Łukasz Nowak, Urszula Tokarczyk, Maciej Sroczyński, Monika Sępek, Agata Dudek, Karolina Sutkowska-Stępień, Katarzyna Kiliś-Pstrusińska, Agnieszka Matera-Witkiewicz, et al.
Assessment of Gastrointestinal Symptoms and Dyspnea in Patients Hospitalized due to COVID-19: Contribution to Clinical Course and Mortality
Reprinted from: *J. Clin. Med.* **2022**, *11*, 1821, doi:10.3390/jcm11071821 75

Nonthalee Pausawasdi, Ekawat Manomaiwong, Uayporn Kaosombatwattana, Khemajira Karaketklang and Phunchai Charatcharoenwitthaya
The Effects of COVID-19 on Clinical Outcomes of Non-COVID-19 Patients Hospitalized for Upper Gastrointestinal Bleeding during the Pandemic
Reprinted from: *J. Clin. Med.* **2022**, *11*, 2461, doi:10.3390/jcm11092461 93

Ji Eun Ryu, Sung-Goo Kang, Sung Hoon Jung, Shin Hee Lee and Sang-Bum Kang
Psychological Effects and Medication Adherence among Korean Patients with Inflammatory Bowel Disease during the Coronavirus Disease 2019 Pandemic: A Single-Center Survey
Reprinted from: *J. Clin. Med.* **2022**, *11*, 3034, doi:10.3390/jcm11113034 103

Urszula Tokarczyk, Krzysztof Kaliszewski, Anna Kopszak, Łukasz Nowak, Karolina Sutkowska-Stępień, Maciej Sroczyński, Monika Sępek, Agata Dudek, Dorota Diakowska, Małgorzata Trocha, et al.
Liver Function Tests in COVID-19: Assessment of the Actual Prognostic Value
Reprinted from: *J. Clin. Med.* **2022**, *11*, 4490, doi:10.3390/jcm11154490 113

Laure-Alix Clerbaux, Julija Fillipovska, Amalia Muñoz, Mauro Petrillo, Sandra Coecke, Maria-Joao Amorim and Lucia Grenga
Mechanisms Leading to Gut Dysbiosis in COVID-19: Current Evidence and Uncertainties Based on Adverse Outcome Pathways
Reprinted from: *J. Clin. Med.* **2022**, *11*, 5400, doi:10.3390/jcm11185400 131

Laure-Alix Clerbaux, Sally A. Mayasich, Amalia Muñoz, Helena Soares, Mauro Petrillo, Maria Cristina Albertini, Nicolas Lanthier, Lucia Grenga and Maria-Joao Amorim
Gut as an Alternative Entry Route for SARS-CoV-2: Current Evidence and Uncertainties of Productive Enteric Infection in COVID-19
Reprinted from: *J. Clin. Med.* **2022**, *11*, 5691, doi:10.3390/jcm11195691 153

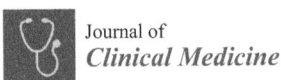

Article

FibroScan-AST Score Predicts 30-Day Mortality or Need for Mechanical Ventilation among Patients Hospitalized with COVID-19

Marko Zelenika [1], Marko Lucijanic [2,3], Tomislav Bokun [1,4], Tonci Bozin [1], Mislav Barisic Jaman [1], Ida Tjesic Drinkovic [1], Frane Pastrovic [1], Anita Madir [3], Ivica Luksic [3,5], Nevenka Piskac Zivkovic [6], Kresimir Luetic [7], Zeljko Krznaric [3,8], Rajko Ostojic [3], Tajana Filipec Kanizaj [3,9], Ivan Bogadi [9], Lucija Virovic Jukic [3,10], Michal Kukla [11] and Ivica Grgurevic [1,3,4,*]

1. Department of Gastroenterology, Hepatology and Clinical Nutrition, University Hospital Dubrava, 10000 Zagreb, Croatia; marko.zelenika@gmail.com (M.Z.); tbokun@gmail.com (T.B.); tbozin@gmail.com (T.B.); mislav.barisic.jaman@gmail.com (M.B.J.); ida.tjesicdrinkovic@gmail.com (I.T.D.); fpastrovic@gmail.com (F.P.)
2. Department of Hematology, University Hospital Dubrava, 10000 Zagreb, Croatia; markolucijanic@yahoo.com
3. School of Medicine, University of Zagreb, 10000 Zagreb, Croatia; anita.madir@gmail.com (A.M.); luksic.ivica@gmail.com (I.L.); zeljko.krznaric1@zg.t-com.hr (Z.K.); rajko.ostojic@gmail.com (R.O.); tajana.filipec@gmail.com (T.F.K.); lucija.jukic@gmail.com (L.V.J.)
4. Faculty of Pharmacy and Biochemistry, University of Zagreb, 10000 Zagreb, Croatia
5. Department of Maxillofacial Surgery, University Hospital Dubrava, 10000 Zagreb, Croatia
6. Department of Pulmology, University Hospital Dubrava, 10000 Zagreb, Croatia; npiskac@gmail.com
7. Department of Gastroenterology and Hepatology, University Hospital Sveti Duh, 10000 Zagreb, Croatia; kresimir.luetic@hlk.hr
8. Department of Gastroenterology and Hepatology, University Hospital Centre Zagreb, 10000 Zagreb, Croatia
9. Department of Gastroenterology and Hepatology, University Hospital Merkur, 10000 Zagreb, Croatia; ivanbogadi08@gmail.com
10. Department of Gastroenterology and Hepatology, University Hospital Sestre Milosrdnice, 10000 Zagreb, Croatia
11. Department of Internal Medicine and Geriatrics, Faculty of Medicine, Jagiellonian University Medical College, 30688 Cracow, Poland; michal.kukla@uj.edu.pl
* Correspondence: ivica.grgurevic@zg.htnet.hr; Tel.: +385-12903434; Fax: +385-12902550

Abstract: Background: Liver involvement in Coronavirus disease 2019 (COVID-19) has been recognised. We aimed to investigate the correlation of non-invasive surrogates of liver steatosis, fibrosis and inflammation using transient elastography (TE) and FibroScan-AST (FAST) score with (a) clinical severity and (b) 30-day composite outcome of mechanical ventilation (MV) or death among patients hospitalized due to COVID-19. Method: Patients with non-critical COVID-19 at admission were included. Liver stiffness measurement (LSM) and controlled attenuation parameter (CAP) were assessed by TE. Clinical severity of COVID-19 was assessed by 4C Mortality Score (4CMS) and need for high-flow nasal cannula (HFNC) oxygen supplementation. Results: 217 patients were included (66.5% males, median age 65 years, 4.6% with history of chronic liver disease). Twenty-four (11.1%) patients met the 30-day composite outcome. Median LSM, CAP and FAST score were 5.2 kPa, 274 dB/m and 0.31, respectively, and neither was associated with clinical severity of COVID-19 at admission. In multivariate analysis FAST > 0.36 (OR 3.19, p = 0.036), 4CMS (OR 1.68, p = 0.002) and HFNC (OR 7.03, p = 0.001) were independent predictors of adverse composite outcome. Conclusion: Whereas LSM and CAP failed to show correlation with COVID-19 severity and outcomes, FAST score was an independent risk factor for 30-day mortality or need for MV.

Keywords: COVID-19; liver; non-alcoholic steatohepatitis; transient elastography; mortality

1. Introduction

Coronavirus disease 2019 (COVID-19) is respiratory disease with multisystem involvement and is responsible for a worldwide pandemic [1]. Reported overall mortality

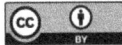

of hospitalized patients is approximately 20%, with considerable variability due to age, comorbidity, level of care and thresholds for hospitalization [2–6]. Risk factors for severe clinical course include older age, male sex, comorbidity, arterial hypertension, diabetes mellitus and obesity [2–7].

Non-alcoholic fatty liver disease (NAFLD) is considered the liver manifestation the metabolic syndrome that includes concomitant presence of obesity, hypertension, diabetes mellitus and dyslipidaemia. NAFLD affects around 25% of adults worldwide, with even greater prevalence among obese individuals (>50%) and those having additional metabolic conditions [8,9]. In line with these facts, the presence of fatty liver might be assumed as the risk factor for more severe forms of COVID-19 and adverse outcomes [10]. In addition, increased hepatic expression of angiotensin-converting enzyme II (ACE2) receptors, as the gate for viral entry in the cells has been demonstrated in patients with non-alcoholic steatohepatitis (NASH) [11]. Several studies have investigated liver involvement in COVID-19, demonstrating worse clinical course of patients with elevated liver functional tests (LFTs) and the presence of cirrhosis [12–14]. On the other hand, patients with non-cirrhotic chronic liver disease (CLD) seem to have comparable survival to patients without CLD. However, more specific data on the prevalence, severity and prognostic impact of liver steatosis, fibrosis and non-alcoholic steatohepatitis (NASH), on the course of COVID-19 are scarce with conflicting results published [15–18]. In fact, there are no specific data considering the impact of NASH, as the inflammatory phenotype of NAFLD, because liver biopsy as the gold standard method to diagnose NASH is rarely performed in the setting of COVID-19. Recently, a non-invasive tool has been developed, called the Fibroscan-AST (FAST) score. This score combines the results of liver stiffness measurement (LSM), steatosis assessment by controlled attenuation parameter (CAP) and aspartate aminotransferase (AST) and has been developed to identify patients with NASH, elevated NAFLD activity score (NAS $\geq$ 4) and significant fibrosis (fibrosis stage F $\geq$ 2) amongst those with NAFLD [19]. In theory, patients who already have liver inflammation due to NASH (as opposed to those with bland steatosis without NASH, and those with a healthy liver) might react with more profound inflammatory response upon contracting COVID-19 and thus have worse clinical outcomes.

In the present study we aimed to investigate the correlation of non-invasive surrogates of liver steatosis, fibrosis and inflammation using transient elastography (TE) and FAST score with (a) severity of clinical presentation and (b) 30-day composite outcome of mechanical ventilation (MV) or death among patients hospitalized with non-critical form of COVID-19 at admission.

2. Patients and Methods

2.1. Patients

This study was performed in the university hospital that was completely re-purposed to serve exclusively as the main regional centre of care for COVID-19 patients during the 2020/2021 pandemic. Those considered for inclusion were non-critically-ill patients admitted to general wards, capable of giving informed consent, over a 3-month period (16 January to 17 April 2021). All patients had positive nasopharyngeal swab for severe acute respiratory syndrome coronavirus 2 (SARS-CoV2) by polymerase chain reaction (PCR) and were admitted following initial examination in the emergency department. Standard work-up in emergency department included blood biochemistry, electrocardiogram, peripheral blood oxygen saturation and chest X-ray. The clinical severity of COVID-19 was initially assessed by using Modified Early Warning Score (MEWS) for each patient [20]. Patients with non-critical form of the disease (MEWS < 5) were admitted to the general ward and those with MEWS $\geq$ 5 were admitted to intensive care unit (ICU). Even if deemed non-critical by MEWS, all patients required oxygen supplementation therapy, and in order to further stratify them, the 4C Mortality Score (4CMS) was calculated for each patient who was hospitalised [21].

Data about the presence of pre-existing chronic liver disease (CLD), including the presence of cirrhosis and previous decompensation, as well as about the alcohol consumption were collected by history taking from each patient and supported by previous medical records. Harmful alcohol intake was considered in patients consuming >30 g/day (males) and >20 g/day (females).

Upon admission to the ward patients were treated by oxygen supplementation by binasal catheters, masks, or high-flow nasal cannula (HFNC) as needed. Other treatment such as dexamethasone or equivalent methylprednisolone dose, remdesivir and low-molecular-weight heparin were instituted according to recommendations by national guidelines [22]. Other therapy was commenced at the discretion of the attending physician, including antibiotics, as well as other medications to treat acute complications and the patients' underlying chronic conditions.

Liver stiffness measurements (LSM) and steatosis assessment by controlled attenuation parameter (CAP) were performed within 72 h from the admission in patients meeting the inclusion criteria: age > 18 years, signed informed consent, non-critical form of COVID-19 at admission (MEWS < 5), and absence of conditions affecting liver stiffness measurement (LSM) (ALT > 5xULN, congestive liver disease, extrahepatic biliary obstruction, infiltrative liver neoplasms) [23].

2.2. Methods
2.2.1. Transient Elastography

Transient elastography (TE) was used to perform LSM and CAP measurements by using Fibroscan device integrated within General Electric Logiq S8 XD Clear ultrasound platform. These examinations were performed in patients after overnight fasting, in the supine position with the right arm in the maximal abduction during the short (3–4 s) apnea period in the neutral breathing position, through the right intercostal approach as recommended by international guidelines [23]. The choice of using Fibroscan M or XL probe was made upon suggestion of automatic probe selection tool embedded within the Fibroscan device [24]. Ten valid LSM had to be performed with the interquartile range of LSM (IQR/Med) < 30%. CAP was automatically measured along with the LSM acquisitions. All examinations were performed by experienced operators (each had previously performed >500 TE examinations).

As the surrogate measure for the presence of significant fibrosis (F $\geq$ 2) in the analysed cohort LSM > 7 kPa was used, whereas LSM $\geq$ 10 kPa was considered representative for advanced fibrosis (F $\geq$ 3) [25,26]. Presence of liver steatosis (S > 0) was considered in patients with CAP > 274 dB/m [27].

2.2.2. Laboratory Tests

Results of blood biochemistry (complete blood counts (CBC), urea, AST, alanine aminotransferase (ALT), gamma glutamyl transferase (GGT), alkaline phosphatase (ALP), bilirubin, prothrombin time (Quick,%), C-reactive protein (CRP)) were obtained no more than 48 h from the time of TE procedure and were recorded for the purpose of this study, except for the patients having HFNC oxygen supplementation in which case we limited this time period to 24 h because of their more unstable clinical course.

FAST score was calculated for each patient using the formula provided by Newsome PN et al.: $FAST = (e^{-1.65 + 1.07 \times \ln(LSM) + 2.66 * 10^{-8} \times CAP^3 - 63.3 \times AST^{-1}})/(1 + e^{-1.65 + 1.07 \times \ln(LSM) + 2.66 * 10^{-8} \times CAP^3 - 63.3 \times AST^{-1}})$ [19]. Using the cut-offs of 0.35 and 0.67, FAST score had $\geq$90 sensitivity and $\geq$90% specificity, respectively to rule-out and rule-in the presence of NASH, elevated NAFLD activity score (NAS $\geq$ 4) and significant fibrosis (fibrosis stage F $\geq$ 2) amongst NAFLD patients in the original study.

As biochemical non-invasive scores for liver fibrosis have also been associated with the outcomes of COVID-19 patients in some reports [28,29], we calculated the following scores according to published formulae in order to compare their prognostic performance to TE:

AST to platelet ratio index (APRI), APRI = ((AST/ULN)/platelet count ($\times 10^9$/L)) $\times$ 100 [30];

Fibrosis-4 index (FIB-4), FIB4 = Age (years) $\times$ AST (IU/L)/platelet count ($\times 10^9$/L) $\times$ ALT (IU/L)1/2 [31];

NAFLD fibrosis score (NFS) = $-1.675 + (0.037 * \text{age (years)}) + (0.094 * \text{BMI (kg/m}^2\text{)}) + (1.13 * \text{Impaired fasting glucose/diabetes (yes = 1, no = 0)}) + (0.99 * \text{AST/ALT ratio}) - (0.013 * \text{platelet count } (\times 10^9/\text{L})) - (0.66 * \text{albumin (g/dL)})$ [32].

2.3. Statistical Analysis

Power analyses were based on assumption of 10% and 25% event rates in the subgroups of interest, type I error of 0.05 and 80% power, suggested that 200 patients had to be included to obtain a statistically significant result. Normality of distribution of numerical variables was tested using the Shapiro–Wilk test. Most of the analysed variables were non-normally distributed and as such all numerical variables are presented as median and interquartile range (IQR) and were compared between groups using the Mann–Whitney U test. Categorical variables are presented as frequencies and percentages and were compared between groups using the X^2 test or the Fisher test where appropriate. Variables acquired by TE (LSM, CAP) and FAST score were compared to the clinically defined outcomes: (a) severity of COVID-19 clinical presentation as assessed by 4CMS or the need for HFNC oxygen supplementation and (b) 30-day mortality or need for MV. ROC curve analysis was used to establish optimal cut-off values of different elastographic measurements for prediction of 30-day mortality. Logistic regression was used to test independent contribution of particular variables to 30-day mortality prediction. p-values < 0.05 were considered statistically significant. All analyses were performed using the MedCalc statistical software version 20 (MedCalc Software Ltd., Ostend, Belgium).

3. Results

3.1. Patient Characteristics

Of 230 patients considered eligible, 217 patients with a non-critical form of COVID-19 at admission (MEWS < 5) were included in the study. In 13/230 patients, LSM was not possible due to obesity or dyspnoea. There were 144/217 (66.4%) males, median age was 65 years, IQR (55–70), median BMI was 28.3 kg/m^2, IQR (25.4–31.5), 70/217 (32.3%) of patients had diabetes and 118/217 (54.4%)—arterial hypertension. Among the participants, 45 (21.1%), 89 (41.8%) and 79 (37.1%) patients had BMI < 25 kg/m^2, 25–30 kg/m^2 and >30 kg/m^2, respectively. History of liver disease was present in 10/217 (4.6%) patients (4 with non-alcoholic fatty liver disease (NAFLD), 4 with alcoholic liver disease (ALD) including 1 with cirrhosis, and 2 patients with chronic hepatitis B). Bilirubin, AST, ALT, GGT and ALP were elevated in 11.5%, 55.3%, 42.4%, 44.2% and 6% patients, respectively. Median time from the initial COVID-19 symptoms to admission was 5 days IQR (1–9). All patients required oxygen supplementation, including 24/217 (11.1%) patients who required HFNC. Median 4C COVID-19 mortality score was 7, IQR (5–9) with 24/217 (11.1%) patients requiring ICU admission and mechanical ventilation (MV) and 22/217 (10.1%) patients dying within 30 days of admission. Patient characteristics and outcomes are summarized in Table 1.

Table 1. Patient characteristics in overall cohort and stratified according to the composite outcome of mechanical ventilation or 30-day mortality.

	Overall	MV or Death No	MV or Death Yes	p-Value
Total number	217	192	25	-
Age (years)	65 IQR (55–70)	64 IQR (55–70)	70 IQR (62–75)	0.014

Table 1. Cont.

	Overall	MV or Death No	MV or Death Yes	p-Value
Sex Male Female	144/217 (66.4%) 73/217 (33.6%)	123/192 (64.1%) 69/192 (35.9%)	21/25 (84%) 4/25 (16%)	0.047
BMI (kg/m^2)	28.3 IQR (25.4–31.5)	28.4 IQR (25.4–31.6)	26.9 IQR (25.65–30.9)	0.342
Probe type M XL	140/217 (64.5%) 77/217 (35.5%)	121/192 (63%) 71/192 (37%)	19/25 (76%) 6/25 (24%)	0.203
SCD (mm)	21 IQR (19–25)	22 IQR (18–25.25)	20 IQR (19–23)	0.652
Chronic liver disease	10/217 (4.6%)	8/192 (4.2%)	2/25 (8%)	0.323
LSM (kPa)	5.2 IQR (4.1–6.5)	5.1 IQR (4.18–6.53)	5.3 IQR (4.1–6.3)	0.873
LSM IQR (%)	13 IQR (9–20)	13 IQR (9–20)	13 IQR (8–18)	0.419
CAP (dB/m)	274 IQR (232–321)	273 IQR (233.5–322)	284 IQR (228–301)	0.643
CAP IQR (dB/m)	31 IQR (22–43)	31 IQR (22–43)	31 IQR (20–38)	0.487
FAST score	0.31 IQR (0.16–0.45)	0.3 IQR (0.14–0.45)	0.4 IQR (0.25–0.47)	0.112
WBC ($\times 10^9$/L)	7.8 IQR (5.45–11.1)	8 IQR (5.53–11.1)	6.9 IQR (3.8–10.9)	0.545
RBC ($\times 10^{12}$/L)	4.5 IQR (4.14–4.89)	4.5 IQR (4.14–4.88)	4.5 IQR (4.12–4.9)	0.872
Platelets ($\times 10^9$/L)	237 IQR (173–327.5)	243.5 IQR (178.25–334)	204 IQR (144–264)	0.087
PT (Quick, %)	101 IQR (90–108)	101.5 IQR (92–108)	89 IQR (76–107)	0.059
Bilirubin (umol/L)	10.6 IQR (8.6–15.4)	10.6 IQR (8.6–15.45)	10.7 IQR (8.1–15.2)	0.979
AST (IU/L)	39 IQR (27–61)	38 IQR (26–57)	58 IQR (35–84)	0.014
ALT (IU/L)	38 IQR (24–63)	37.5 IQR (23.25–62)	41 IQR (27–67)	0.614
ALP (IU/L)	62 IQR (51–78.5)	61 IQR (50–77)	64 IQR (58–86)	0.166
GGT (IU/L)	42 IQR (25.5–82)	43 IQR (27–85.75)	37 IQR (24–56)	0.165
CRP (mg/L)	71.8 IQR (31.2–128.3	69.5 IQR (28.03–122.23)	100.4 IQR (48.8–138.2)	0.072
Albumin (g/L)	32.5 IQR (30–35)	33 IQR (30–35)	32 IQR (30–34)	0.433
4C mortality score	7 IQR (5–9)	7 IQR (4.5–9)	10 IQR (8.75–11)	<0.001
HFNC oxygenation (N, %)	24/217 (11.1%)	14/192 (7.3%)	10/25 (40%)	<0.001

Table legend: BMI, body mass index; CAP, controlled attenuation parameter; FAST, FibroScan-AST score; LSM, liver stiffness measurement; IQR, interquartile range; SCD, skin-to-liver capsule distance; CRP, C-reactive protein; HFNC, high-flow nasal cannula; MV, mechanical ventilation; ALT, alanine transaminase; AST, aspartate aminotransferase; ALP, alkaline phosphatase; GGT, gamma glutamyl transferase; PT, prothrombin time; RBC, red blood cells; WBC, white blood cells.

3.2. Correlations of LSM and CAP with Demographic, Biochemical and Clinical Parameters

Median LSM was 5.2 kPa, with 41/217 (18.9%) patients presenting with LSM of >7 kPa and 12/217 (5.5%) patients with LSM ≥ 10 kPa. LSM was higher in males (5.3 vs. 4.9; $p = 0.026$), patients with history of chronic liver disease (8.05 vs. 5.1; $p = 0.004$), lower PT (Rho = −0.15; $p = 0.029$), higher bilirubin (Rho = 0.2; $p = 0.004$) and higher GGT (Rho = 0.21; $p = 0.002$).

Median CAP was 274 dB/m and 109/217 (50.3%) patients had CAP > 274 dB/m. CAP was significantly associated with higher BMI (Rho = 0.42; $p < 0.001$). No significant associations of CAP with other laboratory and clinical parameters presented in Table 1 were found ($p > 0.05$ for all analyses).

There was no significant correlation between LSM and CAP in the overall cohort of patients. However, in the subgroup of patients with chronic liver disease, a strong negative correlation between LSM and CAP (Rho = −0.81; $p = 0.005$) was observed. Regarding the patients with LSM > 7 kPa, 22/41 (53.7%) had CAP > 274 dB/m, indicative of the presence of liver steatosis.

LSM and CAP were not associated with the severity of clinal presentation of COVID19 as defined by 4CMS or need for HFNC oxygen supplementation ($p > 0.05$).

3.3. Correlations of FAST Score with Demographic, Biochemical and Clinical Parameters

Median FAST score was 0.31, with 119 (55.3%), 85 (39.5%) and 11 (5.1%) of patients having FAST values < 0.35, 0.35–0.67 and >0.67, respectively. FAST was expectedly associated with LSM (Rho = 0.36; $p < 0.001$), CAP (Rho = 0.4; $p < 0.001$) and AST (Rho = 0.81; $p < 0.001$), but also with higher values of ALT (Rho = 0.59; $p < 0.001$), GGT (Rho = 0.41; $p < 0.001$), CRP (Rho = 0.28; $p < 0.001$) and BMI (Rho = 0.21; $p = 0.003$). FAST score was not significantly associated with the severity of clinical presentation of COVID-19 as defined by 4CMS or HFNC oxygen supplementation ($p > 0.05$).

3.4. Relationships between LSM, CAP, FAST Score and 30-Day Clinical Outcomes

When analysed as a continuous variable, higher FAST score was significantly associated with the need for MV (median 0.4 vs. 0.29 in patients with and without MV use, $p = 0.046$) but no significant association with death or composite outcome of MV or death was present ($p > 0.05$ for both analyses). Neither LSM, nor CAP, evaluated as continuous variables, showed a significant association with adverse outcomes ($p > 0.05$ for all analyses).

However, by using ROC curve analysis, we were able to establish optimal cut-offs for FAST of >0.36 (AUROC 0.632) for prediction of 30-day mortality or need of MV. Patients presenting with FAST > 0.36 (85/217 (39.2%)) experienced significantly higher risk of mechanical ventilation (OR = 4.39; $p = 0.002$), death (OR = 3.01; $p = 0.018$) and composite outcome of MV or death (OR = 3.81; $p = 0.003$). Thirty-day mechanical ventilation or death rates in patients with FAST > 0.36 and ≤0.36 were 19.8% and 6.2%, respectively (Figure 1). No similar cut-off level could be established for LSM and CAP.

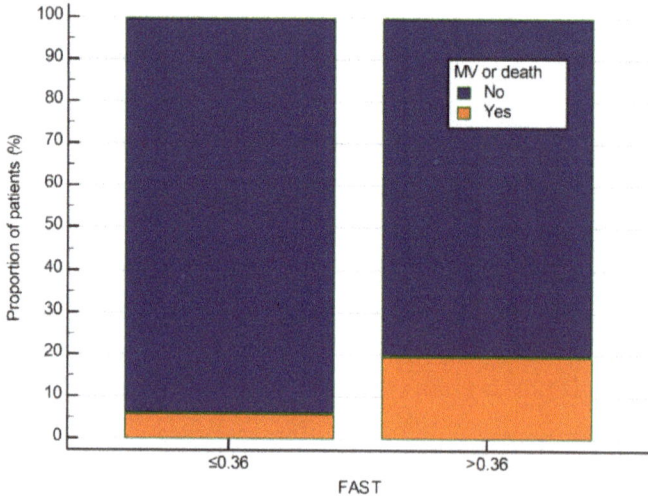

Figure 1. Thirty-day mechanical ventilation or death rates stratified according to the FAST > 0.36. MV, mechanical ventilation; FAST, FibroScan-AST score.

We further investigated the relationship of FAST > 0.36 with reduced survival, need for MV and the composite outcome of MV or death in a series of multivariate logistic regression models. In the first set of models adjusted for age and sex, FAST > 0.36 remained significantly associated with higher occurrence of death (FAST > 0.36 OR 3.2, $p = 0.021$; age OR 1.07, $p = 0.006$; male sex $p = 0.075$), higher need for MV (FAST > 0.36 OR 4.49, $p = 0.003$; age OR 1.05, $p = 0.024$; male sex OR 3.98, $p = 0.030$) and higher occurrence of composite outcome (FAST > 0.36 OR 3.86, $p = 0.005$; age OR 1.06, $p = 0.011$; male sex OR 4.3, $p = 0.021$).

In the second set of models presented in Table 2, after further adjusting for 4CMS and HFNC, FAST > 0.36 showed significant prognostic properties for predicting the need of MV and composite outcome of MV or death, independently of 4CMS and HFNC.

Table 2. Multivariate logistic regression models adjusted for age, sex and COVID-19 severity (4C mortality score, use of HFNC oxygenation) investigating association of FAST score with 30-day mortality, mechanical ventilation and mechanical ventilation or death.

	30-Day Mortality p-Value and OR with 95% C.I.	Mechanical Ventilation p-Value and OR with 95% C.I.	Mechanical Ventilation or Death p-Value and OR with 95% C.I.
FAST > 0.36	p = 0.285 OR = 1.79 (0.61–5.23)	p = 0.019 * OR = 3.78 (1.24–11.5)	p = 0.036 * OR = 3.11 (1.08–8.97)
Age (years)	p = 0.321 OR = 0.95 (0.88–1.04)	p = 0.136 OR = 0.94 (0.87–1.02)	p = 0.199 OR = 0.95 (0.88–1.03)
Male sex	p = 0.761 OR = 0.83 (0.24–2.81)	p = 0.660 OR = 1.33 (0.36–4.92)	p = 0.542 OR = 1.49 (0.41–5.33)
4C mortality score	p = 0.004 * OR = 1.83 (1.31–2.57)	p = 0.001 * OR = 1.72 (1.25–2.38)	p = 0.001 * OR = 1.71 (1.24–2.35)
HFNC oxygenation	p = 0.002 * OR = 7.4 (2.15–24.44)	p < 0.001 * OR = 7.76 (2.4–25.08)	p < 0.001 * OR = 7.17 (2.24–22.92)

Table legend: BMI, body mass index; FAST, FibroScan-AST score; LSM, liver stiffness measurement; IQR, interquartile range; HFNC, high-flow nasal cannula. * Statistically significant at level p < 0.05.

In addition, we evaluated how FAST > 0.36 would perform after adjusting for non-invasive biochemical scores (APRI, NSF, FIB-4). All three scores were associated with worse 30-day composite clinical outcome in univariate analyses (p < 0.05). However, inclusion of these scores in multivariate regression models did not change the relationships of FAST score, HFNC and 4CMS with clinical outcomes. Neither of the biochemical scores remained independently associated with the adverse composite outcome in this context. Furthermore, FAST score was analysed in the model adjusted for chronic metabolic comorbidities (obesity, diabetes, arterial hypertension, dyslipidaemia) and chronic liver disease, and again, only FAST > 0.36 remained significantly associated with the risk of composite adverse outcome (OR 3.68, 95%CI 1.47–9.21, p = 0.0054). Thus, FAST > 0.36 appears to have better prognostic properties compared to metabolic and chronic liver comorbidities in our cohort of patients.

4. Discussion

Our study demonstrates a lack of association between LSM and CAP as non-invasive surrogates for liver fibrosis and steatosis with the outcomes of COVID-19 defined as (a) severity of clinical presentation of COVID-19 and (b) 30-day mortality or need for MV. Nevertheless, higher FAST score, as a non-invasive surrogate for NASH with significant fibrosis, independently predicted the risk of composite outcome of MV or death.

FAST score was previously demonstrated as a reliable non-invasive tool to identify NASH patients with significant activity and liver fibrosis (19). We hypothesised that FAST score may correlate with more severe outcomes of COVID-19 given that patients with NASH are more likely to be obese with metabolic complications and the resulting liver inflammation may be accentuated by COVID 19 contributing to an adverse prognosis. Although we failed to observe a correlation between FAST score and clinical indicators of COVID-19 severity at admission to hospital, probably as the result of selection bias due to patients with critical illness at presentation being excluded from the study, we found FAST score > 0.36 was independently associated with the risk of MV and the composite adverse outcome of death or MV. However, without histological evidence, apparent linkage between FAST score as a non-invasive indicator of NASH and COVID-19 outcomes, as might be assumed based on current results, should be interpreted cautiously.

Previous investigations have clearly determined risk factors for the development of more severe COVID-19 disease and death, such as older age, male sex, increased blood pressure, presence of metabolic derangements such as diabetes and obesity, as well as some biochemical indicators (2–7). Obese patients are more likely to have fatty liver, which has been previously recognised as a risk factor for further deterioration of the metabolic profile of the affected individuals who are not COVID-19 patients [8,33]. Given the shared risk factors between NAFLD and severe COVID-19 disease, a more severe course of COVID-19 might hypothetically be expected amongst patients with fatty liver. Interestingly, in our cohort, FAST score, but not metabolic comorbidities, was independently associated with the risk of experiencing the composite adverse outcome at 30 days.

Liver involvement in COVID-19 has been proposed due to the high prevalence of elevated aminotransferases observed among the analysed cohorts of patients, but conflicting results were reported in terms of their origin, pathophysiological background, and impact on the course of the disease [12,13]. As transaminase elevations in COVID-19 may be multifactorial, the use of diagnostic tools for liver assessment which are not based on liver aminotransferases would be welcome. Whereas liver biopsy is obviously not acceptable for majority of typical cases of COVID-19, TE might represent reliable alternative. Transient elastography measures liver stiffness, as a surrogate of liver fibrosis which is also affected by liver inflammation, and CAP as the surrogate of liver steatosis [34]. Only a few studies have reported on the clinical utility of LSM and/or CAP in COVID-19 patients. Two studies (one European with 32 patients, and one Asian with 98 patients) reported a more severe clinical picture and higher mortality of COVID-19 patients with higher LSM. CAP was not associated with clinical outcomes, and both studies found correlation between LSM and liver transaminases [15,16]. The authors excluded patients with a history of chronic liver disease (CLD) and liver biopsy was not performed to support the findings obtained by TE. As opposed to these findings, a recent study from Barcelona failed to demonstrate any influence of LSM, CAP, baseline ALT and prior liver disease on the clinical course of COVID-19 in a cohort of 98 hospitalized patients, with 9% of them having CLD [17]. Nevertheless, elevated baseline AST especially in patients aged > 65 years was a strong predictor of adverse clinical outcomes. Recently, LSM and CAP were also investigated among patients with persisting post-acute COVID-19 syndrome and no history of liver disease [35]. LSM but not CAP was higher (but still within the normal range) in patients who suffered from a more severe form of COVID-19 during acute illness (5.08 kPa vs. 4.39 kPa, $p = 0.017$ for LSM, and 291.64 dB/m vs. 266.06 dB/m, $p = 0.062$ for CAP).

In agreement with data from the Campos-Varela study [21], our results demonstrate no association of LSM and CAP, when analysed individually, with the clinical severity and 30-day outcomes of COVID-19. Both LSM and CAP were not influenced by the levels of transaminases (up to $5\times$ ULN as defined by inclusion criteria) nor were they correlated mutually. Consequently, LSM might not be a good individual predictor of clinical outcomes in a typical COVID-19 cohort with the low prevalence of chronic liver disease and normal to moderately elevated transaminases. Amongst the entire cohort of 217 patients analysed here, only 10 (4.6%) had a history of chronic liver disease, whereas a fourfold higher prevalence might have been assumed based on LSM. Indeed, 41/217 (18.9%) patients had LSM > 7 kPa and of them 12 (5.5%) had LSM $\geq$ 10 kPa, suggesting the presence of significant and advanced fibrosis, respectively. This could be due to previously unrecognized chronic liver disease amongst the patients coming from general population, now suffering from COVID-19, but alternatively could be secondary to overestimation of fibrosis stage by TE, as previously reported among patients with NAFLD where only 50% of patients with elevated LSM ($\geq$9.6 kPa, suggestive of advanced fibrosis) had advanced fibrosis as confirmed by liver biopsy [36]. Due to high prevalence of overweight/obesity (almost 80%) and fatty liver (>50% with CAP > 274 dB/m), our cohort is comparable and might also follow this pattern of diagnostic performance of TE. Another reason for the increased proportion of patients with LSM > 7 kPa might be liver involvement in the inflammatory response to COVID-19 resulting in the increased liver stiffness.

We also analysed prognostic properties of biochemical non-invasive tests (APRI, FIB-4 and NFS) with respect to the clinical outcomes of patients with COVID-19. Although significantly different values between the patients with different outcomes could be demonstrated for each test, in multivariate regression analysis they failed to independently predict the risk of MV or death. Non-invasive biochemical tests potentially suffer from limitations in assessing liver health in the setting of COVID-19. In particular, they were invented as the indirect indicators of liver fibrosis in patients with chronic liver disease, and consist of liver aminotransferases, platelets and certain demographic indicators. In the setting of COVID-19, liver aminotransferases are elevated in up to 75% of patients without a history of chronic liver disease, and platelets might be decreased due to direct viral effect, immunological mechanisms or induced by medications such as heparin. Therefore, the use of biochemical non-invasive tests in this setting might not be reliable.

Our study has some limitations: liver biopsy is insufficient to reveal correlation between elastographic measurements and histological changes; TE was performed by several operators and we were not able to assess the interobserver variability of LSM and CAP measurements. On the other hand, this is the largest study thus far to report the performance of LSM and CAP by TE, with regard to their correlation with clinical severity of COVID-19 and 30-day outcome, and is the first to evaluate the FAST score in this regard. A strength of our study is that all patients underwent standardized diagnostic and treatment protocols and our cohort is representative of a typical hospitalised COVID-19 patient cohort with a low prevalence of chronic liver disease.

In conclusion, these data demonstrate that LSM and CAP as non-invasive surrogates for liver fibrosis and steatosis do not correlate with the severity and clinical outcomes of COVID-19 in a typical cohort of hospitalised patients with low prevalence of chronic liver disease and normal or moderately elevated transaminases. FAST score > 0.36 was for the first time demonstrated to independently predict the risk of composite 30-day adverse outcomes. Even after adjustment for the presence of chronic metabolic comorbidities and noninvasive biochemical fibrosis indices, FAST score remained significantly associated with the risk of 30-day composite adverse outcome of mechanical ventilation or death. However, the issue of liver involvement in COVID-19 might not be precisely addressed based on the available results until more histological data are collected.

Author Contributions: M.Z.: acquisition of data; analysis and interpretation of data; drafting of the manuscript; critical revision of the manuscript for important intellectual content; final approval; M.L.: study concept and design; analysis and interpretation of data; drafting of the manuscript; critical revision of the manuscript for important intellectual content; statistical analysis; final approval; T.B. (Tomislav Bokun): acquisition of data; analysis and interpretation of data; critical revision of the manuscript for important intellectual content; final approval; T.B. (Tonci Bozin): acquisition of data; critical revision of the manuscript for important intellectual content; final approval; M.B.J.: acquisition of data; analysis and interpretation of data; critical revision of the manuscript for important intellectual content; final approval; I.T.D.: acquisition of data; analysis and interpretation of data; critical revision of the manuscript for important intellectual content; final approval; F.P.: acquisition of data; analysis and interpretation of data; critical revision of the manuscript for important intellectual content; final approval; A.M.: analysis and interpretation of data; critical revision of the manuscript for important intellectual content; administrative support; final approval; I.L.: analysis and interpretation of data; critical revision of the manuscript for important intellectual content; administrative support; final approval; N.P.Z.: analysis and interpretation of data; critical revision of the manuscript for important intellectual content; final approval; K.L.: analysis and interpretation of data; critical revision of the manuscript for important intellectual content; final approval; Z.K.: analysis and interpretation of data; critical revision of the manuscript for important intellectual content; final approval; R.O.: analysis and interpretation of data; critical revision of the manuscript for important intellectual content; final approval; T.F.K.: analysis and interpretation of data; critical revision of the manuscript for important intellectual content; final approval; I.B.: analysis and interpretation of data; critical revision of the manuscript for important intellectual content; final approval; L.V.J.: analysis and interpretation of data; critical revision of the manuscript for important intellectual content; final approval; M.K.: analysis and interpretation of data; critical revision of the manuscript for important intellectual content; final approval; I.G.: study concept and design; acquisition of data; analysis and interpretation of data; drafting of the manuscript; critical revision of the manuscript for important intellectual content; study supervision; final approval of the version to be published. All authors have read and agreed to the published version of the manuscript.

Funding: The authors disclose no funding sources for this research.

Institutional Review Board Statement: This study was conducted in accordance with the World Medical Association Declaration of Helsinki and the study protocol was approved by the Institutional Ethics Committee, No 2020/1012-09. All patients gave the written consent for the participation in the study.

Informed Consent Statement: Informed consent was obtained from all subjects involved in the study.

Data Availability Statement: The data presented in this study are available from the corresponding author upon reasonable request.

Conflicts of Interest: Ivica Grgurevic received lecture fees from Echosens, Ferring and Gilead, travel support from Abbvie, and he served as an advisory board member for General Electric. The remaining authors have nothing to disclose.

Abbreviations

ACE2	Angiotensin-converting enzyme II
ALP	Alkaline phosphatase
ALT	Alanine aminotransferase
APRI	AST to platelet ratio index
AST	Aspartate aminotransferase
BMI	Body mass index
CAP	Controlled attenuation parameter
COVID-19	Coronavirus disease 2019
CRP	C-reactive protein
FAST	FibroScan-AST score
FIB-4	Fibrosis 4 index
GGT	Gamma glutamyl transferase
HFNC	High flow nasal cannula
IQR	Interquartile range
LSM	Liver stiffness measurement
MV	Mechanical ventilation
NAFLD	Non-alcoholic fatty liver disease
NASH	Non-alcoholic steatohepatitis
NFS	Non-alcoholic fatty liver disease fibrosis score
PT	Prothrombin time
RBC	Red blood cells
SCD	Skin-to-liver capsule distance
WBC	White blood cells

References

1. Wang, C.; Horby, P.W.; Hayden, F.G.; Gao, G.F. A novel coronavirus outbreak of global health concern. *Lancet* **2020**, *395*, 470–473. [CrossRef]
2. Wiersinga, W.J.; Rhodes, A.; Cheng, A.C. Pathophysiology, Transmission, Diagnosis, and Treatment of Coronavirus Disease 2019 (COVID-19): A Review. *JAMA* **2020**, *324*, 782–793. [CrossRef] [PubMed]
3. Richardson, S.; Hirsch, J.S.; Narasimhan, M.; Crawford, J.M.; McGinn, T.; Davidson, K.W.; Barnaby, D.P.; Becker, L.B.; Chelico, J.D.; Cohen, S.L.; et al. Presenting Characteristics, Comorbidities, and Outcomes Among 5700 Patients Hospitalized With COVID-19 in the New York City Area. *JAMA* **2020**, *323*, 2052–2059. [CrossRef] [PubMed]
4. Docherty, A.B.; Harrison, E.M.; Green, C.A.; Hardwick, H.E.; Pius, R.; Norman, L.; Holden, K.A.; Read, J.; Dondelinger, F.; Carson, G.; et al. Features of 20 133 UK patients in hospital with COVID-19 using the ISARIC WHO Clinical Characterisation Protocol: Prospective observational cohort study. *BMJ* **2020**, *369*, m1985. [CrossRef] [PubMed]
5. Liu, Z.; Xing Bing, X.; Za, X.Z. Epidemiology Working Group for NCIP Epidemic Response, Chinese Center for Disease Control and PreventionThe epidemiological characteristics of an outbreak of 2019 novel coronavirus diseases (COVID-19) in China. *Zhonghua Liu Xing Bing Xue Za Zhi* **2020**, *41*, 145–151.
6. Hu, B.; Guo, H.; Zhou, P. Characteristics of SARS-CoV-2 and COVID-19. *Nat. Rev. Microbiol.* **2021**, *19*, 141–154. [CrossRef]
7. Kuehn, B.M. More Severe Obesity Leads to More Severe COVID-19 in Study. *JAMA* **2021**, *325*, 1603. [CrossRef]
8. Dufour, J.-F.; Scherer, R.; Balp, M.-M.; McKenna, S.J.; Janssens, N.; Lopez, P.; Pedrosa, M. The global epidemiology of nonalcoholic steatohepatitis (NASH) and associated risk factors–A targeted literature review. *Endocr. Metab. Sci.* **2021**, *3*, 100089. [CrossRef]

9. Subichin, M.; Clanton, J.; Makuszewski, M.; Bohon, A.; Zografakis, J.G.; Dan, A. Liver disease in the morbidly obese: A review of 1000 consecutive patients undergoing weight loss surgery. *Surg. Obes. Relat. Dis.* **2015**, *11*, 137–141. [CrossRef] [PubMed]
10. Mahamid, M.; Nseir, W.; Khoury, T.; Mahamid, B.; Nubania, A.; Sub-Laban, K.; Schifter, J.; Mari, A.; Sbeit, W.; Goldin, E. Nonalcoholic fatty liver disease is associated with COVID-19 severity independently of metabolic syndrome. *Eur. J. Gastroenterol. Hepatol.* **2020**. [CrossRef] [PubMed]
11. Fondevila, M.F. Obese patients with NASH have increased hepatic expression of SARS-CoV-2 critical entry points. *J. Hepatol.* **2021**, *74*, 469–471. [CrossRef]
12. Cai, Q.; Huang, D.; Yu, H.; Zhu, Z.; Xia, Z.; Su, Y.; Li, Z.; Zhou, G.; Gou, J.; Qu, J.; et al. COVID-19: Abnormal liver function tests. *J. Hepatol.* **2020**, *73*, 566–574. [CrossRef] [PubMed]
13. Wang, Y.; Liu, S.; Liu, H. SARS-CoV-2 infection of the liver directly contributes to hepatic impairment in patients with COVID-19. *J. Hepatol.* **2020**, *73*, 807–816. [CrossRef]
14. Kim, D.; Adeniji, N.; Latt, N.; Kumar, S.; Bloom, P.P.; Aby, E.S.; Perumalswami, P.; Roytman, M.; Li, M.; Vogel, A.S.; et al. Predictors of Outcomes of COVID-19 in Patients With Chronic Liver Disease: US Multi-center Study. *Clin. Gastroenterol. Hepatol.* **2021**, *19*, 1469–1479e19. [CrossRef] [PubMed]
15. Effenberger, M.; Grander, C.; Fritsche, G.; Bellmann-Weiler, R.; Hartig, F.; Wildner, S.; Seiwald, S.; Adolph, T.E.; Zoller, H.; Weiss, G.; et al. Liver stiffness by transient elastography accompanies illness severity in COVID-19. *BMJ Open Gastroenterol.* **2020**, *7*, e000445. [CrossRef] [PubMed]
16. Demirtas, C.O.; Keklikkiran, C.; Ergenc, I.; Sengel, B.E.; Eskidemir, G.; Cinel, I.; Odabasi, Z.; Korten, V.; Yilmaz, Y. Liver stiffness is associated with disease severity and worse clinical scenarios in coronavirus disease 2019: A prospective transient elastography study. *Int. J. Clin. Pract.* **2021**, e14363. [CrossRef]
17. Campos-Varela, I.; Villagrasa, A.; Simon-Talero, M.; Riveiro-Barciela, M.; Ventura-Cots, M.; Aguilera-Castro, L.; Alvarez-Lopez, P.; Nordahl, E.A.; Anton, A.; Bañares, J.; et al. The role of liver steatosis as measured with transient elastography and transaminases on hard clinical outcomes in patients with COVID-19. *Ther. Adv. Gastroenterol.* **2021**, *14*. [CrossRef] [PubMed]
18. Ji, D.; Qin, E.; Xu, J.; Zhang, D.; Cheng, G.; Wang, Y.; Lau, G. Non-alcoholic fatty liver diseases in patients with COVID-19: A retrospective study. *J. Hepatol.* **2020**, *73*, 451–453. [CrossRef]
19. Newsome, P.N.; Sasso, M.; Deeks, J.J. FibroScan-AST (FAST) score for the non-invasive identification of patients with non-alcoholic steatohepatitis with significant activity and fibrosis: A prospective derivation and global validation study. *Lancet Gastroenterol. Hepatol.* **2020**, *5*, 362–373. [CrossRef]
20. Subbe, C.; Kruger, M.; Rutherford, P.; Gemmel, L. Validation of a modified Early Warning Score in medical admissions. *QJM Int. J. Med.* **2001**, *94*, 521–526. [CrossRef] [PubMed]
21. Knight, S.R.; Ho, A.; Pius, R. ISARIC4C investigators Risk stratification of patients admitted to hospital with COVID-19 using the ISARIC WHO Clinical Characterisation Protocol: Development and validation of the 4C Mortality Score. *BMJ* **2020**, *370*, m3339. [CrossRef]
22. The Ministry of Health of the Republic of Croatia. Guidelines for Treatment of Patients with COVID-19, Version 2, 19 November 2020. Available online: https://zdravlje.gov.hr/UserDocsImages//2020%20CORONAVIRUS//Smjernice%20za%20lije%C4%8Denje%20oboljelih%20od%20koronavirusne%20bolesti%202019%20(COVID-19),%20verzija%202%20od%2019.%20studenoga%202020.pdf (accessed on 21 June 2021).
23. Dietrich, C.F.; Bamber, J.; Berzigotti, A. EFSUMB Guidelines and Recommendations on the Clinical Use of Liver Ultrasound Elastography, Update 2017 (Long Version). *Ultraschall Med.* **2017**, *38*, e16–e47.
24. Berger, A.; Shili, S.; Zuberbuhler, F.; Hiriart, J.B.; Lannes, A.; Chermak, F.; Hunault, G.; Foucher, J.; Oberti, F.; Fouchard-Hubert, I.; et al. Liver Stiffness Measurement With FibroScan: Use the Right Probe in the Right Conditions! *Clin. Transl. Gastroenterol.* **2019**, *10*, e00023. [CrossRef] [PubMed]
25. Tsochatzis, E.; Gurusamy, K.; Ntaoula, S.; Cholongitas, E.; Davidson, B.; Burroughs, A. Elastography for the diagnosis of severity of fibrosis in chronic liver disease: A meta-analysis of diagnostic accuracy. *J. Hepatol.* **2010**, *54*, 650–659. [CrossRef]
26. de Franchis, R.; Baveno, V.I. Faculty Expanding consensus in portal hypertension: Report of the Baveno VI Consensus Workshop: Stratifying risk and individualizing care for portal hypertension. *J. Hepatol.* **2015**, *63*, 743–752. [CrossRef] [PubMed]
27. Eddowes, P.; Sasso, M.; Allison, M.; Tsochatzis, E.; Anstee, Q.M.; Sheridan, D.; Guha, I.N.; Cobbold, J.F.; Deeks, J.; Paradis, V.; et al. Accuracy of FibroScan Controlled Attenuation Parameter and Liver Stiffness Measurement in Assessing Steatosis and Fibrosis in Patients with Nonalcoholic Fatty Liver Disease. *Gastroenterology* **2019**, *156*, 1717–1730. [CrossRef]
28. Targher, G.; Mantovani, A.; Byrne, C.D.; Wang, X.-B.; Yan, H.-D.; Sun, Q.-F.; Pan, K.-H.; Zheng, K.-I.; Chen, Y.-P.; Eslam, M.; et al. Risk of severe illness from COVID-19 in patients with metabolic dysfunction-associated fatty liver disease and increased fibrosis scores. *Gut* **2020**, *69*, 1545–1547. [CrossRef] [PubMed]
29. Romero-Cristóbal, M.; Clemente-Sánchez, A.; Piñeiro, P.; Cedeño, J.; Rayón, L.; del Río, J.; Ramos, C.; Hernández, D.-A.; Cova, M.; Caballero, A.; et al. Possible unrecognised liver injury is associated with mortality in critically ill COVID-19 patients. *Ther. Adv. Gastroenterol.* **2021**, *14*. [CrossRef]
30. Wai, C.; Greenson, J.K.; Fontana, R.J.; Kalbfleisch, J.D.; Marrero, J.A.; Conjeevaram, H.S.; Lok, A.S.-F. A simple noninvasive index can predict both significant fibrosis and cirrhosis in patients with chronic hepatitis C. *Hepatology* **2003**, *38*, 518–526. [CrossRef] [PubMed]

31. Vallet-Pichard, A.; Mallet, V.; Nalpas, B.; Verkarre, V.; Nalpas, A.; Dhalluin-Venier, V.; Fontaine, H.; Pol, S. FIB-4: An inexpensive and accurate marker of fibrosis in HCV infection comparison with liver biopsy and fibrotest. *Hepatology* **2007**, *46*, 32–36. [CrossRef]
32. Angulo, P.; Hui, J.M.; Marchesini, G.; Bugianesi, E.; George, J.; Farrell, G.C.; Enders, F.; Saksena, S.; Burt, A.; Bida, J.P.; et al. The NAFLD fibrosis score: A noninvasive system that identifies liver fibrosis in patients with NAFLD. *Hepatology* **2007**, *45*, 846–854. [CrossRef] [PubMed]
33. Mustapic, S.; Ziga, S.; Matic, V.; Bokun, T.; Radic, B.; Lucijanic, M.; Marusic, S.; Babic, Z.; Grgurevic, I. Ultrasound Grade of Liver Steatosis Is Independently Associated with the Risk of Metabolic Syndrome. *Can. J. Gastroenterol. Hepatol.* **2018**, *2018*, 1–10. [CrossRef]
34. Tapper, E.B.; Afdhal, N.H. Vibration-controlled transient elastography: A practical approach to the noninvasive assessment of liver fibrosis. *Curr. Opin. Gastroenterol.* **2015**, *31*, 192–198. [CrossRef] [PubMed]
35. Bende, F.; Tudoran, C.; Sporea, I.; Fofiu, R.; Bâldea, V.; Cotrău, R.; Popescu, A.; Sirli, R.; Ungureanu, B.; Tudoran, M. A Multidisciplinary Approach to Evaluate the Presence of Hepatic and Cardiac Abnormalities in Patients with Post-Acute COVID-19 Syndrome—A Pilot Study. *J. Clin. Med.* **2021**, *10*, 2507. [CrossRef] [PubMed]
36. Kwok, R.; Choi, K.C.; Wong, G.L.-H.; Zhang, Y.; Chan, H.L.-Y.; Luk, A.O.-Y.; Shu, S.S.-T.; Chan, A.; Yeung, M.W.; Chan, J.; et al. Screening diabetic patients for non-alcoholic fatty liver disease with controlled attenuation parameter and liver stiffness measurements: A prospective cohort study. *Gut* **2015**, *65*, 1359–1368. [CrossRef] [PubMed]

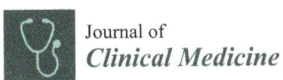

Review

Liver Injury in Patients with Coronavirus Disease 2019 (COVID-19)—A Narrative Review

Liliana Łykowska-Szuber *, Karolina Wołodźko, Anna Maria Rychter *, Aleksandra Szymczak-Tomczak, Iwona Krela-Kaźmierczak and Agnieszka Dobrowolska

Department of Gastroenterology, Dietetics and Internal Diseases, Poznan University of Medical Sciences, 60-355 Poznań, Poland; karolina.wolodzko@gmail.com (K.W.); aleksandra.szymczak@o2.pl (A.S.-T.); krela@op.pl (I.K.-K.); agdob@ump.edu.pl (A.D.)
* Correspondence: lszuber@wp.pl (L.Ł.-S.); a.m.rychter@gmail.com (A.M.R.); Tel.: +48-869-1343 (L.Ł.-S.); Fax: +48-869-189-8459 (L.Ł.-S.)

Abstract: While respiratory symptoms are prevalent in SARS-CoV-2 infected patients, growing evidence indicates that COVID-19 affects a wide variety of organs. Coronaviruses affect not only the respiratory system, but also the circulatory, nervous and digestive systems. The most common comorbidities in COVID-19 patients are hypertension, followed by diabetes, cardiovascular, and respiratory disease. Most conditions predisposing to SARS-CoV-2 infection are closely related to the metabolic syndrome. Obesity and chronic diseases, including liver disease, are associated with the induction of pro-inflammatory conditions and a reduction in immune response disorders, leading to the suspicion that these conditions may increase the susceptibility to SARS-CoV2 infection and the risk of complications. The definition of liver damage caused by COVID-19 has not yet been established. COVID-19 may contribute to both primary and secondary liver injury in people with pre-existing chronic disease and impaired liver reserves, leading to exacerbation of underlying disease, liver decompensation, or acute chronic liver failure. Therefore, many researchers have interpreted it as clinical or laboratory abnormalities in the course of the disease and treatment in patients with or without pre-existing liver disease. The research results available so far indicate that patients with liver disease require special attention in the event of COVID-19 infection.

Keywords: COVID-19; liver disease; clinical manifestations

1. Introduction

It has been over a year since China reported first cases of a mysterious new strain of pneumonia to the World Health Organization and 18 months since it was declared pandemic. We are now vaccinating patients with the fastest vaccine ever developed. The International Committee on Taxonomy of Viruses named the new virus severe acute respiratory distress syndrome coronavirus-2 (SARS-CoV-2) and the condition caused by it, coronavirus infectious disease 2019 (COVID-19) [1]. By the time of this article, WHO has reported over 220 million confirmed cases of COVID-19 of which 55% have fully recovered and 2% have died [2,3].

Although respiratory symptoms with widely varying severity dominate in patients infected with SARS-CoV-2, a growing amount of data highlight the impact of COVID-19 on multiple organs, as it was in the case of SARS-CoV and MERS-CoV. Liver impairment, mainly in the form of biochemical abnormalities, has also been frequently reported as a common manifestation. It is important to determine the clinical and prognostic significance of these disorders and the implications of this new disease for patients with pre-existing liver diseases, such as viral hepatitis, alcoholic liver disease, non-alcoholic fatty liver disease (NAFLD), autoimmune hepatitis and cirrhosis.

2. Clinical Manifestations of COVID-19

SARS-CoV-2 is an enveloped positive-sense single-stranded RNA virus that belongs to the Coronaviridae family and Betacoronavirus genus [4]. Numerous coronaviruses have been found in animals, but only seven are pathogenic to humans, including three that have caused major epidemics of severe pneumonia in the previous two decades. SARS-CoV induced an outbreak of severe acute respiratory syndrome (SARS) in China in 2002. MERS-CoV was identified as the cause of Middle East respiratory syndrome (MERS) in 2012 [4].

Since SARS-CoV-2 belongs to the same Coronaviridae family and its genome sequence is approximately 80% homologous to SARS-CoV, and 50% to MERS-CoV, they share similarities in structure and pathogenicity [4].

All three coronaviruses affect not only the respiratory tract, but also the cardiovascular, nervous and digestive systems.

Most patients present mild symptoms, such as fever, fatigue, dry cough, and myalgia, accompanied by less common symptoms: diarrhea, vomiting and loss of the sense of taste or smell. Symptoms of severe disease—dyspnea and signs of hypoxemia, usually occurring a week after onset of illness—indicate severe pneumonia that can lead to acute respiratory distress syndrome (ARDS), multiple organ dysfunction syndromes (MODS) and death [5].

After an outbreak of severe acute respiratory syndrome (SARS) in 2002, research on the pathogenesis of SARS-Cov revealed that the virus was internalized into the host cells through the functional angiotensin-converting enzyme 2 receptor (ACE2) [6,7]. The same receptor is functional for the novel coronavirus, as both betacoronaviruses belong to genetic lineage B [7]. The virion's envelope spike consisting of glycoprotein (S protein), specifically its receptor-binding domain (RBD), is a ligand that binds with the host cell surface ACE2 receptor facilitating membrane fusion, virus entry and replication [7,8]. However, SARS-Cov-2 binds to the ACE2 with 10-fold to 20-fold higher affinity, compared to SARS-CoV, which may explain its fast transmission rate among humans [9].

The target receptor is highly expressed in lung type II pneumocytes, but prevalence of the extra-pulmonary symptoms suggests that other organs may be also affected by SARS-CoV-2. Transcriptomics and immunohistochemistry studies have proved the presentation of the highest proportion (>1%) of the ACE2 receptor in the lower respiratory tract, lungs, heart, ileum, esophagus, kidneys, and bladder. Organs with lower ACE2 expression levels are, among others, the liver, stomach, pancreas, brain, vessels endothelium, testis, uterus, ovary, breast, oral and nasal mucosa [10].

3. COVID-19 and Comorbidities

COVID-19 affects all age groups with a median age of 47 years, and it is more prevalent in men and those with comorbidities [11].

Moreover, older age and the presence of additional disease were more common among patients with severe course of infection.

A meta-analysis involving 46,248 patients showed that the most common comorbidities in COVID-19 patients are hypertension (14–22%), followed by diabetes mellitus (6–11%), cardiovascular diseases (4–7%) and respiratory disease (1–3%). The same conditions are associated with higher mortality [12]—49% in comparison to overall case fatality rate at 2–5% [11,12].

Three studies from New York associated overweight and obesity with higher prevalence of COVID-19 and greater risk of hospitalization in intensive care units [13–15].

Most of the conditions predisposing to SARS-CoV-2 infection are closely related to metabolic syndrome. The liver, as an organ crucial for lipid and glucose metabolism, is a key determinant of metabolic abnormalities. Therefore, it is not surprising to observe that some research linked severe course of COVID-19 to non-alcoholic fatty liver disease (lately referred as metabolic dysfunction-associated fatty liver disease—MAFLD [12]), which is likely seen as a cause or consequence of metabolic syndrome [13]. It remains unclear whether the risk is specific to NAFLD or results from coexisting metabolic conditions.

Obesity and chronic disorders, including liver diseases, are associated with the induction of proinflammatory states and the attenuation of disturbances in the immune response, leading to suspicion that these conditions may increase the susceptibility to SARS-CoV2 infection as well as the risk of complications.

4. COVID-19 and Liver Disease

A review of 12,882 confirmed COVID-19 patients hospitalized until the end of June 2020 showed that overall prevalence of hepatic comorbidities in this group was 2–11% and it was not associated with poorer outcomes of infection [14,16]. However, according to an American study focusing on patients with preexisting liver diseases (9% of 2780 individuals), they are at higher risk of death (12% vs. 4%) and increased hospitalization days [15]. However, in this group, the percentage of mortality was the highest. It is also worth noting that in this cohort, patients with underlying hepatic conditions were older with a larger proportion of other comorbidities, such as hypertension (68%) or diabetes (48%)—even in comparison to data from the meta-analysis mentioned above [15].

The hepatic distribution of the SARS-CoV-2 target receptor discussed above is heterogeneous. Many reviews have confirmed its presence on cholangiocytes and absence on Kupffer cells, or sinusoidal endothelial cells [16,17].

Hamming and colleagues, who used immunohistochemistry for evaluation, reported that hepatocytes are negative for the ACE2 receptor [18]. However, other studies performed with the use of scRNA-seq identified low frequency of ACE2 expression on the same cells [19,20]. Moreover, in the same research, Chai et al. showed that the level of ACE2 expression cholangiocytes was found to be similar to that of type II pneumocytes [19]. These findings suggest that hepatocytes might not be targeted directly by the virus, contrary to the biliary epithelium. The finding does not explain why the majority of patients with COVID-19-related liver injury tend to present with abnormal AST and/or ALT, but not a cholestasis picture.

The definition of COVID-19-induced hepatic damage has not been established yet. That is why many researchers interpret it as any liver-related clinical or laboratory abnormality occurring during the course of the disease and treatment in patients with or without pre-existing liver condition.

Similar to SARS and MERS, patients have shown various degrees of liver impairment, most commonly presented as mild-to-moderate aminotransferase elevation, in some cases accompanied by a slight increase in serum bilirubin and decrease in albumin levels [21]. Disfunction of the liver among COVID-19 patients ranged from 14.8% up to 53% and is significantly higher in patients with a more serious infection, reaching 58–78% among death. Coincidence of hypoalbuminemia has been reported to be an independent predictive factor for poor prognosis [22]. The predominant type of liver injury is the hepatocellular pattern. It is worth mentioning that damage of skeletal or cardiac muscle, also occurring in COVID-19, could also result in the elevation of serum transaminase along with LDH levels.

According to the study by Kaneko S. et al. the predictors of liver impairment presented by transaminases elevation are C-reactive protein (CRP) at baseline, oxygenation, intubation, and gastrointestinal symptoms, such as appetite loss, diarrhea and nausea [23]. This confirmed conclusions from a couple months before when Jin X et al. had found that liver impairment occurred more frequently in patients presenting gastrointestinal signs. The same research showed that the coexistence of underlying liver disease also is associated with digestive tract symptoms [24].

In retrospective studies, it was also observed that low testosterone concentration in younger men (<65 years of age) may be an independent factor predisposing to acute liver failure in the course of COVID-19. In people over 65 years of age, the gender difference did not affect the occurrence of this complication [25,26]. It may result from the fact that testosterone deficiency is associated with obesity, metabolic syndrome, type 2 diabetes and their clinical consequences, such as fatty liver and atherosclerosis. In younger women, female sex hormones are protective in this regard [27].

The pathogenesis of liver injury caused by SARS-CoV-2 is still unclear. Several possible mechanisms are taken under consideration: direct cytopathic effect of the virus through the ACE2 receptor, immune-mediated hepatitis as a result of uncontrolled inflammatory response following COVID-19 infection, leading to cytokine storm syndrome, anoxia as a cause of hypoxic hepatitis due to pneumonia and respiratory failure and drug-induced liver injury secondary to medications used for the treatment, among others, as well as antipyretic drugs or antiviral agents (Figure 1) [19,28–30].

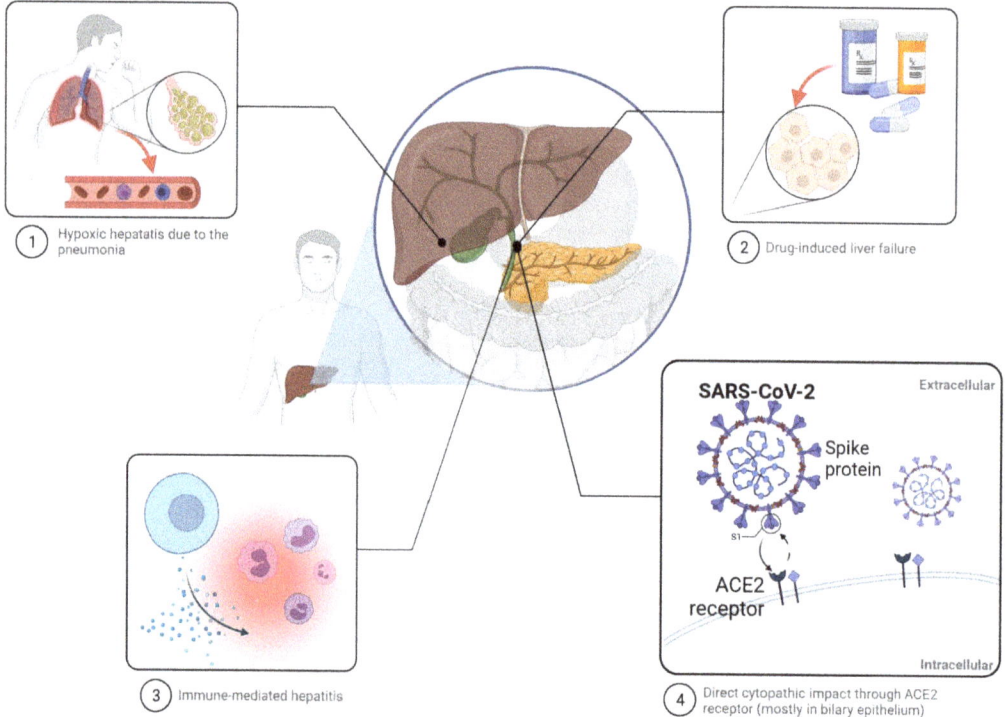

Figure 1. Probable pathogenesis of liver injury caused by SARS-CoV-2.

The Mechanisms of Liver Injury in COVID-19

It can be suspected that a combination of these mechanisms results in the acute liver injury observed in COVID-19 patients, especially in those with a severe course of the disease, experiencing severe pneumonia, SIRS, sepsis or MODS.

Moreover, COVID-19 may contribute to additional hepatic impairment in people with pre-existing chronic liver conditions and compromised hepatic reserves, leading to exacerbation of the underlying disease, hepatic decompensation or acute-on-chronic liver failure.

Post-mortem examination of 44 cases revealed signs of a pre-existing liver disorder in 18 cases (n = 14 steatosis, and n = 4 cirrhosis) [31]. Liver histology results have varied depending on the study. The main findings were congestive hepatopathy and moderate microvascular steatosis. In some cases, patchy hepatic necrosis, mild lobular lymphocytic infiltration and nuclear glycogen deposition were reported [31,32]. None of the findings are specific for direct viral injury, even though the presence of viral RNA was detected through RT-PCR in the liver parenchyma, as it was in the case of the SARS-CoV genome [32,33].

Currently, there are insufficient data regarding the impact of SARS-CoV-2 infection on the course of pre-existing chronic liver conditions. As mentioned above, the overall prevalence of hepatic comorbidities among COVID-19 patients was reported to reach 2–11% with a predominance of NAFLD (MAFLD), whose presence increased the risk of disease progression, abnormal liver function and longer viral shedding time, compared to patients without NAFLD [15]. In another study, MAFLD was associated with more than 2-fold higher prevalence of severe infection, but only in patients younger than 60 years. The mechanisms of the age-dependent relationship are unclear (See Table 1) [16].

Another risk factor for COVID-19 exacerbation is the presence of fibrosis in MAFLD/NAFLD, established with the use of the non-invasive evaluation of FIB-4 or nonalcoholic fatty liver disease fibrosis (NFS) scores, independently of metabolic comorbidities [34].

A case-control study from the U.S.A. confirmed that patients with chronic liver disease had significantly higher odds of developing COVID-19, compared to those without hepatic comorbidity, even after adjusting for COVID-19 risk factors (however, authors showed that age and gender had no additional effect on the risk of acquiring COVID-19 among patients with chronic liver disease, in contrast to the race). The strongest correlation concerned non-alcoholic liver disease and non-alcoholic cirrhosis, followed by patients with chronic hepatitis C, alcoholic liver damage, alcoholic liver cirrhosis, and chronic hepatitis B. Furthermore, patients with both SARS-CoV-2 infection and pre-existing liver disease had higher rates of hospitalization and death than others [35].

Table 1. Liver statistics and outcomes.

Data/Location	Statistics/Outcomes			
	Liver disease statistics			
Sharma et al. meta-analysis 2020 [16]	Acute LD	Comorbid chronic LD	Elevated AST	Elevated ALT
	26.5%	2.6%	41.1%	29.1%
	Poor outcomes, odds ratio			
	1.68	0.96 (insignificant)	1.85	2.98
Singh et al. 2020 Multicenter Research Network Study, U.S.A. [17]	Mortality, relative risk			
	Preexisting liver disease		Cirrhosis	
	2.8		4.6	
Ji et al. 2020 China [15]	Liver disease statistics			
	Admission		Hospitalization	
	50%		75.2%	
	COVID-19 progression, odds ratio			
	Higher BMI		NAFLD	
	1.3		6.4	
Shalimar et al. 2020 India [36]	Liver disease statistics (total 3.7%, $n = 28$)			
	Liver cirrhosis, $n = 26$	NAFLD, $n = 1$		EHPVO, $n = 1$
	Mortality, %			
	Cirrhosis		Without cirrhosis	
	42.3%		23.1%	
Marjot et al. 2021 International registry study, U.K. [37]	Mortality, %			
	Cirrhosis		Without cirrhosis	
	32.00%		8.00%	
	Mortality, odds ratio			
	Child–Pugh A	Child–Pugh B	Child–Pugh C	Cirrhosis and alcohol-related diseases
	1.9	4.14	9.32	1.79

LD—liver disease; AST—aspartate aminotransferase; ALT—alanine aminotransferase; BMI—body-mass index; NAFLD—non-alcoholic fatty liver disease.

Cirrhotic patients were reported to be more susceptible to the novel coronavirus infection, which has led, in almost half of cases, to hepatic decompensation of cirrhosis and eventually to the development of acute-on-chronic liver failure, due to potential impairment of the innate immune system in encounters with a cytokine storm [36,37]. Additionally, the mortality rate is higher in COVID-19 patients with alcohol-related liver disease and cirrhosis, increasing in line with the Child–Pugh class (A [19%], B [35%], C [51%] reaching up to 100% in patients presenting as acute-on-chronic liver failure [36,37]. However, the main cause of death is respiratory failure [37]. Therefore, the suggestion that cirrhosis patients presenting with signs of decompensation of the liver disease should be evaluated for SARS-CoV-2 infection is advisable (Table 1) [36].

After a year of pandemic, data on correlation between COVID-19 and less common chronic liver diseases are limited. A few studies concerning AIH patients have shown that incidence of SARS-CoV-2 infection in this group was similar to that of the general population [38]. Moreover, adverse outcomes, such as hospitalization, ICU admission, mechanical ventilation and death, are comparable between AIH patients and those with other chronic liver diseases, including PSC and PBC patients, or without any hepatic comorbidity [39]. Baseline stadium of cirrhosis and age are independent determinants of death, while immunosuppressive therapy is not associated with an increased risk of severe course of infection or mortality [39,40].

5. SARS-CoV-2 Infection and Liver Transplantation

Another population affected by the pandemic are liver transplant patients. Management of waiting list candidates and post-transplant patients as well as the possibility of performing surgical procedures have been impeded for over one and a half years, due to limitations on elective and non-urgent surgery, and the reduced availability of hospital and intensive care beds, medical staff, blood products and personal protective equipment, but also uncertainty about the safety of transplantation during the SARS-CoV-2 pandemic.

Analysis of 128 surveys completed by transplant centers from all over the world revealed a decrease in the number of performed liver transplants and wait-listed candidates with higher mortality among this group in comparison to 2019 [41].

The main symptoms of SARS-CoV-2 infection among this group are same as in the general population—fever, cough and shortness of breath. The incidence of gastrointestinal symptoms, such as diarrhea, was reported to be more common in post-transplant patients than in the control group [42,43].

Up to this point, it is not fully confirmed whether organ transplant recipients are at higher risk for severe course of COVID-19 or mortality. Based on several studies, it appears that liver transplantation is not an independent predictive factor for poor prognosis, but combined with immunosuppression, underlying diseases and elderly age increases that risk [44].

The presence of non-liver cancer, older age and higher baseline serum creatinine are factors associated with death [43].

As mentioned before, data collected during three coronavirus epidemics suggest that immunosuppression is not among the risk factors of severe course of the disease or higher mortality [45].

On the one hand, immunosuppressants used to reduce the risk of transplant rejection may increase susceptibility to COVID-19, but on the other, they potentially impair the uncontrolled inflammatory response following SARS-CoV-2 infection. Furthermore, long-term use of immunosuppressants may prolong the period of viral shedding and may, therefore, prolong the duration of the communicable period [46].

Another issue raises the question of donor-derived coronavirus infection. Although RNA of SARS-CoV, MERS-CoV and SARS-CoV-2 were detected in blood samples from a certain percentage of affected patients and residual SARS-CoV-2 viral antigens were found in the hepatic tissues of convalescents, no documented cases of coronavirus transmission through transplantation have been reported [47,48].

COVID-19 patients were not considered potential living or deceased donors, as long as the risk of virus transmission was not eliminated [49].

Most societies recommend the restriction of transplantation to patients with acute liver failure (ALF/ACLF), high model for end-stage liver disease (MELD) score or hepatocellular carcinoma (HCC) at the upper limits of the Milan criteria. Moreover, organ donors and recipients should be tested for SARS-CoV-2 [50].

6. Consensus World Gastroenterology Organization for the Care of Patients with COVID-19 and Liver Disease

As the pandemic spreads, our understanding of how the virus affects our patients grows. Knowing already the negative impact of SARS-CoV-2 virus on the liver and the risk of liver damage, many scientific societies have presented their views on the care of patients with liver diseases. Below, we present the position of the World Gastroenterology Organization (WGO). It is important to clarify when and which group of patients require liver function tests. The WGO states that in the absence of underlying liver disease, outpatients with COVID-19 do not require routine biochemical analysis. In contrast, all hospitalized patients should undergo laboratory evaluation, including ALT, AST, GGT, ALP, and bilirubin. It is unclear whether patients with HCV or HBV infection are at higher risk of liver damage from COVID-19. In this group of patients, antiviral therapy should not be interrupted, under no circumstances. Undoubtedly, patients with liver cirrhosis have a worse prognosis, including the risk of acute liver decompensation. Patients with autoimmune hepatitis, due to the immunosuppressive treatment, constitute a group of particularly high risk. During the SARS-CoV-2 infection, it is not recommended to reduce immunosuppressive therapy, as it may lead to exacerbation of the underlying disease and the need for glucocorticoids. However, in the course of COVID-19, lymphopenia is also observed in patients. In such a situation, a reduction in azathioprine dosage may be necessary. Patients with a poor short-term prognosis, e.g., patients with a high MELD score, acute liver failure, or HCC should be eligible for liver transplantation. Both donors and recipients should have rapid PCR tests for SARS-CoV-2 virus. Given the possible complications of COVID-19 for patients with liver disease, stable patients should be encouraged to telemedicine whenever possible. This will minimize the potential risk of infection [3].

7. COVID-19 Vaccinations in Patients with Liver Disease

The development of vaccines against SARS-CoV-2 has raised questions about their effectiveness and safety in the general population as well as in the population of patients with coexisting diseases. People with comorbidities require special attention in times of COVID-19 pandemic; therefore, vaccination prophylaxis is particularly important for them. Patients with underlying liver diseases may present a lower immune response to vaccination as was indicated in the previous studies on the response to vaccination against hepatitis A, hepatitis B and seasonal flu. Immunosuppressive drugs commonly used by autoimmune hepatitis patients contribute to a reduced response to vaccination [51–53].

The pace of the development of vaccines against SARS-CoV-2 has been undoubtedly unprecedented. According to the WHO COVID-19 vaccine tracer, since the beginning of pandemic up to now, 126 different vaccines have been included into clinical development. Seven of them have been approved by WHO for use. The most commonly administered are BNT162b2 (Pfizer-Bio NTech) and mRNA-1273 (Moderna), which are based on mRNA encoding SARS-CoV-2 spiny glycoprotein variants. The two remaining are adenoviral vector–based vaccines: ChAdOx1 nCov-19 (AZD1222, also known as the Oxford-AstraZeneca) is a replication-free chimpanzee adenoviral vector containing a full-length, codon-optimized gene encoding the SARS-CoV-2 spike protein; and Ad26.COV2.S (Johnson & Johnson/Janssen) is a recombinant human adenovirus type 26 vector encoding SARS-CoV-2 spike protein. None of the three vaccines contain any living virus and consequently cannot replicate, even in immunocompromised individuals [54]. Introducing a new vaccine is always accompanied by concerns about the occurrence of complications. The COVID-19 vaccines can cause mild side effects after the first or second dose; the main ones include temperature rise, general fatigue, and pain at the injection site, but in a small percentage of cases, severe adverse events, such as an anaphylactic shock, may occur [55]. Another issue regarding new vaccines is related to the potential ability to induce autoimmune conditions. Both patients and clinicians are concerned about the potential risk for relapse or worsening of autoimmune diseases mainly because of insufficient data. So far, such a correlation has not been unequivocally proven for any of the vaccines used [56]. It should be noted that clinical trials of vaccines also included patients with stable chronic liver disease. The data on COVID-19 vaccines in patients with chronic liver disease are limited, but until now, there was no higher frequency or severity of adverse events noted in these subgroups [57]. While we do not have data on the long-term safety of SARS-CoV-2 vaccinations, it is important to consider the risks of gains and losses when deciding whether to vaccinate. This is particularly important in the groups of patients where the risk of complications and mortality due to COVID-19 is much higher than in the general population. There is currently no approved commercial test to measure neutralizing antibody responses to SARS CoV-2. Therefore, we are not able to unequivocally assess the responses to the used vaccination. Research in this area is ongoing. Meanwhile, we should note that the benefits of authorized vaccines outweigh the potential risks of adverse events [58].

8. Consensus American Association for the Study of Liver Diseases and European Association the Study of the Liver on COVID-19 Vaccination

The American Association for the Study of Liver Diseases and European Association the Study of the Liver suggest that COVID-19 vaccines should be administered to all adult patients with chronic liver disease and liver transplantation. In addition, patients with chronic liver disease who receive antiviral drugs for hepatitis B or hepatitis C should not withhold their medications while receiving COVID-19 vaccines. For patients with hepatocellular carcinoma undergoing locoregional or systemic therapy, vaccination should also be considered without interruption in their treatment. For liver transplant candidates, COVID-19 vaccination should be continued, even if liver transplant occurs before the second dose is given. The second dose should be administered at the earliest appropriate time after transplantation (e.g., 6 weeks post-transplant). It is recommended that people with a known history of previous COVID-19 infection wait a minimum of 90 days before receiving a COVID-19 vaccine, due to concerns about an overly exaggerated immune response. However, there may be special circumstances under which prior vaccination may occur.

While co-administration of vaccines is usually safe, we do not have much data on whether co-administration reduces the immune response. Vaccinations against COVID-19 have become a challenge for contemporary global health protection. Given that flu season is approaching, researchers asked themselves whether it would be possible to safely administer both vaccines at the same time. This would undoubtedly reduce the costs of vaccinations and increase the number of vaccinations received. It is important to establish whether co-administration reduces the immune response to either vaccine, taking into account the importance of complete protection against both infections. During the COVID-19 pandemic, we realized the importance of cellular immunity and immune memory in evaluating vaccine responses, and antibodies are only one aspect of the immune response. Based on the currently available studies, it can be concluded that the concomitant administration of the influenza vaccine with either a booster dose or a second dose of COVID-19 vaccine is safe. More research is ongoing [59–61].

9. Conclusions

In summary, based on the observations so far of patients with a history of COVID-19, coexisting liver injuries are usually mild and do not require special treatment. In cases of severe hepatic injury reported in the literature, underlying liver disease or ischemic hepatitis is most likely to be present. It cannot be ruled out that the drugs used may influence the degree of liver damage. Their number in more severe course of infection is much greater [62].

Despite the fact that the amount of data on COVID-19 and its consequences is increasing every day, understanding of the long-term health effects of the disease and assessing its impact on patients with comorbidities require further research.

Studies on patients with underlying chronic liver diseases, referred to in this article, included small groups of individuals, given the total number of COVID-19 confirmed cases. In addition, it is difficult to separate liver disease patients from those with coexisting hypertension, cardiovascular disease, diabetes mellitus or obesity, which are known to be associated with COVID-19 increased susceptibility and risk of severe course of the disease. Therefore, larger studies with detailed evaluation and long-term follow-up will provide more information in this area.

However, the results of studies available so far indicate that patients with liver diseases require special attention in the case of COVID-19 infection [26]. At the same time, it should be remembered that patients at risk with chronic liver disease should be vaccinated against COVID-19 first.

Author Contributions: Conceptualization, L.Ł.-S. and A.D.; writing—original draft preparation, K.W., L.Ł.-S., A.M.R.; writing—review and editing, A.D., A.S.-T., I.K.-K., L.Ł.-S., K.W.; visualization, L.Ł.S. and I.K.-K.; supervision, A.D. and I.K.-K. All authors have read and agreed to the published version of the manuscript.

Funding: This research received no external funding.

Institutional Review Board Statement: Not applicable.

Informed Consent Statement: Not applicable.

Data Availability Statement: Data are available and publicly accessible. The data presented in this study are openly available in the Medline and PubMed databases and on the publisher's website. The keywords that were used include "SARS-CoV2 infection", "COVID-19", "liver disease", "Coronaviridae", "respiratory symptoms". All data in the text are quoted and all works used are listed in the bibliography along with DOI and reference numbers.

Conflicts of Interest: The authors declare no conflict of interest.

References

1. Merola, E.; Pravadelli, C.; de Pretis, G. Prevalence of Liver Injury in Patients with Coronavirus Disease 2019 (COVID-19): A Systematic Review and Meta-Analysis. *Acta Gastroenterol. Belg.* **2020**, *83*, 454–460. [PubMed]
2. WHO Coronavirus (COVID-19) Dashboard. Available online: https://covid19.who.int (accessed on 24 March 2021).
3. COVID-19 Map. Available online: https://coronavirus.jhu.edu/map.html (accessed on 7 September 2021).
4. Lu, R.; Zhao, X.; Li, J.; Niu, P.; Yang, B.; Wu, H.; Wang, W.; Song, H.; Huang, B.; Zhu, N.; et al. Genomic Characterisation and Epidemiology of 2019 Novel Coronavirus: Implications for Virus Origins and Receptor Binding. *Lancet* **2020**, *395*, 565–574. [CrossRef]
5. Wu, Z.; McGoogan, J.M. Characteristics of and Important Lessons From the Coronavirus Disease 2019 (COVID-19) Outbreak in China: Summary of a Report of 72 314 Cases From the Chinese Center for Disease Control and Prevention. *JAMA* **2020**, *323*, 1239. [CrossRef]
6. Li, F.; Li, W.; Farzan, M.; Harrison, S.C. Structure of SARS Coronavirus Spike Receptor-Binding Domain Complexed with Receptor. *Science* **2005**, *309*, 1864–1868. [CrossRef]
7. Letko, M.; Marzi, A.; Munster, V. Functional Assessment of Cell Entry and Receptor Usage for SARS-CoV-2 and Other Lineage B Betacoronaviruses. *Nat. Microbiol.* **2020**, *5*, 562–569. [CrossRef]
8. Wu, F.; Zhao, S.; Yu, B.; Chen, Y.-M.; Wang, W.; Song, Z.-G.; Hu, Y.; Tao, Z.-W.; Tian, J.-H.; Pei, Y.-Y.; et al. A New Coronavirus Associated with Human Respiratory Disease in China. *Nature* **2020**, *579*, 265–269. [CrossRef]
9. Wrapp, D.; Wang, N.; Corbett, K.S.; Goldsmith, J.A.; Hsieh, C.-L.; Abiona, O.; Graham, B.S.; McLellan, J.S. Cryo-EM Structure of the 2019-NCoV Spike in the Prefusion Conformation. *Science* **2020**, *367*, 1260–1263. [CrossRef] [PubMed]
10. Beyerstedt, S.; Casaro, E.B.; Rangel, É.B. COVID-19: Angiotensin-Converting Enzyme 2 (ACE2) Expression and Tissue Susceptibility to SARS-CoV-2 Infection. *Eur. J. Clin. Microbiol. Infect. Dis.* **2021**, *40*, 905–919. [CrossRef]
11. Guan, W.; Ni, Z.; Hu, Y.; Liang, W.; Ou, C.; He, J.; Liu, L.; Shan, H.; Lei, C.; Hui, D.S.C.; et al. Clinical Characteristics of Coronavirus Disease 2019 in China. *N. Engl. J. Med.* **2020**, *382*, 1708–1720. [CrossRef]

12. Huang, C.; Wang, Y.; Li, X.; Ren, L.; Zhao, J.; Hu, Y.; Zhang, L.; Fan, G.; Xu, J.; Gu, X.; et al. Clinical Features of Patients Infected with 2019 Novel Coronavirus in Wuhan, China. *Lancet* **2020**, *395*, 497–506. [CrossRef]
13. Argenziano, M.G.; Bruce, S.L.; Slater, C.L.; Tiao, J.R.; Baldwin, M.R.; Barr, R.G.; Chang, B.P.; Chau, K.H.; Choi, J.J.; Gavin, N.; et al. Characterization and Clinical Course of 1000 Patients with Coronavirus Disease 2019 in New York: Retrospective Case Series. *BMJ* **2020**, *369*, m1996. [CrossRef]
14. Eslam, M.; Sanyal, A.J.; George, J. International Consensus Panel MAFLD: A Consensus-Driven Proposed Nomenclature for Metabolic Associated Fatty Liver Disease. *Gastroenterology* **2020**, *158*, 1999–2014. [CrossRef]
15. Ji, D.; Qin, E.; Xu, J.; Zhang, D.; Cheng, G.; Wang, Y.; Lau, G. Non-Alcoholic Fatty Liver Diseases in Patients with COVID-19: A Retrospective Study. *J. Hepatol.* **2020**, *73*, 451–453. [CrossRef] [PubMed]
16. Sharma, A.; Jaiswal, P.; Kerakhan, Y.; Saravanan, L.; Murtaza, Z.; Zergham, A.; Honganur, N.-S.; Akbar, A.; Deol, A.; Francis, B.; et al. Liver Disease and Outcomes among COVID-19 Hospitalized Patients-A Systematic Review and Meta-Analysis. *Ann. Hepatol.* **2021**, *21*, 100273. [CrossRef] [PubMed]
17. Singh, S.; Khan, A. Clinical Characteristics and Outcomes of Coronavirus Disease 2019 Among Patients With Preexisting Liver Disease in the United States: A Multicenter Research Network Study. *Gastroenterology* **2020**, *159*, 768–771.e3. [CrossRef] [PubMed]
18. Hamming, I.; Timens, W.; Bulthuis, M.L.C.; Lely, A.T.; Navis, G.J.; van Goor, H. Tissue Distribution of ACE2 Protein, the Functional Receptor for SARS Coronavirus. A First Step in Understanding SARS Pathogenesis. *J. Pathol.* **2004**, *203*, 631–637. [CrossRef] [PubMed]
19. Chai, X.; Hu, L.; Zhang, Y.; Han, W.; Lu, Z.; Ke, A.; Zhou, J.; Shi, G.; Fang, N.; Fan, J.; et al. Specific ACE2 Expression in Cholangiocytes May Cause Liver Damage After 2019-NCoV Infection. *bioRxiv* **2020**. [CrossRef]
20. Pirola, C.J.; Sookoian, S. SARS-CoV-2 Virus and Liver Expression of Host Receptors: Putative Mechanisms of Liver Involvement in COVID-19. *Liver Int.* **2020**, *40*, 2038–2040. [CrossRef] [PubMed]
21. Xu, L.; Liu, J.; Lu, M.; Yang, D.; Zheng, X. Liver Injury during Highly Pathogenic Human Coronavirus Infections. *Liver Int.* **2020**, *40*, 998–1004. [CrossRef]
22. Huang, J.; Cheng, A.; Kumar, R.; Fang, Y.; Chen, G.; Zhu, Y.; Lin, S. Hypoalbuminemia Predicts the Outcome of COVID-19 Independent of Age and Co-Morbidity. *J. Med. Virol.* **2020**, *92*, 2152–2158. [CrossRef]
23. Kaneko, S.; Kurosaki, M.; Nagata, K.; Taki, R.; Ueda, K.; Hanada, S.; Takayama, K.; Suzaki, S.; Harada, N.; Sugiyama, T.; et al. Liver Injury with COVID-19 Based on Gastrointestinal Symptoms and Pneumonia Severity. *PLoS ONE* **2020**, *15*, e0241663. [CrossRef] [PubMed]
24. Jin, X.; Lian, J.-S.; Hu, J.-H.; Gao, J.; Zheng, L.; Zhang, Y.-M.; Hao, S.-R.; Jia, H.-Y.; Cai, H.; Zhang, X.-L.; et al. Epidemiological, Clinical and Virological Characteristics of 74 Cases of Coronavirus-Infected Disease 2019 (COVID-19) with Gastrointestinal Symptoms. *Gut* **2020**, *69*, 1002. [CrossRef] [PubMed]
25. Naaraayan, A.; Nimkar, A.; Hasan, A.; Pant, S.; Durdevic, M.; Elenius, H.; Nava Suarez, C.; Jesmajian, S. Analysis of Male Sex as a Risk Factor in Older Adults With Coronavirus Disease 2019: A Retrospective Cohort Study from the New York City Metropolitan Region. *Cureus* **2020**, *12*, e9912. [CrossRef] [PubMed]
26. Cichoż-Lach, H.; Michalak, A. Liver Injury in the Era of COVID-19. *World J. Gastroenterol.* **2021**, *27*, 377–390. [CrossRef] [PubMed]
27. Kelly, D.M.; Akhtar, S.; Sellers, D.J.; Muraleedharan, V.; Channer, K.S.; Jones, T.H. Testosterone Differentially Regulates Targets of Lipid and Glucose Metabolism in Liver, Muscle and Adipose Tissues of the Testicular Feminised Mouse. *Endocrine* **2016**, *54*, 504–515. [CrossRef]
28. Liu, J.; Li, S.; Liu, J.; Liang, B.; Wang, X.; Wang, H.; Li, W.; Tong, Q.; Yi, J.; Zhao, L.; et al. Longitudinal Characteristics of Lymphocyte Responses and Cytokine Profiles in the Peripheral Blood of SARS-CoV-2 Infected Patients. *EBioMedicine* **2020**, *55*, 102763. [CrossRef]
29. Huang, H.; Li, H.; Chen, S.; Zhou, X.; Dai, X.; Wu, J.; Zhang, J.; Shao, L.; Yan, R.; Wang, M.; et al. Prevalence and Characteristics of Hypoxic Hepatitis in COVID-19 Patients in the Intensive Care Unit: A First Retrospective Study. *Front. Med. (Lausanne)* **2021**, *7*, 607206. [CrossRef]
30. Yang, R.-X.; Zheng, R.-D.; Fan, J.-G. Etiology and Management of Liver Injury in Patients with COVID-19. *World J. Gastroenterol.* **2020**, *26*, 4753–4762. [CrossRef]
31. Polak, S.B.; Van Gool, I.C.; Cohen, D.; von der Thüsen, J.H.; van Paassen, J. A Systematic Review of Pathological Findings in COVID-19: A Pathophysiological Timeline and Possible Mechanisms of Disease Progression. *Mod. Pathol.* **2020**, *33*, 2128–2138. [CrossRef]
32. Remmelink, M.; De Mendonça, R.; D'Haene, N.; De Clercq, S.; Verocq, C.; Lebrun, L.; Lavis, P.; Racu, M.-L.; Trépant, A.-L.; Maris, C.; et al. Unspecific Post-Mortem Findings despite Multiorgan Viral Spread in COVID-19 Patients. *Crit. Care* **2020**, *24*, 495. [CrossRef]
33. Farcas, G.A.; Poutanen, S.M.; Mazzulli, T.; Willey, B.M.; Butany, J.; Asa, S.L.; Faure, P.; Akhavan, P.; Low, D.E.; Kain, K.C. Fatal Severe Acute Respiratory Syndrome Is Associated with Multiorgan Involvement by Coronavirus. *J. Infect. Dis.* **2005**, *191*, 193–197. [CrossRef] [PubMed]
34. Targher, G.; Mantovani, A.; Byrne, C.D.; Wang, X.-B.; Yan, H.-D.; Sun, Q.-F.; Pan, K.-H.; Zheng, K.I.; Chen, Y.-P.; Eslam, M.; et al. Risk of Severe Illness from COVID-19 in Patients with Metabolic Dysfunction-Associated Fatty Liver Disease and Increased Fibrosis Scores. *Gut* **2020**, *69*, 1545–1547. [CrossRef]

35. Wang, Q.; Davis, P.B.; Xu, R. COVID-19 Risk, Disparities and Outcomes in Patients with Chronic Liver Disease in the United States. *EClinicalMedicine* **2021**, *31*, 100688.
36. Shalimar; Elhence, A.; Vaishnav, M.; Kumar, R.; Pathak, P.; Soni, K.D.; Aggarwal, R.; Soneja, M.; Jorwal, P.; Kumar, A.; et al. Poor Outcomes in Patients with Cirrhosis and Corona Virus Disease-19. *Indian J. Gastroenterol.* **2020**, *39*, 285–291. [CrossRef]
37. Marjot, T.; Moon, A.M.; Cook, J.A.; Abd-Elsalam, S.; Aloman, C.; Armstrong, M.J.; Pose, E.; Brenner, E.J.; Cargill, T.; Catana, M.-A.; et al. Outcomes Following SARS-CoV-2 Infection in Patients with Chronic Liver Disease: An International Registry Study. *J. Hepatol.* **2021**, *74*, 567–577. [CrossRef]
38. Di Giorgio, A.; Nicastro, E.; Speziani, C.; De Giorgio, M.; Pasulo, L.; Magro, B.; Fagiuoli, S.; D' Antiga, L. Health Status of Patients with Autoimmune Liver Disease during SARS-CoV-2 Outbreak in Northern Italy. *J. Hepatol.* **2020**, *73*, 702–705. [CrossRef] [PubMed]
39. Marjot, T.; Buescher, G.; Sebode, M.; Barnes, E.; Barritt, A.S., 4th; Armstrong, M.J.; Baldelli, L.; Kennedy, J.; Mercer, C.; Ozga, A.-K.; et al. SARS-CoV-2 Infection in Patients with Autoimmune Hepatitis. *J. Hepatol.* **2021**, *74*, 1335–1343. [CrossRef] [PubMed]
40. Gerussi, A.; Rigamonti, C.; Elia, C.; Cazzagon, N.; Floreani, A.; Pozzi, R.; Pozzoni, P.; Claar, E.; Pasulo, L.; Fagiuoli, S.; et al. Coronavirus Disease 2019 in Autoimmune Hepatitis: A Lesson From Immunosuppressed Patients. *Hepatol. Commun.* **2020**, *4*, 1257–1262. [CrossRef] [PubMed]
41. Russo, F.P.; Izzy, M.; Rammohan, A.; Kirchner, V.A.; Di Maira, T.; Belli, L.S.; Berg, T.; Berenguer, M.C.; Polak, W.G. Global Impact of the First Wave of COVID-19 on Liver Transplant Centers: A Multi-Society Survey (EASL-ESOT/ELITA-ILTS). *J. Hepatol.* **2021**. [CrossRef] [PubMed]
42. Imam, A.; Abukhalaf, S.A.; Merhav, H.; Abu-Gazala, S.; Cohen-Arazi, O.; Pikarsky, A.J.; Safadi, R.; Khalaileh, A. Prognosis and Treatment of Liver Transplant Recipients in the COVID-19 Era: A Literature Review. *Ann. Transplant.* **2020**, *25*, e926196. [CrossRef]
43. Heimbach, J.K.; Taner, T. SARS-CoV-2 Infection in Liver Transplant Recipients: Collaboration in the Time of COVID-19. *Lancet Gastroenterol. Hepatol.* **2020**, *5*, 958–960. [CrossRef]
44. Pereira, M.R.; Mohan, S.; Cohen, D.J.; Husain, S.A.; Dube, G.K.; Ratner, L.E.; Arcasoy, S.; Aversa, M.M.; Benvenuto, L.J.; Dadhania, D.M.; et al. COVID-19 in Solid Organ Transplant Recipients: Initial Report from the US Epicenter. *Am. J. Transplant.* **2020**, *20*, 1800–1808. [CrossRef]
45. Azzi, Y.; Bartash, R.; Scalea, J.; Loarte-Campos, P.; Akalin, E. COVID-19 and Solid Organ Transplantation: A Review Article. *Transplantation* **2021**, *105*, 37–55. [CrossRef]
46. Sahin, T.T.; Akbulut, S.; Yilmaz, S. COVID-19 Pandemic: Its Impact on Liver Disease and Liver Transplantation. *World J. Gastroenterol.* **2020**, *26*, 2987–2999. [CrossRef] [PubMed]
47. Kates, O.S.; Fisher, C.E.; Rakita, R.M.; Reyes, J.D.; Limaye, A.P. Use of SARS-CoV-2-Infected Deceased Organ Donors: Should We Always "Just Say No?". *Am. J. Transplant.* **2020**, *20*, 1787–1794. [CrossRef] [PubMed]
48. Gaussen, A.; Hornby, L.; Rockl, G.; O'Brien, S.; Delage, G.; Sapir-Pichhadze, R.; Drews, S.J.; Weiss, M.J.; Lewin, A. Evidence of SARS-CoV-2 Infection in Cells, Tissues, and Organs and the Risk of Transmission Through Transplantation. *Transplantation* **2021**, *105*, 1405–1422. [CrossRef]
49. Tuncer, A.; Akbulut, S.; Baskiran, A.; Karakas, E.E.; Baskiran, D.Y.; Carr, B.; Yilmaz, S. A Recipient and Donor Both Have COVID-19 Disease. Should We Perform a Liver Transplant? *J. Gastrointest. Cancer* **2021**, *52*, 1143–1147. [CrossRef] [PubMed]
50. Care of Patients with Liver Disease during the COVID-19 Pandemic: EASL-ESCMID Position Paper. *EASL-Home Hepatol.* **2020**, *2*, 100113.
51. Mendenhall, C.; Roselle, G.A.; Lybecker, L.A.; Marshall, L.E.; Grossman, C.J.; Myre, S.A.; Weesner, R.E.; Morgan, D.D. Hepatitis B Vaccination. Response of Alcoholic with and without Liver Injury. *Dig. Dis. Sci.* **1988**, *33*, 263–269. [CrossRef]
52. Wörns, M.A.; Teufel, A.; Kanzler, S.; Shrestha, A.; Victor, A.; Otto, G.; Lohse, A.W.; Galle, P.R.; Höhler, T. Incidence of HAV and HBV Infections and Vaccination Rates in Patients with Autoimmune Liver Diseases. *Am. J. Gastroenterol.* **2008**, *103*, 138–146. [CrossRef]
53. Effectiveness of Influenza Vaccines in Adults with Chronic Liver Disease: A Systematic Review and Meta-Analysis | BMJ Open. Available online: https://bmjopen.bmj.com/content/9/9/e031070 (accessed on 20 October 2021).
54. Motamedi, H.; Ari, M.M.; Dashtbin, S.; Fathollahi, M.; Hossainpour, H.; Alvandi, A.; Moradi, J.; Abiri, R. An Update Review of Globally Reported SARS-CoV-2 Vaccines in Preclinical and Clinical Stages. *Int. Immunopharmacol.* **2021**, *96*, 107763. [CrossRef] [PubMed]
55. Chen, M.; Yuan, Y.; Zhou, Y.; Deng, Z.; Zhao, J.; Feng, F.; Zou, H.; Sun, C. Safety of SARS-CoV-2 Vaccines: A Systematic Review and Meta-Analysis of Randomized Controlled Trials. *Infect. Dis. Poverty* **2021**, *10*, 94. [CrossRef] [PubMed]
56. Genovese, C.; La Fauci, V.; Squeri, A.; Trimarchi, G.; Squeri, R. HPV Vaccine and Autoimmune Diseases: Systematic Review and Meta-Analysis of the Literature. *J. Prev. Med. Hyg.* **2018**, *59*, E194–E199. [CrossRef] [PubMed]
57. Sharma, A.; Patnaik, I.; Kumar, A.; Gupta, R. COVID-19 Vaccines in Patients With Chronic Liver Disease. *J. Clin. Exp. Hepatol.* **2021**. [CrossRef]
58. Walsh, E.E.; Frenck, R.W.; Falsey, A.R.; Kitchin, N.; Absalon, J.; Gurtman, A.; Lockhart, S.; Neuzil, K.; Mulligan, M.J.; Bailey, R.; et al. Safety and Immunogenicity of Two RNA-Based Covid-19 Vaccine Candidates. *N. Engl. J. Med.* **2020**, *383*, 2439–2450. [CrossRef]

59. Lazarus, R.; Baos, S.; Cappel-Porter, H.; Carson-Stevens, A.; Clout, M.; Culliford, L.; Emmett, S.R.; Garstang, J.; Gbadamoshi, L.; Hallis, B.; et al. The Safety and Immunogenicity of Concomitant Administration of COVID-19 Vaccines (ChAdOx1 or BNT162b2) with Seasonal Influenza Vaccines in Adults: A Phase IV, Multicentre Randomised Controlled Trial with Blinding (ComFluCOV). *Lancet* **2021**, 1–36. Available online: https://papers.ssrn.com/sol3/papers.cfm?abstract_id=3931758 (accessed on 20 October 2021).
60. Fix, O.K.; Blumberg, E.A.; Chang, K.-M.; Chu, J.; Chung, R.T.; Goacher, E.K.; Hameed, B.; Kaul, D.R.; Kulik, L.M.; Kwok, R.M.; et al. American Association for the Study of Liver Diseases Expert Panel Consensus Statement: Vaccines to Prevent Coronavirus Disease 2019 Infection in Patients With Liver Disease. *Hepatology* **2021**, *74*, 1049–1064. [CrossRef] [PubMed]
61. Cornberg, M.; Buti, M.; Eberhardt, C.S.; Grossi, P.A.; Shouval, D. EASL Position Paper on the Use of COVID-19 Vaccines in Patients with Chronic Liver Diseases, Hepatobiliary Cancer and Liver Transplant Recipients. *J. Hepatol.* **2021**, *74*, 944–951. [CrossRef]
62. Guan, W.; Liang, W.; Zhao, Y.; Liang, H.; Chen, Z.; Li, Y.; Liu, X.; Chen, R.; Tang, C.; Wang, T.; et al. Comorbidity and Its Impact on 1590 Patients with Covid-19 in China: A Nationwide Analysis. *Eur. Respir J.* **2020**, 2000547. [CrossRef]

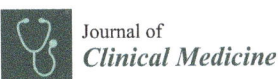

Article

An Unprecedented Challenge: The North Italian Gastroenterologist Response to COVID-19

Gian Eugenio Tontini [1,2,*], Giovanni Aldinio [1,2], Nicoletta Nandi [1,2], Alessandro Rimondi [1,2], Dario Consonni [3], Massimo Iavarone [4], Paolo Cantù [2], Angelo Sangiovanni [4], Pietro Lampertico [2,4] and Maurizio Vecchi [1,2]

1. Gastroenterology and Endoscopy Unit, Fondazione IRCCS Ca' Granda Ospedale Maggiore Policlinico, 20100 Milan, Italy; giovanni.aldinio@unimi.it (G.A.); nicoletta.nandi@unimi.it (N.N.); alessandro.rimondi@unimi.it (A.R.); maurizio.vecchi@unimi.it (M.V.)
2. Department of Pathophysiology and Organ Transplantation, University of Milan, 20100 Milan, Italy; paolo.cantu@policlinico.mi.it (P.C.); pietro.lampertico@unimi.it (P.L.)
3. Epidemiology Unit, Fondazione IRCCS Ca' Granda Ospedale Maggiore Policlinico, 20100 Milan, Italy; dario.consonni@policlinico.mi.it
4. Gastroenterology and Hepatology Unit, Fondazione IRCCS Ca' Granda Ospedale Maggiore Policlinico, 20100 Milan, Italy; massimo.iavarone@policlinico.mi.it (M.I.); angelo.sangiovanni@policlinico.mi.it (A.S.)
* Correspondence: gianeugeniotontini@gmail.com

Abstract: Background: COVID-19 pandemic has profoundly changed the activities and daily clinical scenarios, subverting organizational requirements of our Gastroenterology Units. AIM: to evaluate the clinical needs and outcomes of the gastroenterological ward metamorphosis during the COVID-19 outbreaks in a high incidence scenario. Methods: we compared the pertinence of gastroenterological hospitalization, modality of access, mortality rate, days of hospitalization, diagnostic and interventional procedures, age, Charlson comorbidity index, and frequency of SARS-CoV-2 infections in patients and healthcare personnel across the first and the second COVID-19 outbreaks in a COVID-free gastroenterological ward in the metropolitan area of Milan, that was hit first and hardest during the first COVID-19 outbreak since March 2020. Results: pertinence of gastroenterological hospitalization decreased both during the first and, to a lesser degree, the second SARS-CoV2 waves as compared to the pre-COVID era (43.6, 85.4, and 96.2%, respectively), as occurred to the admissions from domicile, while age, comorbidities, length of stay and mortality increased. Endoscopic and interventional radiology procedures declined only during the first wave. Hospitalized patients resulted positive to a SARS-CoV-2 nasopharyngeal swab in 10.2% of cases during the first COVID-19 outbreak after a median of 7 days since admission (range 1–15 days) and only 1 out of 318 patients during the second wave (6 days after admission). During the first wave, 19.5% of healthcare workers tested positive for SARS-CoV-2. Conclusions: a sudden metamorphosis of the gastroenterological ward was observed during the first COVID-19 outbreak with a marked reduction in the gastroenterological pertinence at the admission, together with an increase in patients' age and multidisciplinary complexity, hospital stays, and mortality, and a substantial risk of developing a SARS-CoV-2 test positivity. This lesson paved the way for the efficiency of hospital safety protocols and admission management, which contributed to the improved outcomes recorded during the second COVID-19 wave.

Keywords: COVID-19; SARS-CoV-2; gastroenterology; hepatology; endoscopy; delivery of healthcare

1. Introduction

COVID-19 pandemic has profoundly changed the activities and daily clinical scenarios, subverting essential clinical and organizational requirements of all hospital units. As of today, there are only a few studies describing the features and consequences of COVID-related re-organization of Gastroenterology departments [1,2], but there are no experiences describing both the changes that occurred in these settings, as well as the consequent adjustments applied and their impact on hospitalized patients and healthcare personnel.

During the firsts SARS-CoV2 outbreak, the Internal Medicine Units and other specialized units were suddenly converted into COVID Units, while other specialized Units, such as Gastroenterology Units and the Nephrology Units, became COVID-free wards with dedicated safety protocols to guarantee adequate inpatients assistance for a broad range of clinical presentations.

We evaluated the clinical needs and outcomes of a COVID-free gastroenterological ward of a hospital in the metropolitan area of Milan that was hit first and hardest during the first COVID-19 outbreak since March 2020 [3], before the availability of the first SARS-CoV-2 vaccinations (27 December 2020 for healthcare workers and only afterward for the general population).

We hypothesized a sudden metamorphosis of the gastroenterological clinical practice towards a situation that resembles an Internal Medicine and a Geriatric Unit in the pre-COVID era, with a marked reduction in the gastroenterological pertinence and elective admissions, together with an increase in hospital stays and mortality.

2. Material and Methods

Hospital charts related to hospitalized patients in January and February 2020 were used as a model for the pre-COVID era. Patients admitted between March and April, in September and from October to December 2020 represent, respectively, the first wave, the transition period, and the second wave of COVID-19 pandemic according to the regional epidemiological trends in the general population.

First, we assessed and compared the pertinence of hospitalization within the gastroenterological ward during different periods across the first and the second SARS-CoV2 outbreaks.

Secondly, we evaluated modality of access, mortality, days of hospitalization, gastroenterological diagnostic and operative procedures, age, Charlson comorbidity index (CCI), and frequency of SARS-CoV-2 infections in patients and healthcare personnel within the gastroenterological ward based on a molecular test performed on a nasopharyngeal swab. This monocentric retrospective cohort study was performed in the gastroenterological ward of a tertiary referral university hospital located in the city center of Milan (Italy), which encompasses a Gastroenterology and Endoscopy Unit and a Gastroenterology and Hepatology Unit.

Safety measures adopted in the gastroenterological ward to face the COVID-19 outbreak and protect both patients and healthcare workers were reported in detail in the Supplementary Methods.

The inclusion criteria were adult age (>18 years old), being hospitalized in the Gastroenterology Units from 1 January 1 2020 to 30 April 2020 and from 1 September 2020 to 31 December 2020.

In the absence of a validated definition in literature, the gastroenterological pertinence of the diagnoses was defined a priori as "any primary or secondary condition that determines a clinically significant dysfunction of the gastrointestinal system."

For each patient, the following data were collected: sex, age, entry and exit dates in the Unit; modality of access (collected as 2 categories: from domicile and others including Emergency Department, other Units, other Hospitals); discharge diagnosis; CCI [4,5], date of the positive nasopharyngeal swab for SARS-CoV-2; endoscopic and other interventional procedures (e.g., trans-arterial chemoembolization, TACE) performed throughout the hospitalization period in our Units.

In June 2020, healthcare workers received a questionnaire assessing their involvement in the Gastroenterological ward from 1 January 2020 to 30 April 2020 to weigh their potential worker exposure to SARS-CoV2 infection during the first wave (i.e., hours per week with direct involvement within the Gastroenterological ward).

Descriptive data were expressed as counts and percentages for categorical variables, as medians and ranges for continuous variables. The chi-squared test was used to analyze dichotomous variables. Univariate log-binomial regression models were used to calculate prevalence ratios (PR) and 95% confidence intervals (CI) for different periods vs. the pre-COVID period. The Kruskal–Wallis test was applied for the analysis of quantitative variables in the 4 periods. Statistical analyses were performed using Stata 17 (StataCorp., College Station, TX, USA, 2021).

The study was carried out in accordance with the Declaration of Helsinki adopted in 1964, incorporating all later amendments after formal approbation from the local Ethical Committee (Comitato Etico Milano Area 2, 19 May 2020; ID1588). All participants gave informed consent to participate in the study according to the study protocol.

3. Results

The total number of recruited patients in the study periods was 699, of which 426 males and 273 females, with a median age of 68 years (range 17 to 98 years) (Table 1). From March to April 2020, 39 out of 381 patients (10.2%) resulted positive to SARS-CoV-2 testing with a molecular nasopharyngeal swab after a median length of stay of 7 days (range 1–200) (Figure 1). From September to December 2020, only 1 out of 318 patients (0.003%) resulted positive to SARS-CoV-2 after 6 days spent in the gastroenterological ward. Notably, most of them (35/40) had at least one molecular nasopharyngeal swab negative for SARS-CoV-2 performed before ward admission (i.e., emergency room or pre-hospital triage), while 4 cases occurred in patients admitted a few days before the adoption of a systematic SARS-CoV-2 pre-hospital triage when the first COVID19 outbreak was already in progress but still largely unexpected. Among the 40 patients who tested positive for SARS-CoV-2, 27 (67.5%) had respiratory symptoms (at least one among cough, dyspnea, and mild respiratory insufficiency) at the time of hospital admission, 7 (17.5%) developed respiratory symptoms during the hospital stay, and 6 (15.0%) had no respiratory symptom. No false positive or false negative tests were found during the first and the second wave.

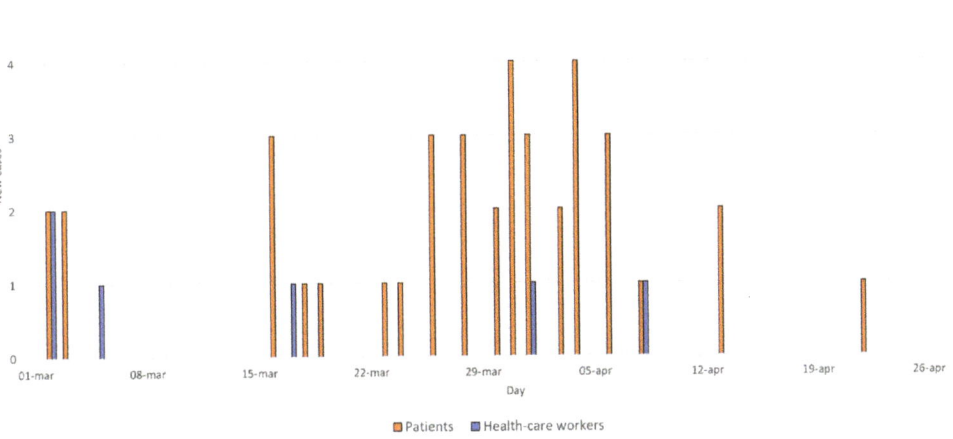

Figure 1. Daily incidence of SARS-CoV-2 during the first wave (SARS-CoV-2 molecular nasopharyngeal swab positive tests).

Table 1. Study population.

Outcome	Pre-COVID (N = 209) No. (%) of Patients	First Wave (N = 172)		Transition (N = 85)		Second Wave (N = 233)	
		No. (%) of Patients	Prevalence Ratio (95% CI)	No. (%) of Patients	Prevalence Ratio (95% CI)	No. (%) of Patients	Prevalence Ratio (95% CI)
Sex							
Female	72 (34.5)	70 (40.7)		32 (37.7)		99 (42.5)	
Male	157 (65.5)	102 (59.3)	0.90 (0.77 to 1.06)	53 (62.3)	0.95 (0.78 to 1.15)	134 (57.5)	0.88 (0.76 to 1.02)
Pertinent GE diagnoses	201 (96.2)	75 (43.6)	0.45 (0.38 to 0.54)	79 (92.9)	0.97 (0.91 to 1.03)	199 (85.4)	0.89 (0.84 to 0.94)
Admissions from domicile	124 (59.3)	27 (15.7)	0.26 (0.18 to 0.38)	38 (44.7)	0.75 (0.58 to 0.98)	95 (40.8)	0.69 (0.57 to 0.83)
Mortality	1 (0.5)	7 (4.1)	8.51 (1.06 to 68.5)	3 (3.5)	7.38 (0.78 to 69.9)	13 (5.6)	11.66 (1.54 to 88.4)
Patients undergoing ≥ 1 endoscopic procedure	98 (46.9)	31 (18.0)	0.38 (0.27 to 0.55)	44 (51.8)	1.10 (0.86 to 1.42)	96 (41.2)	0.88 (0.71 to 1.08)
IR procedure	69 (33.0)	26 (15.1)	0.46 (0.31 to 0.69)	29 (34.1)	1.03 (0.73 to 1.47)	67 (28.8)	0.87 (0.66 to 1.15)

During the first wave, among the 36 physicians that answered the questionnaire, 6 (16.7%) resulted positive to a nasopharyngeal swab and 1 (2.8%) to the serologic tests (Figure 1). No correlation was found between such SARS-CoV-2 testing and the healthcare workers attending the gastroenterological ward activities.

Compared to the pre-COVID era (96.1%), the gastroenterological pertinence of hospitalized patients decreased both during the first (43.6%) and the second (85.4) COVID-19 wave, while it was similar to the pre-COVID era during the transition period (92.9%) (Figure 2, Table 1). The same trend was observed for admissions from domiciles (Supplementary Figure S1, Table 1). Endoscopic and interventional radiology procedures dropped during the first wave, going back to normal levels during the transition period and the second wave (Supplementary Figure S7, Table 1). The median age at the admission raised during the first and the second wave as well (Supplementary Figure S3, Table 2), while the median CCI raised only during the first wave (Supplementary Figure S5, Table 2). Compared to the pre-COVID era, mortality and the median length of stay increased during all the following periods (Supplementary Figures S2 and S6, Tables 1 and 2). For the discharge diagnoses of the deceased patients, see Supplementary Table S1.

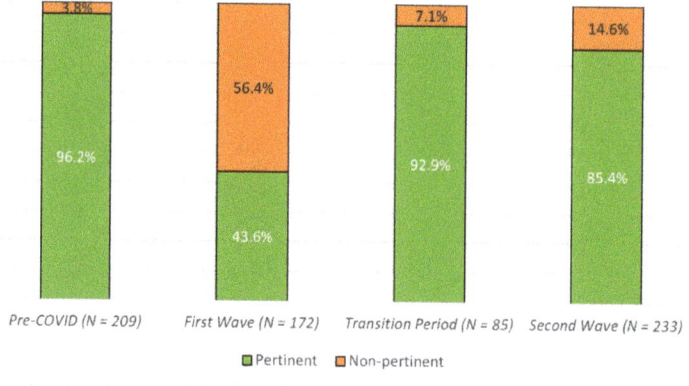

Figure 2. Proportions of pertinent gastroenterological discharge diagnoses.

Table 2. Length of stay and Charlson comorbidity index.

Outcome	Pre-COVID (N = 209) Median (Range)	First Wave (N = 172) Median (Range)	Transition (N = 85) Median (Range)	Second Wave (N = 233) Median (Range)	Total Median (Range)	p
Age (years)	65.0 (22.5 to 92.2)	73.0 (18.8 to 98.9)	64.0 (17.0 to 88.0)	69.0 (18.5 to 96.0)	68.0 (17.0 to 98.9)	<0.001
Length of stay (days)	4.0 (0.0 to 201.0)	5.5 (0.0 to 40.0)	7.0 (1.0 to 61.0)	6.0 (0.0 to 52.0)	5.0 (0.0 to 201.0)	0.001
Charlson comorbidity index	5.0 (0.0 to 12.0)	6.0 (0.0 to 16.0)	5.0 (0.0 to 11.0)	5.0 (0.0 to 11.0)	5.0 (0.0 to 16.0)	0.02

4. Discussion

This report clearly shows a remarkable metamorphosis of a COVID-free gastroenterological ward in the area with the highest European SARS-CoV-2 incidence during the first COVID-19 outbreak. Hospitalized patients were older, with more comorbidities, and they were mostly affected by Internal and Geriatric disorders. Hospitalizations were longer and characterized by higher mortality compared to the pre-COVID era. Coherently, elective admissions and endoscopic or dedicated interventional radiological procedures decreased, reflecting the cancellation of all deferrable procedures [6–9] and the relocation of most gastroenterological resources (beds, facilities, instrumentations, healthcare personnel) to the prevaricating care needs linked to the pandemic. Another aspect highlighted in our study is the importance and efficacy of regular active surveillance of patients and healthcare personnel with nasopharyngeal swabs and the use of second-level single-use PPE. Indeed, these strategies learned from experience during the first wave, once applied routinely when the second wave began, have led to a significant decrease in the positive cases among patients admitted in our units (in-hospital positive test within day 9) and in the rate of COVID positivity during hospitalization (possible hospital-acquired infection from day 10 to 14, definite hospital-acquired infection from day 15; Supplementary Table S2 and Supplementary Figure S8) along with the decrease in healthcare personnel infection. Notably, when the first SARS-CoV2 wave invested in the metropolitan area of Milan (March 2020), there were no developed isolation protocols nor recommendations on the systematic use of PPE and SARS-CoV2 testing for patients and healthcare personnel with no history of direct contact with confirmed cases regardless of the presence of respiratory symptoms [10]. Consistently, the first measures adopted to face the COVID-19 outbreak in that area (Supplementary methods) were the result of expert consensus based on limited real-life or published evidence and were updated or refined almost day-by-day and with heterogeneity across different hospitals according to the changing availability of human (e.g., intensive care personnel) and instrumental resources (e.g., PPE, respirators, COVID-free facilities). This reflects the scenario of the sudden and unexpected metamorphosis of any hospital protocols that shocked at any level the clinical practice with remarkable impacts on either hospitalized patients' outcomes, outpatient care continuity, or healthcare personnel daily practice and safety. Moreover, the implementation of preventive measures allowed a satisfactory recovery of elective admissions, endoscopic and interventional radiology procedures during the second wave. This was reflected in the rise of pertinent gastroenterological discharge diagnoses in the transition period and in the second wave compared with the first wave, despite a non-inferior impact of COVID-19 cases on the regional healthcare system [11].

As with all retrospective studies, the present one allows for rapid analysis of the outcomes to find answers for the current scientific needs present in a state of emergency at a global level. One limitation is the possible heterogeneity of data not systematically collected by multiple healthcare professionals. Moreover, considering the unique geographical and temporal setting, no generalization of these results can be made.

5. Conclusions

Overall, our study suggests that active surveillance with repeated SARS-CoV-2 testing and the systematic adoption of second-level single-use PPE when visiting patients are effective measures to control the spread of the virus in a hospital setting. In addition, our experience clearly demonstrates the nonobvious ability to maintain a balance between the need for beds to hospitalize COVID-19 patients and the necessity of continuing practicing medicine during the pandemic to avoid the effects that postponing the activities left behind would have on specific frail populations (e.g., those affected by cancer, cardiovascular, or other chronic conditions).

Supplementary Materials: The following are available online at https://www.mdpi.com/article/10.3390/jcm11010109/s1, Figure S1: Modalities of access. Figure S2: Length of stay in the Gastroenterological Unit. Figure S3: Age at the admission. Figure S4: Gender distribution. Figure S5: Charlson comorbidity index. Figure S6: Mortality. Figure S7: Patients attending at least one diagnostic procedure. Figure S8: Days from admission to diagnosis of SARS-CoV-2 infection. Figure S9: Days from the admission in the Gastroenterological Unit to the diagnosis of COVID-19 shown for each case. Table S1: Discharge diagnoses of deceased patients. Table S2: Days from the admission to the Unit to the diagnosis of COVID-19 during the first wave.

Author Contributions: G.E.T.: study concept, interpretation of data, drafting of the manuscript, critical revision of the manuscript, study supervision; G.A.: study concept, acquisition of data, interpretation of data, drafting of the manuscript, critical revision of the manuscript, statistical analysis; N.N. and A.R.: acquisition of data, interpretation of data, critical revision of the manuscript; D.C.: statistical analysis, interpretation of data, critical revision of the manuscript; P.C., M.I., A.S. and P.L.: interpretation of data, critical revision of the manuscript; M.V.: study concept, interpretation of data, drafting of the manuscript, critical revision of the manuscript, study supervision. All authors have read and agreed to the published version of the manuscript.

Funding: This spontaneous search has received no funding.

Institutional Review Board Statement: The study was conducted according to the guidelines of the Declaration of Helsinki, and approved by the Ethics Committee of Milano Area 2 (protocol code 1588; date of approval 19 May 2020).

Informed Consent Statement: All participants gave informed consent to participate in the study according to the study protocol.

Conflicts of Interest: The authors declare that there is no conflict of interest.

References

1. Priori, A.; Baisi, A.; Banderali, G.; Biglioli, F.; Bulfamante, G.; Canevini, M.P.; Cariati, M.; Carugo, S.; Cattaneo, M.; Cerri, A.; et al. The Many Faces of COVID-19 at a Glance: A University Hospital Multidisciplinary Account From Milan, Italy. *Front. Public Health* **2021**, *8*, 575029. [CrossRef]
2. Danese, S.; Ran, Z.H.; Repici, A.; Tong, J.; Omodei, P.; Aghemo, A.; Malesci, A. Gastroenterology department operational reorganisation at the time of COVID-19 outbreak: An Italian and Chinese experience. *Gut* **2020**, *69*, 981–983. [CrossRef]
3. Tunesi, S.; Murtas, R.; Riussi, A.; Sandrini, M.; Andreano, A.; Greco, M.T.; Gattoni, M.E.; Guido, D.; Gervasi, F.; Consolazio, D.; et al. Describing the epidemic trends of COVID-19 in the area covered by agency for health protection of the metropolitan area of Milan. *Epidemiol. Prev.* **2020**, *44*, 95–103. [CrossRef] [PubMed]
4. Charlson, M.E.; Pompei, P.; Ales, K.L.; MacKenzie, C.R. A new method of classifying prognostic comorbidity in longitudinal studies: Development and validation. *J. Chronic Dis.* **1987**, *40*, 373–383. [CrossRef]
5. Quan, H.; Li, B.; Couris, C.M.; Fushimi, K.; Graham, P.; Hider, P.; Januel, J.M.; Sundararajan, V. Updating and Validating the Charlson Comorbidity Index and Score for Risk Adjustment in Hospital Discharge Abstracts Using Data from 6 Countries. *Am. J. Epidemiol.* **2011**, *173*, 676–682. [CrossRef]
6. Elli, L.; Tontini, G.E.; Filippi, E.; Scaramella, L.; Cantù, P.; Vecchi, M.; Bertè, R.; Baldassarri, A.; Penagini, R. Efficacy of endoscopic triage during the COVID-19 outbreak and infective risk. *Eur. J. Gastroenterol. Hepatol.* **2020**, *32*, 1301–1304. [CrossRef]
7. Repici, A.; Pace, F.; Gabbiadini, R.; Colombo, M.; Hassan, C.; Dinelli, M.; Maselli, R.; Spadaccini, M.; Mutignani, M.; Gabbrielli, A.; et al. Endoscopy Units and the Coronavirus Disease 2019 Outbreak: A Multicenter Experience from Italy. *Gastroenterology* **2020**, *159*, 363–366.e3. [CrossRef]

8. Iavarone, M.; Antonelli, B.; Ierardi, A.M.; Topa, M.; Sangiovanni, A.; Gori, A.; Oggioni, C.; Rossi, G.; Carrafiello, G.; Lampertico, P. Reshape and secure HCC managing during COVID-19 pandemic: A single center analysis of four periods in 2020 versus 2019. *Liver Int.* **2021**. online ahead of print. [CrossRef] [PubMed]
9. Elli, L.; Tontini, G.E.; Scaramella, L.; Cantù, P.; Topa, M.; Dell'Osso, B.; Muscatello, A.; Gori, A.; Neumann, H.; Vecchi, M.; et al. Reopening Endoscopy after the COVID-19 Outbreak: Indications from a High Incidence Scenario. *J. Gastrointestin. Liver Dis.* **2020**, *29*, 295–299. [CrossRef]
10. World Health Organization. *Infection Prevention and Control during Health Care When COVID-19 Is Suspected: Interim Guidance, 19 March 2020*; World Health Organization: Geneva, Switzerland, 2020.
11. Bongiovanni, M.; Arienti, R.; Bini, F.; Bodini, B.D.; Corbetta, E.; Gianturco, L. Differences between the waves in Northern Italy: How the characteristics and the outcome of COVID-19 infected patients admitted to the emergency room have changed. *J. Infect.* **2021**, *83*, e32–e33. [CrossRef]

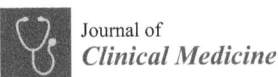

Review

Acute Mesenteric Ischemia in COVID-19 Patients

Dragos Serban [1,2,*,†], Laura Carina Tribus [3,4,†], Geta Vancea [1,5,†], Anca Pantea Stoian [1], Ana Maria Dascalu [1,*,†], Andra Iulia Suceveanu [6], Ciprian Tanasescu [7,8], Andreea Cristina Costea [9], Mihail Silviu Tudosie [1], Corneliu Tudor [2], Gabriel Andrei Gangura [1,10], Lucian Duta [2] and Daniel Ovidiu Costea [6,11,†]

1. Faculty of Medicine, "Carol Davila" University of Medicine and Pharmacy, 020021 Bucharest, Romania; geta.vancea@umfcd.ro (G.V.); ancastoian@yahoo.com (A.P.S.); mihail.tudosie@umfcd.ro (M.S.T.); gabriel.gangura@umfcd.ro (G.A.G.)
2. Fourth Surgery Department, Emergency University Hospital Bucharest, 050098 Bucharest, Romania; lulutudor@gmail.com (C.T.); lucian.duta@gmail.com (L.D.)
3. Faculty of Dental Medicine, "Carol Davila" University of Medicine and Pharmacy, 020021 Bucharest, Romania; laura.tribus@umfcd.ro
4. Department of Internal Medicine, Ilfov Emergency Clinic Hospital Bucharest, 022104 Bucharest, Romania
5. "Victor Babes" Infectious and Tropical Disease Hospital Bucharest, 030303 Bucharest, Romania
6. Faculty of Medicine, Ovidius University Constanta, 900470 Constanta, Romania; andrasuceveanu@yahoo.com (A.I.S.); Daniel.costea@365.univ-ovidius.ro (D.O.C.)
7. Faculty of Medicine, Lucian Blaga University of Sibiu, 550024 Sibiu, Romania; ciprian.tanasescu@ulbsibiu.ro
8. Department of Surgery, Emergency County Hospital Sibiu, 550245 Sibiu, Romania
9. Department of Nephrology, Diaverum Clinic Constanta, 900612 Constanta, Romania; acostea2021@gmail.com
10. Second Surgery Department, Emergency University Hospital Bucharest, 050098 Bucharest, Romania
11. General Surgery Department, Emergency County Hospital Constanta, 900591 Constanta, Romania
* Correspondence: dragos.serban@umfcd.ro (D.S.); ana.dascalu@umfcd.ro (A.M.D.); Tel.: +40-72-330-0370 (D.S.); +40-72-740-2495 (A.M.D.)
† These authors contributed equally to this work.

Abstract: Acute mesenteric ischemia is a rare but extremely severe complication of SARS-CoV-2 infection. The present review aims to document the clinical, laboratory, and imaging findings, management, and outcomes of acute intestinal ischemia in COVID-19 patients. A comprehensive search was performed on PubMed and Web of Science with the terms "COVID-19" and "bowel ischemia" OR "intestinal ischemia" OR "mesenteric ischemia" OR "mesenteric thrombosis". After duplication removal, a total of 36 articles were included, reporting data on a total of 89 patients, 63 being hospitalized at the moment of onset. Elevated D-dimers, leukocytosis, and C reactive protein (CRP) were present in most reported cases, and a contrast-enhanced CT exam confirms the vascular thromboembolism and offers important information about the bowel viability. There are distinct features of bowel ischemia in non-hospitalized vs. hospitalized COVID-19 patients, suggesting different pathological pathways. In ICU patients, the most frequently affected was the large bowel alone (56%) or in association with the small bowel (24%), with microvascular thrombosis. Surgery was necessary in 95.4% of cases. In the non-hospitalized group, the small bowel was involved in 80%, with splanchnic veins or arteries thromboembolism, and a favorable response to conservative anticoagulant therapy was reported in 38.4%. Mortality was 54.4% in the hospitalized group and 21.7% in the non-hospitalized group ($p < 0.0001$). Age over 60 years ($p = 0.043$) and the need for surgery ($p = 0.019$) were associated with the worst outcome. Understanding the mechanisms involved and risk factors may help adjust the thromboprophylaxis and fluid management in COVID-19 patients.

Keywords: acute mesenteric ischemia; COVID-19; thromboemboembolism; SARS-CoV-2; endothelitis; cytokines; hypercoagulability

Citation: Serban, D.; Tribus, L.C.; Vancea, G.; Stoian, A.P.; Dascalu, A.M.; Suceveanu, A.I.; Tanasescu, C.; Costea, A.C.; Tudosie, M.S.; Tudor, C.; et al. Acute Mesenteric Ischemia in COVID-19 Patients. *J. Clin. Med.* **2022**, *11*, 200. https://doi.org/10.3390/jcm11010200

Academic Editor: Hiroki Tanabe

Received: 9 December 2021
Accepted: 27 December 2021
Published: 30 December 2021

Publisher's Note: MDPI stays neutral with regard to jurisdictional claims in published maps and institutional affiliations.

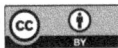

Copyright: © 2021 by the authors. Licensee MDPI, Basel, Switzerland. This article is an open access article distributed under the terms and conditions of the Creative Commons Attribution (CC BY) license (https://creativecommons.org/licenses/by/4.0/).

1. Introduction

Acute mesenteric ischemia (AMI) is a major abdominal emergency, characterized by a sudden decrease in the blood flow to the small bowel, resulting in ischemic lesions of the intestinal loops, necrosis, and if left untreated, death by peritonitis and septic shock. In non-COVID patients, the etiology may be mesenteric arterial embolism (in 50%), mesenteric arterial thrombosis (15–25%), venous thrombosis (5–15%), or less frequent, from non-occlusive causes associated with low blood flow [1]. Several systemic conditions, such as arterial hypertension, atrial fibrillation, atherosclerosis, heart failure, or valve disease are risk factors for AMI. Portal vein thrombosis and mesenteric vein thrombosis can be seen with celiac disease [2], appendicitis [3], pancreatitis [4], and, in particular, liver cirrhosis and hepatocellular cancer [5].

Acute intestinal ischemia is a rare manifestation during COVID-19 disease, but a correct estimation of its incidence is challenging due to sporadic reports, differences in patients' selection among previously published studies, and also limitations in diagnosis related to the strict COVID-19 regulations for disease control and difficulties in performing imagistic investigations in the patients in intensive care units. COVID-19 is known to cause significant alteration of coagulation, causing thromboembolic acute events, of which the most documented were pulmonary embolism, acute myocardial infarction, and lower limb ischemia [6].

Gastrointestinal features in COVID-19 disease are relatively frequently reported, varying from less than 10% in early studies from China [7,8] to 30–60%, in other reports [9,10]. In an extensive study on 1992 hospitalized patients for COVID-19 pneumonia from 36 centers, Elmunzer et al. [7] found that the most frequent clinical signs reported were mild and self-limited in up to 74% of cases, consisting of diarrhea (34%), nausea (27%), vomiting (16%), and abdominal pain (11%). However, severe cases were also reported, requiring emergency surgery for acute bowel ischemia or perforation [5,8].

The pathophysiology of the digestive features in COVID-19 patients involves both ischemic and non-ischemic mechanisms. ACE2 receptors are present at the level of the intestinal wall, and enterocytes may be directly infected by SARS-CoV-2. The virus was evidenced in feces and enteral walls in infected subjects [4,11–13]. In a study by Xu et al., rectal swabs were positive in 8 of 10 pediatric patients, even after the nasopharyngeal swabs became negative [14]. However, the significance of fecal elimination of viral ARN is still not fully understood in the transmission chain of the SARS-CoV-2 infection. On the other hand, disturbance of lung-gut axis, prolonged hospitalization in ICU, and the pro coagulation state induced by SARS-CoV-2 endothelial damage was incriminated for bowel ischemia, resulting in intestinal necrosis and perforation [8,9,15]. Early recognition and treatment of gastrointestinal ischemia are extremely important, but it is often challenging in hospitalized COVID-19 patients with severe illness.

The present review aims to document the risk factors, clinical, imagistic, and laboratory findings, management, and outcomes of acute intestinal ischemic complications in COVID-19 patients.

2. Materials and Methods

A comprehensive search was performed on PubMed and Web of Science with the terms "COVID-19" AND ("bowel ischemia" OR "intestinal ischemia" OR "mesenteric ischemia" OR "mesenteric thrombosis"). All original papers and case reports, in the English language, for which full text could be obtained, published until November 2021, were included in the review. Meeting abstracts, commentaries, and book chapters were excluded. A hand search was performed in the references of the relevant reviews on the topic.

2.1. Data Extraction and Analysis

The review is not registered in PROSPERO. A PRISMA flowchart was employed to screen papers for eligibility (Figure 1) and a PRISMA checklist is presented as a Supplementary File S1. A data extraction sheet was independently completed by two researchers, with strict adherence to PRISMA guidelines.

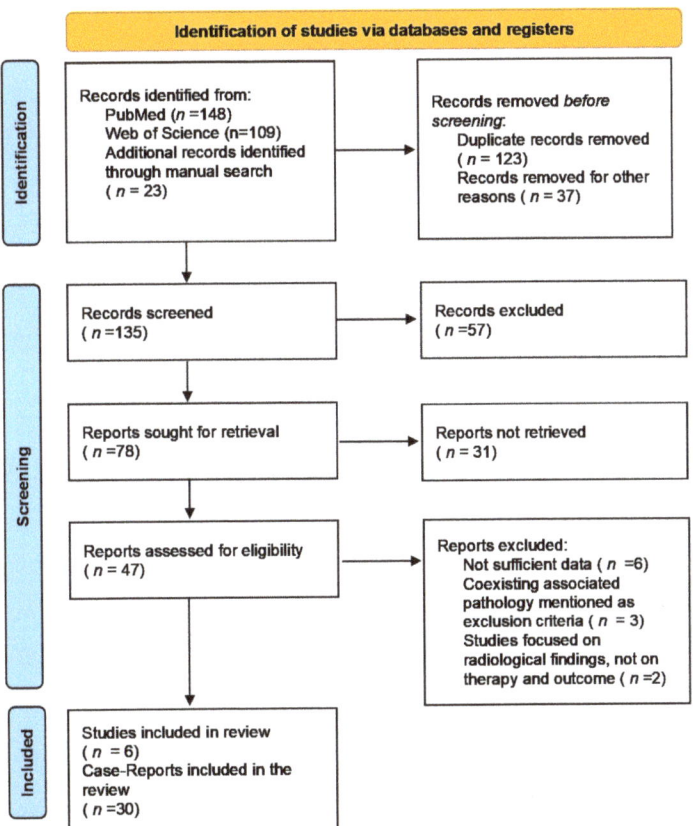

Figure 1. PRISMA 2020 flowchart for the studies included in the review.

The relevant data abstracted from these studies are presented in Tables 1–3. COVID-19 diagnosis was made by PCR assay in all cases. All patients reported with COVID-19 disease and mesenteric ischemia were documented in terms of age, sex, comorbidities, time from SARS-CoV-2 infection diagnosis, presentation, investigations, treatment, and outcome. A statistical analysis of the differences between acute intestinal ischemia in previously non-hospitalized vs. previously hospitalized patients was performed. The potential risk factors for an adverse vital prognosis were analyzed using SciStat® software (www.scistat.com (accessed on 25 November 2021)).

Papers that did not provide sufficient data regarding evaluation at admission, documentation of SARS-CoV-2 infection, or treatment were excluded. Patients suffering from other conditions that could potentially complicate intestinal ischemia, such as liver cirrhosis, hepatocellular carcinoma, intraabdominal infection (appendicitis, diverticulitis), pancreatitis, and celiac disease were excluded. Any disagreement was solved by discussion.

Table 1. Patients with intestinal ischemia in retrospective studies on hospitalized COVID-19 patients.

Study	No of Patients with Gastrointestinal Ischemia (Total No of COVID-19 Patients in ICU)	Sex (M; F)	Age (Mean)	BMI	Time from Admission to Onset (Days)	Abdominal CT Signs	Intraoperative/Endoscopic Findings	Treatment	Outcomes
Kaafarani HMA [16]	5 (141); 3.8%	1;3	62.5	32.1	51.5 (18–104) days	NA	Cecum-1—patchy necrosis Cecum_ileon-1 Small bowel-3; yellow discoloration on the antimesenteric side of the small bowel; 1 case + liver necrosis	Surgical resection	NA
Kraft M [17]	4 (190); 2.1%	NA	NA	NA	NA	NA	Bowel ischemia + perforation (2) Bowel ischemia + perforation (1) MAT+massive bowel ischemia (1)	Right hemicolectomy (2) Transverse colectomy (1) Conservative, not fit for surgery	Recovery (3) Death (1)
Yang C [18]	20 (190 in ICU; 582 in total); 10.5%	15;5	69	31.2	26.5 (17–42)	Distension Wall thickness Pneumatosis intestinalis Perforation SMA or celiac thrombosis	no info	Right hemicolectomy 7(35%) Sub/total colectomy12 (60%) Ileocecal resection 1(5%)	Recovery (11) Death (9)
Hwabejire J [19]	20	13;7	58.7	32.5	13 (1–31)	Pneumatosis intestinalis 42% Portal venous gas (33%) Mesenteric vessel patency 92%	large bowel ischemia (8) small bowel ischemia (4) both (8) yellow discoloration of the ischemic bowel	resection of the ischemic segment abdomen left open + second look (14)	Recovery (10) Death (10)
O'Shea A [20]	4 (142); 2.8%	NA	NA	NA	NA	bowel ischemia, portal vein gas, colic pneumatosis	NA	NA	NA
Qayed E [21]	2 (878); 0.22%	NA	NA	NA	NA	NA	diffuse colonic ischemia (1) Small + large bowel ischemia and pneumatosis (1)	Total colectomy (1) Extensive resection (1)	Recovery (1) Death (1)

NA: not acknowledged; MAT: mesenteric artery thrombosis; SMA: superior mesenteric artery.

Table 2. Case reports and case series presenting gastrointestinal ischemia in hospitalized COVID-19 patients under anticoagulant medication.

Article	Sex	Age	Comorbidities	Time from COVID-19 Diagnosis; Time from Admission (Days)	ICU; Type of Ventilation	Clinical Signs at Presentation	Leukocytes (/mm³)	CRP (mg/L)	Lactat mmol/L	Ferritin (ng/mL)	LDH (U/L)	Thrombocytes (/mm3)	D-Dimers (ng/mL)	Abdominal CT Signs	Treatment	Outcome
Azouz E [22]	M	56	none	1; 2 (hospitalized for acute ischemic stroke)	No info	abdominal pain and vomiting	No info	-	-	-	-	-	-	Multiple arterial thromboembolic complications: AMS, right middle cerebral artery, a free-floating clot in the aortic arch	Anticoagulation (no details), endovascular thrombectomy Laparotomy + resection of necrotic small bowel loops	No info
Al Mahruqi G [23]	M	51	none	26; 24	yes, intubated	Fever, metabolic acidosis, required inotropes	30,000	-	7	687	-	-	2.5	Non-occlusive AMI Hypoperfused small bowel, permeable aorta, SMA, IMA + deep lower limb thrombosis	enoxaparin 40 mg/day from admission; surgery refused by family	death
Ucpinar BA [24]	F	82	Atrial fibrillation, hypertension, chronic kidney disease	3; 3	no	-	14,800	196	5.1	-	-	-	1600	SMA thrombosis; distended small bowel, with diffuse submucosal pneumatosis portomesenteric gas	fluid resuscitation; continued ceftriaxone, enoxaparin 0.4cc twice daily; not operable due to fulminant evolution	Death
Karna ST [25]	F	61	DM, hypertension	4; 4	Yes, HFNO	diffuse abdominal pain with distention	21,400	421.6	1.4	-	-	464,000	No	thrombosis of the distal SMA with dilated jejunoileal loops and normal enhancing bowel wall	Iv heparin 5000 ui, followed by 1000 ui, Ecospin and clopidogrel Laparotomy after 10 days with segmental enterectomy of the necrotic bowel	Death by septic shock and acute renal failure
Singh B [26]	F	82	Hypertension, T2DM	32; 18	Yes, Ventilator support	severe diffuse abdominal distension and tenderness	22,800	308	2.5	136	333	146,000	1.3	SMA—colic arteries thrombosis pneumatosis intestinalis affecting the ascending colon and cecum	laparotomy, ischemic colon resection, ileostomy; heparin in therapeutic doses pre- and post-surgery	slow recovery

Table 2. *Cont.*

Article	Sex	Age	Comorbidities	Time from COVID-19 Diagnosis; Time from Admission (Days)	ICU; Type of Ventilation	Clinical Signs at Presentation	Leukocytes (/mm³)	CRP (mg/L)	Lactat mmol/L	Ferritin (ng/mL)	LDH (U/L)	Thrombocytes (/mm3)	D-Dimers (ng/mL)	Abdominal CT Signs	Treatment	Outcome
Nakatsutmi K [27]	F	67	DM, diabetic nephropathy requiring dialysis, angina, post-resection gastric cancer	16; 12	ICU, intubation	hemodynamic deterioration, abdominal distension	15,100	32.14	-	-	-	-	26.51	edematous transverse colon; abdominal vessels with sclerotic changes	laparotomy, which revealed vascular micro thrombosis of transverse colon—right segment resection of the ischemic colonic segment, ABTHERA management, second look, and closure of the abdomen after 24 h	death
Dinoto E [28]	F	84	DM, hypertension, renal failure	2; 2	no	Acute abdominal pain and distension;	18,000	32.47	-	-	431	-	6937	SMA origin stenosis and occlusion at 2 cm from the origin, absence of bowel enhancement	Endovascular thrombectomy of SMA; surgical transfemoral thrombectomy and distal superficial femoral artery stenting	Death due to respiratory failure
Kiwango F [29]	F	60	DM, hypertension	12; 3	no	Sudden onset abdominal pain	7700	-	-	-	-	-	23.8	Not performed	Not performed due to rapid oxygen desaturation Massive bowel acute ischemia	death

Table 3. Case reports and case series presenting gastrointestinal ischemia in non-hospitalized COVID-19 patients.

Article	Sex	Age	Comorbidities	Time from COVID-19 Diagnosis (Days)	Clinical Signs at Presentation	Leukocyte Count (/mm³)	CRP (mg/L)	Lactate mmol/L	Ferritin (ng/mL)	LDH (U/L)	Thrombocytes (/mm³)	D-Dimers (ng/mL)	Abdominal CT Signs	Treatment	Outcome
Sevella, P [30]	M	44	none	10	Acute abdominal pain constipation, vomiting	23,400	-	-	-	1097	360,000	1590	Viable jejunum, ischemic bowel, peritoneal thickening with fat stranding; free fluid in the peritoneal cavity	LMWH 60 mg daily Piperacillin 4g/day Tazobactam 500 mg/day Extensive small bowel + right colon resection	death
Nasseh S [31]	M	68	no info	First diagnosis	epigastric pain and diarrhea for 4 days	17,660	125	-	-	-	-	6876	terminal segment of the ileocolic artery thrombosis; thickening of the right colon wall and the last 30 cm of the small bowel	unfractioned heparin laparoscopy -no bowel resection needed	recovery
Aleman W [32]	M	44	none	20	severe abdominopelvic pain	36,870	-	-	456.23	-	574,000	263.87	absence of flow at SMV, splenic, portal vein; Small bowel loop dilatation and mesenteric fat edema	enoxaparin and pain control medication 6 days, then switched to warfarin 6 months	recovery
Jeilani M [33]	M	68	Alzheimer disease, COPD	9	Sharp abdominal pain +distension	12,440	307	-	-	-	318,000	897	a central venous filling defect within the portal vein extending to SMV; no bowel wall changes	LMWH, 3 months	recovery
Randhawa J [34]	F	62	none	First diagnosis	right upper quadrant pain and loss of appetite for 14 days	Normal limits	-	-	-	346	-	-	large thrombus involving the SMV, the main portal vein with extension into its branches	Fondaparinux 2.5. mg 5 days, then warfarin 4 mg (adjusted by INR), 6 months	recovery
Cheung S [35]	M	55	none	12 (discharged for 7 days)	Nausea, vomiting and worsening generalized abdominal pain with guarding	12,446	-	0.68	-	-	-	-	low-density clot, 1.6 cm in length, causing high-grade narrowing of the proximal SMA	continuous heparin infusion continued 8 h postoperative. Laparotomy with SMA thromboembolectomy and enterectomy (small bowel)	recovery

Table 3. Cont.

Article	Sex	Age	Comorbidities	Time from COVID-19 Diagnosis (Days)	Clinical Signs at Presentation	Leukocyte Count (/mm³)	CRP (mg/L)	Lactate mmol/L	Ferritin (ng/mL)	LDH (U/L)	Thrombocytes (/mm³)	D-Dimers (ng/mL)	Abdominal CT Signs	Treatment	Outcome
Beccara L [36]	M	52	none	22 (5 days after discharge and cessation prophylactic LMWH)	vomiting and abdominal pain, tenderness in epigastrium and mesogastrium	30,000	222	-	-	-	-	-	arterial thrombosis of vessels efferent of the SMA with bowel distension	Enterectomy (small bowel) LMWH plus aspirin 100 mg/day at discharge	recovery
Vulliamy P [37]	M	75	none	14	abdominal pain and vomiting for 2 days	18,100	3.2	-	-	-	497,000	320	intraluminal thrombus was present in the descending thoracic aorta with embolic occlusion of SMA	Catheter-directed thrombolysis, enterectomy (small bowel)	recovery
De Barry O [38]	F	79	none	First diagnosis	Epigastric pain, diarrhea, fever for 8 days, acute dyspnea	12600	125	5.36	-	-	-	-	SMV, portal vein, SMA, and jejunal artery thrombosis Distended loops, free fluid	anticoagulation Resection of affected colon+ ileum, SMA thrombolysis, thrombectomy	death
Romero MCV [39]	M	73	smoker, DM, hypertension	14	severe abdominal pain, nausea, fecal emesis, peritoneal irritation	18,000	-	-	-	-	120,000	>5000	RX: distention of intestinal loops, inter-loop edema, intestinal pneumatosis	enoxaparin (60 mg/0.6 mL), antibiotics (no info) enterectomy, anastomotic fistula, reintervention	death
Posada Arango [40]	M F F	62 22 65	None Appendectomy 7 days before left nephrectomy.	5 3 15	colicative abdominal pain at food intake; unsystematized gastrointestinal symptoms; abdominal pain in the upper hemiabdomen	20,100 - -	- - -	- - -	1536 - -	534 - -	- - -	- - -	Case 1: thrombus in distal SMA and its branches, intestinal loops dilatation, hydroaerical levels, free fluid Case 2: SMV thrombosis and adjacent fat edema Case 3: thrombi in the left jejunal artery branch with infarction of the corresponding jejunal loops	Case 1: Laparotomy; extensive jejunum + ileum ischemia; surgery could not be performed Case 2: Anticoagulation analgesic and antibiotics Case 3: segmental enterectomy	Case 1: death Case 2: recovery Case 3: recovery

Table 3. Cont.

Article	Sex	Age	Comorbidities	Time from COVID-19 Diagnosis (Days)	Clinical Signs at Presentation	Leukocyte Count (/mm³)	CRP (mg/L)	Lactate mmol/L	Ferritin (ng/mL)	LDH (U/L)	Thrombocytes (/mm³)	D-Dimers (ng/mL)	Abdominal CT Signs	Treatment	Outcome
Pang JHQ [41]	M	30	none	First diagnosis	colicky abdominal pain, vomiting	-	-	-	-	-	-	20	SMV thrombosis with diffuse mural thickening and fat stranding of multiple jejunal loops	conservative, anticoagulation with LMWH 1 mg/kc, twice daily, 3 months; readmitted and operated for congenital adherence causing small bowel obstruction	recovery
Lari E [42]	M	38	none	First diagnosis	abdominal pain, nausea, intractable vomiting, and shortness of breath	Mild leukocytosis	-	2.2	-	-	-	2100	extensive thrombosis of the portal, splenic, superior, and inferior mesenteric veins + mild bowel ischemia	Anticoagulation, resection of the affected bowel loop	No info
Carmo Filho A [43]	M	33	Obesity (BMI: 33), other not reported	7	severe low back pain radiating to the hypogastric region	-	58.2	-	1570	-	-	879	enlarged inferior mesenteric vein not filled by contrast associated with infiltration of the adjacent adipose planes	enoxaparin 5 days, followed by long term oral warfarin	recovery
Hanif M [44]	F	20	none	8	abdominal pain and abdominal distension	15,900	62	-	1435.3	825	633,000	2340	not performed	evidence of SMA thrombosis; enterectomy with exteriorization of both ends	recovery
Amaravathi U [45]	M	45	none	5	Acute epigastric and peri-umbilical pain	-	Normal value	1.3	324.3	-	-	5.3	SMA and SMV thrombus	i.v. heparin; Laparotomy with SMA thrombectomy; 48 h Second look: resection of the gangrenous bowel segment	No info
Al Mahruqi G [23]	M	51	none	4	generalized abdominal pain, nausea, vomiting	16,000	-	-	619	-	-	10	SMA thrombosis and non-enhancing proximal ileal loops consistent with small bowel ischemia	unfractionated heparin, thrombectomy + repeated resections of the ischemic bowel at relook (jejunum+ileon+cecum)	Case 2: recovery

Table 3. Cont.

Article	Sex	Age	Comorbidities	Time from COVID-19 Diagnosis (Days)	Clinical Signs at Presentation	Leukocyte Count (/mm³)	CRP (mg/L)	Lactate mmol/L	Ferritin (ng/mL)	LDH (U/L)	Thrombocytes (/mm³)	D-Dimers (ng/mL)	Abdominal CT Signs	Treatment	Outcome
Goodfellow M [46]	F	36	RYGB, depression, asthma	6	epigastric pain, irradiating back, nausea	9650	1.2	0.7	-	-	-	-	abrupt cut-off of the SMV in the proximal portion; diffuse infiltration of the mesentery, wall thickening of small bowel	IV heparin infusion, followed by 18,000 UI delteparin after 72 h	recovery
Abeysekera KW [26]	M	42	Hepatitis B	14	right hypochondrial pain, progressively increasing for 9 days	-	-	-	-	-	-	-	enhancement of the entire length of the portal vein and a smaller thrombus in the mid-superior mesenteric vein, mural edema of the distal duodenum, distal small bowel, and descending colon	factor Xa inhibitor apixaban 5 mg ×2/day, 6 months	recovery
Rodriguez-Nakamura RM [27]	M F	45 42	-vitiligo -obesity	14	severe mesogastric pain, nausea, diaphoresis	16,400 18,800	367 239	- -	970 -	- -	685,000 -	1450 14,407	Case 1: SMI of thrombotic etiology with partial rechanneling through the middle colic artery, and hypoxic-ischemic changes in the distal ileum and the cecum Case 2: thrombosis of the portal and mesenteric veins and an abdominopelvic collection in the mesentery with gas	Case 1: resection with entero-enteral anastomosis; rivaroxaban 10 mg/day, 6 months Case 2: Loop resection, entero-enteral manual anastomosis, partial omentectomy, and cavity wash (fecal peritonitis)	Case 1: Recovery Case 2: death
Plotz B [47]	F	27	SLE with ITP	First diagnosis	acute onset nausea, vomiting, and non-bloody diarrhea	-	-	-	-	-	-	5446	diffuse small bowel edema	enoxaparin, long term apixaban at discharge	recovery

Table 3. *Cont.*

Article	Sex	Age	Comorbidities	Time from COVID-19 Diagnosis (Days)	Clinical Signs at Presentation	Leukocyte Count (/mm³)	CRP (mg/L)	Lactate mmol/L	Ferritin (ng/mL)	LDH (U/L)	Thrombocytes (/mm³)	D-Dimers (ng/mL)	Abdominal CT Signs	Treatment	Outcome
Chiu CY [48]	F	49	Hypertension, DM, chronic kidney disease	28	diffuse abdominal pain melena and hematemesis	-	-	-	-	-	-	12,444	distended proximal jejunum with mural thickening	laparotomy, proximal jejunum resection	no info
Farina D [49]	M	70	no info	3	abdominal pain, nausea	15,300	149	-	-	-	-	-	acute small bowel hypoperfusion, SMA thromboembolism	not operable due to general condition	Death

SMA: superior mesenteric artery; SMV: superior mesenteric vein; DM: diabetes mellitus; T2DM: type 2 diabetes mellitus; AMI: acute mesenteric ischemia; IMV: inferior mesenteric vein; RYGB: Roux-en-Y gastric bypass (bariatric surgery).

2.2. Risk of Bias

The studies analyzed in the present review were comparable in terms of patient selection, methodology, therapeutic approach, and the report of final outcome. However, there were differences in the reported clinical and laboratory data. The sample size was small, most of them being case reports or case series, which may be a significant source of bias. Therefore, studies were compared only qualitatively.

3. Results

After duplication removal, a total of 36 articles were included in the review, reporting data on a total of 89 patients. Among these, we identified 6 retrospective studies [16–21], documenting intestinal ischemia in 55 patients admitted to intensive care units (ICU) with COVID-19 pneumonia for whom surgical consult was necessary (Table 1).

We also identified 30 case reports or case series [22–51] presenting 34 cases of acute bowel ischemia in patients positive for SARS-CoV-2 infection in different clinical settings. 8 cases were previously hospitalized for COVID-19 pneumonia and under anticoagulant medication (Table 2). In 26 cases, the acute ischemic event appeared as the first symptom of COVID-19 disease, or in mild forms treated at home, or after discharge for COVID -19 pneumonia and cessation of the anticoagulant medication (Table 3).

3.1. Risk Factors of Intestinal Ischemia in COVID-19 Patients

Out of a total of 89 patients included in the review, 63 (70.7%) were hospitalized for severe forms of COVID-19 pneumonia at the moment of onset. These patients were receiving anticoagulant medication when reported, consisting of low molecular weight heparin (LMWH) at prophylactic doses. The incidence of acute intestinal ischemia in ICU patients with COVID-19 varied widely between 0.22–10.5% (Table 1). In a study by O'Shea et al. [20], 26% of hospitalized patients for COVID-19 pneumonia who underwent imagistic examination, presented results positive for coagulopathy, and in 22% of these cases, the thromboembolic events were with multiple locations.

The mean age was 56.9 years. We observed a significantly lower age in non-hospitalized COVID-19 patients presenting with acute intestinal ischemia when compared to the previously hospitalized group ($p < 0.0001$).

There is a slight male to female predominance (M:F = 1:68). Obesity might be considered a possible risk factor, with a reported mean BMI of 31.2–32.5 in hospitalized patients [16,18,19]. However, this association should be regarded with caution, since obesity is also a risk factor for severe forms of COVID-19. Prolonged stay in intensive care, intubation, and the need for vasopressor medication was associated with increased risk of acute bowel ischemia [8,18,19].

Diabetes mellitus and hypertension were the most frequent comorbidities encountered in case reports (8 in 34 patients, 23%), and 7 out of 8 patients presented both (Table 4). There was no information regarding the comorbidities in the retrospective studies included in the review.

3.2. Clinical Features in COVID-19 Patients with Acute Mesenteric Ischemia

Abdominal pain, out of proportion to physical findings, is a hallmark of portomesenteric thrombosis, typically associated with fever and leukocytosis [4]. Abdominal pain was encountered in all cases, either generalized from the beginning, of high intensity, or firstly localized in the epigastrium or the mezogastric area. In cases of portal vein thrombosis, the initial location may be in the right hypochondrium, mimicking biliary colic [26,34].

Fever is less useful in COVID-19 infected patients, taking into consideration that fever is a general sign of infection, and on the other hand, these patients might be already under antipyretic medication.

Table 4. Demographic data of the patients included in the review.

Nr. of Patients	89
M	48 (61.5% *)
F	30 (38.5% *)
NA	11
The first sign of COVID-19	6 (6.7%)
Home treated	17 (19.1%)
Hospitalized	63 (70.7%)
• ICU	58 (92% of hospitalized patients)
Discharged	3 (3.3%)
Time from diagnosis of COVID-19 infection	
• Non-Hospitalized	8.7 ± 7.4 (1–28 days)
• Hospitalized (*when mentioned)	9.6 ± 8.3 (1–26 days)
Time from admission in hospitalized patients	1–104 days
Age (mean)	59.3 ± 12.7 years
• Hospitalized	62 ± 9.6 years. ($p < 0.0001$)
• Non-hospitalized	52.8 ± 16.4 years.
BMI	31.2–32.5
Comorbidities	
• Hypertension	8
• DM	7
• smokers	2
• Atrial fibrillation	1
• COPD	2
• Cirrhosis	1
• RYGB	1
• Vitiligo	1
• Recent appendicitis	1
• Operated gastric cancer	1
• Alzheimer disease	1
• SLE	1

*: percentage calculated in known information group; BMI: body mass index; COPD: chronic obstructive pulmonary disease; SLE: systemic lupus erythematosus.

Other clinical signs reported were nausea, anorexia, vomiting, and food intolerance [23,31,38,45]. However, these gastrointestinal signs are encountered in 30–40% of patients with SARS-CoV-2 infection. In a study by Kaafarani et al., up to half of the patients with gastrointestinal features presented some degrees of intestinal hypomotility, possibly due to direct viral invasion of the enterocytes and neuro-enteral disturbances [16].

Physical exam evidenced abdominal distension, reduced bowel sounds, and tenderness at palpation. Guarding may be evocative for peritonitis due to compromised vascularization of bowel loops and bacterial translocation or franc perforation [35,39].

A challenging case was presented by Goodfellow et al. [25] in a patient with a recent history of bariatric surgery with Roux en Y gastric bypass, presenting with acute abdominal pain which imposed the differential diagnosis with an internal hernia.

Upcinar et al. [24] reported a case of an 82-years female that also associated atrial fibrillation. The patient was anticoagulated with enoxaparin 0.4 cc twice daily before admission and continued the anticoagulant therapy during hospitalization for COVID-19 pneumonia. Bedside echocardiography was performed to exclude atrial thrombus. Although SMA was reported related to COVID-19 pneumonia, atrial fibrillation is a strong risk factor for SMA of non-COVID-19 etiology.

In ICU patients, acute bowel ischemia should be suspected in cases that present acute onset of digestive intolerance and stasis, abdominal distension, and require an increase of vasopressor medication [19].

3.3. Imagistic and Lab Test Findings

D-dimer is a highly sensitive investigation for the prothrombotic state caused by COVID-19 [45] and, when reported, was found to be above the normal values. Leukocytosis and acute phase biomarkers, such as fibrinogen and CRP were elevated, mirroring the intensity of inflammation and sepsis caused by the ischemic bowel. However, there was no significant statistical correlation between either the leukocyte count ($p = 0.803$) or D-dimers ($p = 0.08$) and the outcome. Leucocyte count may be within normal values in case of early presentation [34]. Thrombocytosis and thrombocytopenia have been reported in published cases with mesenteric ischemia [30,35,42,46,50].

Lactate levels were reported in 9 cases, with values higher than 2 mmol/L in 5 cases (55%). LDH was determined in 6 cases, and it was found to be elevated in all cases, with a mean value of 594+/−305 U/L.

Ferritin is another biomarker of potential value in mesenteric ischemia, that increases due to ischemia-reperfusion cellular damage. In the reviewed studies, serum ferritin was raised in 7 out of 9 reported cases, with values ranging from 456 to 1570 ng/mL. However, ferritin levels were found to be correlated also with the severity of pulmonary lesions in COVID-19 patients [52]. Due to the low number of cases in which lactate, LDH, and ferritin were reported, no statistical association could be performed with the severity of lesions or with adverse outcomes.

The location and extent of venous or arterial thrombosis were determined by contrast-enhanced abdominal CT, which also provided important information on the viability of the intestinal segment whose vascularity was affected.

Radiological findings in the early stages included dilated intestinal loops, thickening of the intestinal wall, mesenteric fat edema, and air-fluid levels. Once the viability of the affected intestinal segment is compromised, a CT exam may evidence pneumatosis as a sign of bacterial proliferation and translocation in the intestinal wall, pneumoperitoneum due to perforation, and free fluid in the abdominal cavity. In cases with an unconfirmed diagnosis of COVID-19, examination of the pulmonary basis during abdominal CT exam can add consistent findings to establish the diagnosis.

Venous thrombosis affecting the superior mesenteric vein and or portal vein was encountered in 40.9% of reported cases of non-hospitalized COVID-19 patients, and in only one case in the hospitalized group (Table 5). One explanation may be the beneficial role of thrombotic prophylaxis in preventing venous thrombosis in COVID-19 patients, which is routinely administered in hospitalized cases, but not reported in cases treated at home with COVID-19 pneumonia.

In ICU patients, CT exam showed in most cases permeable mesenteric vessels and diffuse intestinal ischemia affecting the large bowel alone (56%) or in association with the small bowel (24%), suggesting pathogenic mechanisms, direct viral infection, small vessel thrombosis, or "nonocclusive mesenteric ischemia" [16].

3.4. Management and Outcomes

The management of mesenteric ischemia includes gastrointestinal decompression, fluid resuscitation, hemodynamic support, anticoagulation, and broad antibiotics.

Once the thromboembolic event was diagnosed, heparin, 5000IU iv, or enoxaparin or LMWH in therapeutic doses was initiated, followed by long-term oral anticoagulation and/or anti-aggregating therapy. Favorable results were obtained in 7 out of 9 cases (77%) of splanchnic veins thrombosis and in 2 of 7 cases (28.5%) with superior mesenteric artery thrombosis. At discharge, anticoagulation therapy was continued either with LMWH, for a period up to 3 months [33,36,41], either, long term warfarin, with INR control [32,34,41] or apixaban 5 mg/day, up to 6 months [26,47]. No readmissions were reported.

Table 5. Comparative features in acute intestinal ischemia encountered in previously hospitalized and previously non-hospitalized COVID-19 patients.

Parameter	Hospitalized (63)	Non-Hospitalized (26)	p * Value
Type of mesenteric ischemia:			
• Arterial	5 (14.7% *)	10 (38.4%)	
• Venous	1 (2.9%)	11 (42.3%)	
• Mixt (A + V)	0	2 (7.6%)	$p < 0.0001$
• Diffuse microthrombosis	30 (88.2%)	3 (11.5%)	
• Multiple thromboembolic locations	2 (5.8%)	1 (3.8%)	
• NA	29	0	
Management:			
• Anticoagulation therapy only	0	10 (38.4%)	
• Endovascular thrombectomy	2 (1 + surgery) (3%)	2 (+surgery)	$p < 0.0001$
• Laparotomy with ischemic bowel resection	60 (95.4%)	15 (57.6%)	
• None (fulminant evolution)	2 (3%)	1 (3.8%)	
Location of the resected segment:			
• Colon	35 (56%)	0	
• Small bowel	10 (16%)	12 (80%)	$p < 0.0001$
• Colon+small bowel	15 (24%)	3 (20%)	
• NA	6	0	
Outcomes:			
• Recovery	26 (46.4%)	17 (79.3%)	
• Death	30 (54.4%)	5 (21.7%)	$p = 0.013$
• NA	7	3	

* calculated for Chi-squared test.

Antibiotic classes should cover anaerobes including *F. necrophorum* and include a combination of beta-lactam and beta-lactamase inhibitor (e.g., piperacillin-tazobactam), metronidazole, ceftriaxone, clindamycin, and carbapenems [4].

In early diagnosis, during the first 12 h from the onset, vascular surgery may be tempted, avoiding the enteral resection [25,53]. Endovascular management is a minimally invasive approach, allowing quick restoration of blood flow in affected vessels using techniques such as aspiration, thrombectomy, thrombolysis, and angioplasty with or without stenting [40].

Laparotomy with resection of the necrotic bowel should be performed as quickly as possible to avoid perforation and septic shock. In cases in which intestinal viability cannot be established with certainty, a second look laparotomy was performed after 24–48 h [43] or the abdominal cavity was left open, using negative pressure systems such as ABTHERA [51], and successive segmentary enterectomy was performed.

Several authors described in acute bowel ischemia encountered in ICU patients with COVID-19, a distinct yellowish color, rather than the typical purple or black color of ischemic bowel, predominantly located at the antimesenteric side or circumferentially with affected areas well delineated from the adjacent healthy areas [18,19]. In these cases, patency of large mesenteric vessels was confirmed, and the histopathological reports showed endothelitis, inflammation, and microvascular thrombosis in the submucosa or transmural. Despite early surgery, the outcome is severe in these cases, with an overall mortality of 45–50% in reported studies and up to 100% in patients over 65 years of age according to Hwabejira et al. [19].

In COVID-19 patients non hospitalized at the onset of an acute ischemic event, with mild and moderate forms of the disease, the outcome was less severe, with recovery in 77% of cases.

We found that age over 60 years and the necessity of surgical treatment are statistically correlated with a poor outcome in the reviewed studies (Table 6). According to the type of mesenteric ischemia, the venous thrombosis was more likely to have a favorable outcome (recovery in 80% of cases), while vascular micro thrombosis lead to death in 66% of cases.

Table 6. Risk factors for severe outcome.

Parameters	Outcome: Death	p-Value
Age • Age < 60 • Age > 60	27.2% 60%	0.0384 * 0.043 **
Surgery • No surgery • surgery	0% 60%	0.019 **
Type of mesenteric ischemia • Arterial • Venous • Micro thrombosis	47% 20% 66%	0.23 **
D dimers	Wide variation	0.085 * 0.394 **
Leucocytes	Wide variation (9650–37,000/mmc)	0.803 0.385 **

* One-way ANOVA test; ** Chi-squared test (SciStat® software, www.scistat.com (accessed on 25 November 2021)).

4. Discussions

Classically, acute mesenteric ischemia is a rare surgical emergency encountered in the elderly with cardiovascular or portal-associated pathology, such as arterial hypertension, atrial fibrillation, atherosclerosis, heart failure, valve disease, and portal hypertension. However, in the current context of the COVID-19 pandemic, mesenteric ischemia should be suspected in any patient presenting in an emergency with acute abdominal pain, regardless of age and associated diseases.

Several biomarkers were investigated for the potential diagnostic and prognostic value in acute mesenteric ischemia. Serum lactate is a non-specific biomarker of tissue hypoperfusion and undergoes significant elevation only after advanced mesenteric damage. Several clinical trials found a value higher than 2 mmol/L was significantly associated with increased mortality in non-COVID-patients. However, its diagnostic value is still a subject of debate. There are two detectable isomers, L-lactate, which is a nonspecific biomarker of anaerobic metabolism, and hypoxia and D-lactate, which is produced by the activity of intestinal bacteria. Higher D-lactate levels could be more specific for mesenteric ischemia due to increased bacterial proliferation at the level of the ischemic bowel, but the results obtained in different studies are mostly inconsistent [53,54].

Several clinical studies found that LDH is a useful biomarker for acute mesenteric ischemia, [55,56]. However, interpretation of the results may be difficult in COVID-19 patients, as both lactate and LDH were also found to be independent risk factors of severe forms of COVID-19 [57,58].

The diagnosis of an ischemic bowel should be one of the top differentials in critically ill patients with acute onset of abdominal pain and distension [50,59]. If diagnosed early, the intestinal ischemia is potentially reversible and can be treated conservatively. Heparin has an anticoagulant, anti-inflammatory, endothelial protective role in COVID-19, which can improve microcirculation and decrease possible ischemic events [25]. The appropriate dose, however, is still a subject of debate with some authors recommending the prophylactic, others the intermediate or therapeutic daily amount [25,60].

We found that surgery is associated with a severe outcome in the reviewed studies. Mucosal ischemia may induce massive viremia from bowel epithelium causing vasoplegic shock after surgery [25]. Moreover, many studies reported poor outcomes in COVID-19 patients that underwent abdominal surgery [61,62].

4.1. Pathogenic Pathways of Mesenteric Ischemia in COVID-19 Patients

The intestinal manifestations encountered in SARS-CoV-2 infection are represented by inflammatory changes (gastroenteritis, colitis), occlusions, ileus, invaginations, and ischemic manifestations. Severe inflammation in the intestine can cause damage to the submucosal vessels, resulting in hypercoagulability in the intestine. Cases of acute cholecystitis, splenic infarction, or acute pancreatitis have also been reported in patients infected with SARS-CoV-2, with microvascular lesions as a pathophysiological mechanism [63].

In the study of O'Shea et al., on 146 COVID-19 hospitalized patients that underwent CT-scan, vascular thrombosis was identified in 26% of cases, the most frequent location being in lungs [20]. Gastrointestinal ischemic lesions were identified in 4 cases, in multiple locations (pulmonary, hepatic, cerebellar parenchymal infarction) in 3 patients. The authors raised awareness about the possibility of underestimation of the incidence of thrombotic events in COVID-19 patients [20].

Several pathophysiological mechanisms have been considered, and they can be grouped into occlusive and non-occlusive causes [64]. The site of the ischemic process, embolism or thrombosis, may be in the micro vascularization, veins, or mesenteric arteries.

Acute arterial obstruction of the small intestinal vessels and mesenteric ischemia may appear due to hypercoagulability associated with SARS-CoV-2 infection, mucosal ischemia, viral dissemination, and endothelial cell invasion vis ACE-2 receptors [65,66]. Viral binding to ACE2Receptors leads to significant changes in fluid-coagulation balance: reduction in Ang 2 degradation leads to increased Il6 levels, and the onset of storm cytokines, such as IL-2, IL-7, IL-10, granulocyte colony-stimulating factor, IgG -induced protein 10, monocyte chemoattractant protein-1, macrophage inflammatory protein 1-alpha, and tumor necrosis factor α [67], but also in the expression of the tissue inhibitor of plasminogen -1, and a tissue factor, and subsequently triggering the coagulation system through binding to the clotting factor VIIa [68]. Acute embolism in small vessels may be caused by the direct viral invasion, via ACE-2 Receptors, resulting in endothelitis and inflammation, recruiting immune cells, and expressing high levels of pro-inflammatory cytokines, such as Il-6 and TNF-alfa, with consequently apoptosis of the endothelial cells [69].

Capillary viscometry showed hyperviscosity in critically ill COVID-19 patients [70,71]. Platelet activation, platelet–monocyte aggregation formation, and Neutrophil external traps (NETs) released from activated neutrophils, constitute a mixture of nucleic DNA, histones, and nucleosomes [59,72] were documented in severe COVID-19 patients by several studies [70,71,73].

Plotz et al. found a thrombotic vasculopathy with histological evidence for lectin pathway complement activation mirroring viral protein deposition in a patient with COVID-19 and SLE, suggesting this might be a potential mechanism in SARS-CoV-2 associated thrombotic disorders [47].

Numerous alterations in fluid-coagulation balance have been reported in patients hospitalized for COVID-19 pneumonia. Increases in fibrinogen, D-dimers, but also coagulation factors V and VIII. The mechanisms of coagulation disorders in COVID-19 are not yet fully elucidated. In a clinical study by Stefely et al. [68] in a group of 102 patients with severe disease, an increase in factor V > 200 IU was identified in 48% of cases, the levels determined being statistically significantly higher than in non-COVID mechanically ventilated or unventilated patients hospitalized in intensive care. This showed that the increased activity of Factor V cannot be attributed to disease severity or mechanical ventilation. Additionally, an increase in factor X activity was shown, but not correlated with an increase in factor V activity, but with an increase in acute phase reactants, suggesting distinct pathophysiological mechanisms [74].

Giuffre et al. suggest that fecal calcoprotein (FC) may be a biomarker for the severity of gastrointestinal complications, by both ischemic and inflammatory mechanisms [75]. They found particularly elevated levels of FC to be well correlated with D-dimers levels in patients with bowel perforations, and hypothesized that the mechanism may be related to a thrombosis localized to the gut and that FC increase is related to virus-related inflammation and thrombosis-induced ischemia, as shown by gross pathology [76].

Non-occlusive mesenteric ischemia in patients hospitalized in intensive care units for SARS-CoV-2 pneumonia requiring vasopressor medication may be caused vasospastic constriction [19,64,65]. Thrombosis of the mesenteric vessels could be favored by hypercoagulability, relative dehydration, and side effects of corticosteroids.

4.2. Question Still to Be Answered

Current recommendations for in-hospital patients with COVID-19 requiring anticoagulation suggest LMWH as first-line treatment has advantages, with higher stability compared to heparin during cytokine storms, and a reduced risk of interaction with antiviral therapy compared to oral anticoagulant medication [77]. Choosing the adequate doses of LMWH in specific cases—prophylactic, intermediate, or therapeutic—is still in debate. Thromboprophylaxis is highly recommended in the absence of contraindications, due to the increased risk of venous thrombosis and arterial thromboembolism associated with SARS-CoV-2 infection, with dose adjustment based on weight and associated risk factors. Besides the anticoagulant role, some authors also reported an anti-inflammatory role of heparin in severe COVID-19 infection [66,78,79]. Heparin is known to decrease inflammation by inhibiting neutrophil activity, expression of inflammatory mediators, and the proliferation of vascular smooth muscle cells [78]. Thromboprophylaxis with enoxaparin could be also recommended to ambulatory patients with mild to moderate forms of COVID-19 if the results of prospective studies show statistically relevant benefits [80].

In addition to anticoagulants, other therapies, such as anti-complement and interleukin (IL)-1 receptor antagonists, need to be explored, and other new agents should be discovered as they emerge from our better understanding of the pathogenetic mechanisms [81]. Several studies showed the important role of Il-1 in endothelial dysfunction, inflammation, and thrombi formation in COVID-19 patients by stimulating the production of Thromboxane A2 (TxA2) and thromboxane B2 (TxB2). These findings may justify the recommendation for an IL-1 receptor antagonist (IL-1Ra) which can prevent hemodynamic changes, septic shock, organ inflammation, and vascular thrombosis in severe forms of COVID-19 patients [80–82].

5. Conclusions

Understanding the pathological pathways and risk factors could help adjust the thromboprophylaxis and fluid management in COVID-19 patients. The superior mesenteric vein thrombosis is the most frequent cause of acute intestinal ischemia in COVID-19 non-hospitalized patients that are not under anticoagulant medication, while non-occlusive mesenteric ischemia and microvascular thrombosis are most frequent in severe cases, hospitalized in intensive care units.

COVID-19 patients should be carefully monitored for acute onset of abdominal symptoms. High-intensity pain and abdominal distension, associated with leukocytosis, raised inflammatory biomarkers and elevated D-dimers and are highly suggestive for mesenteric ischemia. The contrast-enhanced CT exam, repeated, if necessary, offers valuable information regarding the location and extent of the acute ischemic event. Early diagnosis and treatment are essential for survival.

Supplementary Materials: The following supporting information can be downloaded at: https://www.mdpi.com/article/10.3390/jcm11010200/s1, File S1: The PRISMA 2020 statement.

Author Contributions: Conceptualization, D.S., L.C.T. and A.M.D.; methodology, A.P.S., C.T. (Corneliu Tudor); software, G.V.; validation, A.I.S., M.S.T., D.S. and L.D.; formal analysis, A.C.C., C.T. (Ciprian Tanasescu); investigation, G.A.G.; data curation, D.O.C.; writing—original draft preparation, L.C.T., A.M.D., G.V., D.O.C., G.A.G., C.T. (Corneliu Tudor); writing—review and editing, L.D., C.T. (Ciprian Tanasescu), A.C.C., D.S., A.P.S., A.I.S., M.S.T.; visualization, G.V. and L.C.T.; supervision, D.S., A.M.D. and D.S. have conducted the screening and selection of studies included in the review All authors have read and agreed to the published version of the manuscript.

Funding: This research received no external funding.

Conflicts of Interest: The authors declare no conflict of interest.

References

1. Bala, M.; Kashuk, J.; Moore, E.E.; Kluger, Y.; Biffl, W.; Gomes, C.A.; Ben-Ishay, O.; Rubinstein, C.; Balogh, Z.J.; Civil, I.; et al. Acute mesenteric ischemia: Guidelines of the World Society of Emergency Surgery. *World J. Emerg. Surg.* **2017**, *12*, 38. [CrossRef]
2. Dumic, I.; Martin, S.; Salfiti, N.; Watson, R.; Alempijevic, T. Deep Venous Thrombosis and Bilateral Pulmonary Embolism Revealing Silent Celiac Disease: Case Report and Review of the Literature. *Case Rep. Gastrointest. Med.* **2017**, *2017*, 5236918. [CrossRef] [PubMed]
3. Akhrass, F.A.; Abdallah, L.; Berger, S.; Sartawi, R. Gastrointestinal variant of Lemierre's syndrome complicating ruptured appendicitis. *IDCases* **2015**, *2*, 72–76. [CrossRef]
4. Radovanovic, N.; Dumic, I.; Veselinovic, M.; Burger, S.; Milovanovic, T.; Nordstrom, C.W.; Niendorf, E.; Ramanan, P. Fusobacterium necrophorum subsp. necrophorum Liver Abscess with Pylephlebitis: An Abdominal Variant of Lemierre's Syndrome. *Case Rep. Infect. Dis.* **2020**, *2020*, 9237267. [CrossRef]
5. Sogaard, K.K.; Astrup, L.B.; Vilstrup, H.; Gronbaek, H. Portal vein thrombosis; risk factors, clinical presentation and treatment. *BMC Gastroenterol.* **2007**, *7*, 34. [CrossRef] [PubMed]
6. Moradi, H.; Mouzannar, S.; Miratashi Yazdi, S.A. Post COVID-19 splenic infarction with limb ischemia: A case report. *Ann. Med. Surg.* **2021**, *71*, 102935. [CrossRef] [PubMed]
7. Elmunzer, B.J.; Spitzer, R.L.; Foster, L.D.; Merchant, A.A.; Howard, E.F.; Patel, V.A.; West, M.K.; Qayed, E.; Nustas, R.; Zakaria, A.; et al. North American Alliance for the Study of Digestive Manifestations of COVID-19. Digestive Manifestations in Patients Hospitalized With Coronavirus Disease 2019. *Clin. Gastroenterol. Hepatol.* **2021**, *19*, 1355–1365.e4. [CrossRef]
8. Guan, W.J.; Ni, Z.Y.; Hu, Y. Clinical characteristics of coronavirus disease 2019 in China. *N. Engl. J. Med.* **2020**, *382*, 1708–1720. [CrossRef]
9. Estevez-Cerda, S.C.; Saldaña-Rodríguez, J.A.; Alam-Gidi, A.G.; Riojas-Garza, A.; Rodarte-Shade, M.; Velazco-de la Garza, J.; Leyva-Alvizo, A.; Gonzalez-Ruvalcaba, R.; Martinez-Resendez, M.F.; Ortiz de Elguea-Lizarraga, J.I. Severe bowel complications in SARS-CoV-2 patients receiving protocolized care. *Rev. Gastroenterol. Mex. Engl. Ed.* **2021**, *86*, 378–386. [CrossRef]
10. Redd, W.D.; Zhou, J.C.; Hathorn, K.E. Prevalence and characteristics of gastrointestinal symptoms in patients with SARS-CoV-2 infection in the United States: A multicenter cohort study. *Gastroenterology* **2020**, *159*, 765–767.e2. [CrossRef]
11. Hajifathalian, K.; Krisko, T.; Mehta, A. Gastrointestinal and hepatic manifestations of 2019 novel coronavirus disease in a large cohort of infected patients from New York: Clinical implications. *Gastroenterology* **2020**, *159*, 1137–1140.e2. [CrossRef]
12. Kotfis, K.; Skonieczna-Żydecka, K. COVID-19: Gastrointestinal symptoms and potential sources of SARS-CoV-2 transmission. *Anaesthesiol. Intensive Ther.* **2020**, *52*, 171–172. [CrossRef]
13. Xiao, F.; Tang, M.; Zheng, X. Evidence for gastrointestinal infection of SARS-CoV-2. *Gastroenterology* **2020**, *158*, 1831–1833. [CrossRef] [PubMed]
14. Xu, Y.; Li, X.; Zhu, B.; Liang, H.; Fang, C.; Gong, Y.; Guo, Q.; Sun, X.; Zhao, D.; Shen, J.; et al. Characteristics of pediatric SARS-CoV-2 infection and potential evidence for persistent fecal viral shedding. *Nat. Med.* **2020**, *26*, 502–505. [CrossRef] [PubMed]
15. Ludewig, S.; Jarbouh, R.; Ardelt, M.; Mothes, H.; Rauchfuß, F.; Fahrner, R.; Zanow, J.; Settmacher, U. Bowel Ischemia in ICU Patients: Diagnostic Value of I-FABP Depends on the Interval to the Triggering Event. *Gastroenterol. Res. Pract.* **2017**, 2795176. [CrossRef]
16. Kaafarani, H.; El Moheb, M.; Hwabejire, J.O.; Naar, L.; Christensen, M.A.; Breen, K.; Gaitanidis, A.; Alser, O.; Mashbari, H.; Bankhead-Kendall, B.; et al. Gastrointestinal Complications in Critically Ill Patients With COVID-19. *Ann. Surg.* **2020**, *272*, e61–e62. [CrossRef]
17. Kraft, M.; Pellino, G.; Jofra, M.; Sorribas, M.; Solís-Peña, A.; Biondo, S.; Espín-Basany, E. Incidence, features, outcome and impact on health system of de-novo abdominal surgical diseases in patients admitted with COVID-19. *Surg. J. R. Coll. Surg. Edinb. Irel.* **2021**, *19*, e53–e58. [CrossRef]
18. Yang, C.; Hakenberg, P.; Weiß, C.; Herrle, F.; Rahbari, N.; Reißfelder, C.; Hardt, J. Colon ischemia in patients with severe COVID-19: A single-center retrospective cohort study of 20 patients. *Int. J. Colorectal Dis.* **2021**, *36*, 2769–2773. [CrossRef]

19. Hwabejire, J.O.; Kaafarani, H.M.; Mashbari, H.; Misdraji, J.; Fagenholz, P.J.; Gartland, R.M.; Abraczinskas, D.R.; Mehta, R.S.; Paranjape, C.N.; Eng, G.; et al. Bowel Ischemia in COVID-19 Infection: One-Year Surgical Experience. *Am. Surg.* **2021**, *87*, 1893–1900. [CrossRef] [PubMed]
20. O'shea, A.; Parakh, A.; Hedgire, S.; Lee, S.I. Multisystem assessment of the imaging manifestations of coagulopathy in hospitalized patients with coronavirus. *Am. J. Roentgenol.* **2021**, *216*, 1088–1098. [CrossRef] [PubMed]
21. Qayed, E.; Deshpande, A.R.; Elmunzer, B.J.; North American Alliance for the Study of Digestive Manifestations of COVID-19. Low Incidence of Severe Gastrointestinal Complications in COVID-19 Patients Admitted to the Intensive Care Unit: A Large, Multicenter Study. *Gastroenterology* **2021**, *160*, 1403–1405. [CrossRef] [PubMed]
22. Azouz, E.; Yang, S.; Monnier-Cholley, L.; Arrivé, L. Systemic arterial thrombosis and acute mesenteric ischemia in a patient with COVID-19. *Intensive Care Med.* **2020**, *46*, 1464–1465. [CrossRef] [PubMed]
23. Al Mahruqi, G.; Stephen, E.; Abdelhedy, I.; Al Wahaibi, K. Our early experience with mesenteric ischemia in COVID-19 positive patients. *Ann. Vasc. Surg.* **2021**, *73*, 129–132. [CrossRef] [PubMed]
24. Ucpinar, B.A.; Sahin, C. Superior Mesenteric Artery Thrombosis in a Patient with COVID-19: A Unique Presentation. *J. Coll Physicians Surg. Pak.* **2020**, *30*, 112–114. [CrossRef]
25. Karna, S.T.; Panda, R.; Maurya, A.P.; Kumari, S. Superior Mesenteric Artery Thrombosis in COVID-19 Pneumonia: An Underestimated Diagnosis—First Case Report in Asia. *Indian J. Surg.* **2020**, *82*, 1235–1237. [CrossRef]
26. Abeysekera, K.W.; Karteszi, H.; Clark, A.; Gordon, F.H. Spontaneous portomesenteric thrombosis in a non-cirrhotic patient with SARS-CoV-2 infection. *BMJ Case Rep.* **2020**, *13*, e238906. [CrossRef]
27. Rodriguez-Nakamura, R.M.; Gonzalez-Calatayud, M.; Martinez Martinez, A.R. Acute mesenteric thrombosis in two patients with COVID-19. Two cases report and literature review. *Int. J. Surg. Case Rep.* **2020**, *76*, 409–414. [CrossRef]
28. Dinoto, E.; Ferlito, F.; La Marca, M.A.; Mirabella, D.; Bajardi, G.; Pecoraro, F. Staged acute mesenteric and peripheral ischemia treatment in COVID-19 patient: Case report. *Int. J. Surg. Case Rep.* **2021**, *84*, 106105. [CrossRef]
29. Kiwango, F.; Mremi, A.; Masenga, A.; Akrabi, H. Intestinal ischemia in a COVID-19 patient: Case report from Northern Tanzania. *J. Surg. Case Rep.* **2021**, *2021*, rjaa537. [CrossRef]
30. Sevella, P.; Rallabhandi, S.; Jahagirdar, V.; Kankanala, S.R.; Ginnaram, A.R.; Rama, K. Acute Mesenteric Ischemia as an Early Complication of COVID-19. *Cureus* **2021**, *13*, e18082. [CrossRef]
31. Nasseh, S.; Trabelsi, M.M.; Oueslati, A.; Haloui, N.; Jerraya, H.; Nouira, R. COVID-19 and gastrointestinal symptoms: A case report of a Mesenteric Large vessel obstruction. *Clin. Case Rep.* **2021**, *9*, e04235. [CrossRef] [PubMed]
32. Alemán, W.; Cevallos, L.C. Subacute mesenteric venous thrombosis secondary to COVID-19: A late thrombotic complication in a nonsevere patient. *Radiol. Case Rep.* **2021**, *16*, 899–902. [CrossRef] [PubMed]
33. Jeilani, M.; Hill, R.; Riad, M.; Abdulaal, Y. Superior mesenteric vein and portal vein thrombosis in a patient with COVID-19: A rare case. *BMJ Case Rep.* **2021**, *14*, e244049. [CrossRef]
34. Randhawa, J.; Kaur, J.; Randhawa, H.S.; Kaur, S.; Singh, H. Thrombosis of the Portal Vein and Superior Mesenteric Vein in a Patient With Subclinical COVID-19 Infection. *Cureus* **2021**, *13*, e14366. [CrossRef] [PubMed]
35. Cheung, S.; Quiwa, J.C.; Pillai, A.; Onwu, C.; Tharayil, Z.J.; Gupta, R. Superior Mesenteric Artery Thrombosis and Acute Intestinal Ischemia as a Consequence of COVID-19 Infection. *Am. J. Case Rep.* **2020**, *21*, e925753. [CrossRef]
36. Beccara, L.A.; Pacioni, C.; Ponton, S.; Francavilla, S.; Cuzzoli, A. Arterial Mesenteric Thrombosis as a Complication of SARS-CoV-2 Infection. *Eur. J. Case Rep. Intern. Med.* **2020**, *7*, 001690. [CrossRef] [PubMed]
37. Vulliamy, P.; Jacob, S.; Davenport, R.A. Acute aorto-iliac and mesenteric arterial thromboses as presenting features of COVID-19. *Br. J. Haematol.* **2020**, *189*, 1053–1054. [CrossRef]
38. De Barry, O.; Mekki, A.; Diffre, C.; Seror, M.; El Hajjam, M.; Carlier, R.Y. Arterial and venous abdominal thrombosis in a 79-year-old woman with COVID-19 pneumonia. *Radiol. Case Rep.* **2020**, *15*, 1054–1057. [CrossRef]
39. Romero, M.D.C.V.; Cárdenas, A.M.; Fuentes, A.B.; Barragán, A.A.S.; Gómez, D.B.S.; Jiménez, M.T. Acute mesenteric arterial thrombosis in severe SARS-Co-2 patient: A case report and literature review. *Int. J. Surg. Case Rep.* **2021**, *86*, 106307. [CrossRef]
40. Posada-Arango, A.M.; García-Madrigal, J.; Echeverri-Isaza, S.; Alberto-Castrillón, G.; Martínez, D.; Gómez, A.C.; Pinto, J.A.; Pinillos, L. Thrombosis in abdominal vessels associated with COVID-19 Infection: A report of three cases. *Radiol. Case Rep.* **2021**, *16*, 3044–3050. [CrossRef]
41. Pang, J.H.Q.; Tang, J.H.; Eugene-Fan, B. A peculiar case of small bowel stricture in a coronavirus disease 2019 patient with congenital adhesion band and superior mesenteric vein thrombosis. *Ann. Vasc. Surg.* **2021**, *70*, 286–289. [CrossRef]
42. Lari, E.; Lari, A.; AlQinai, S. Severe ischemic complications in COVID-19-a case series. *Int. J. Surg. Case Rep.* **2020**, *75*, 131–135. [CrossRef] [PubMed]
43. Carmo Filho, A.; Cunha, B.D.S. Inferior mesenteric vein thrombosis and COVID-19. *Rev. Soc. Bras. Med. Trop.* **2020**, *53*, e20200412. [CrossRef]
44. Hanif, M.; Ahmad, Z.; Khan, A.W.; Naz, S.; Sundas, F. COVID-19-Induced Mesenteric Thrombosis. *Cureus* **2021**, *13*, e12953. [CrossRef]
45. Amaravathi, U.; Balamurugan, N.; Muthu Pillai, V.; Ayyan, S.M. Superior Mesenteric Arterial and Venous Thrombosis in COVID-19. *J. Emerg. Med.* **2021**, *60*, e103–e107. [CrossRef] [PubMed]
46. Goodfellow, M.; Courtney, M.; Upadhyay, Y.; Marsh, R.; Mahawar, K. Mesenteric Venous Thrombosis Due to Coronavirus in a Post Roux-en-Y Gastric Bypass Patient: A Case Report. *Obes. Surg.* **2021**, *31*, 2308–2310. [CrossRef] [PubMed]

47. Plotz, B.; Castillo, R.; Melamed, J.; Magro, C.; Rosenthal, P.; Belmont, H.M. Focal small bowel thrombotic microvascular injury in COVID-19 mediated by the lectin complement pathway masquerading as lupus enteritis. *Rheumatology* **2021**, *60*, e61–e63. [CrossRef]
48. Chiu, C.Y.; Sarwal, A.; Mon, A.M.; Tan, Y.E.; Shah, V. Gastrointestinal: COVID-19 related ischemic bowel disease. *J. Gastroenterol. Hepatol.* **2021**, *36*, 850. [CrossRef] [PubMed]
49. Farina, D.; Rondi, P.; Botturi, E.; Renzulli, M.; Borghesi, A.; Guelfi, D.; Ravanelli, M. Gastrointestinal: Bowel ischemia in a suspected coronavirus disease (COVID-19) patient. *J. Gastroenterol. Hepatol.* **2021**, *36*, 41. [CrossRef]
50. Singh, B.; Mechineni, A.; Kaur, P.; Ajdir, N.; Maroules, M.; Shamoon, F.; Bikkina, M. Acute Intestinal Ischemia in a Patient with COVID-19 Infection. *Korean J. Gastroenterol.* **2020**, *76*, 164–166. [CrossRef]
51. Nakatsutsumi, K.; Endo, A.; Okuzawa, H.; Onishi, I.; Koyanagi, A.; Nagaoka, E.; Morishita, K.; Aiboshi, J.; Otomo, Y. Colon perforation as a complication of COVID-19: A case report. *Surg. Case Rep.* **2021**, *7*, 175. [CrossRef]
52. Carubbi, F.; Salvati, L.; Alunno, A.; Maggi, F.; Borghi, E.; Mariani, R.; Mai, F.; Paoloni, M.; Ferri, C.; Desideri, G.; et al. Ferritin is associated with the severity of lung involvement but not with worse prognosis in patients with COVID-19: Data from two Italian COVID-19 units. *Sci. Rep.* **2021**, *11*, 4863. [CrossRef]
53. Isfordink, C.J.; Dekker, D.; Monkelbaan, J.F. Clinical value of serum lactate measurement in diagnosing acute mesenteric ischaemia. *Neth. J. Med.* **2018**, *76*, 60–64. [PubMed]
54. Montagnana, M.; Danese, E.; Lippi, G. Biochemical markers of acute intestinal ischemia: Possibilities and limitations. *Ann. Transl. Med.* **2018**, *6*, 341. [CrossRef]
55. Matsumoto, S.; Sekine, K.; Funaoka, H.; Yamazaki MShimizu, M.; Hayashida, K.; Kitano, M. Diagnostic performance of plasma biomarkers in patients with acute intestinal ischaemia. *Br. J. Surg.* **2014**, *101*, 232–238. [CrossRef] [PubMed]
56. Soni, N.; Bhutra, S.; Vidyarthi, S.H.; Sharma, V. Role of serum lactic dehydrogenase, glutamic oxaloacetic transaminase, creatine phosphokinase, alkaline phospatase, serum phosphorus in the cases of bowel Ischaemia in acute abdomen. *Int. Surg. J.* **2017**, *4*, 1997–2001. [CrossRef]
57. Han, Y.; Zhang, H.; Mu, S.; Wei, W.; Jin, C.; Tong, C.; Song, Z.; Zha, Y.; Xue, Y.; Gu, G. Lactate dehydrogenase, an independent risk factor of severe COVID-19 patients: A retrospective and observational study. *Aging* **2020**, *12*, 11245–11258. [CrossRef]
58. Carpenè, G.; Onorato, D.; Nocini, R.; Fortunato, G.; Rizk, J.G.; Henry, B.M.; Lippi, G. Blood lactate concentration in COVID-19: A systematic literature review. *Clin. Chem. Lab. Med.* **2021**. advance online publication. [CrossRef]
59. Singh, B.; Kaur, P.; Maroules, M. Splanchnic vein thrombosis in COVID-19: A review of literature. *Dig. Liver Dis.* **2020**, *52*, 1407–1409. [CrossRef]
60. Jagielski, M.; Piątkowski, J.; Jackowski, M. Challenges encountered during the treatment of acute mesenteric ischemia. *Gastroenterol. Res. Pract.* **2020**, 5316849. [CrossRef] [PubMed]
61. Rasslan, R.; Dos Santos, J.P.; Menegozzo, C.; Pezzano, A.; Lunardeli, H.S.; Dos Santos Miranda, J.; Utiyama, E.M.; Damous, S. Outcomes after emergency abdominal surgery in COVID-19 patients at a referral center in Brazil. *Updates Surg.* **2021**, *73*, 763–768. [CrossRef]
62. Lei, S.; Jiang, F.; Su, W.; Chen, C.; Chen, J.; Mei, W.; Zhan, L.Y.; Jia, Y.; Zhang, L.; Liu, D.; et al. Clinical characteristics and outcomes of patients undergoing surgeries during the incubation period of COVID-19 infection. *EClinicalMedicine* **2020**, *21*, 100331. [CrossRef]
63. Serban, D.; Socea, B.; Badiu, C.D.; Tudor, C.; Balasescu, S.A.; Dumitrescu, D.; Trotea, A.M.; Spataru, R.I.; Vancea, G.; Dascalu, A.M.; et al. Acute surgical abdomen during the COVID 19 pandemic: Clinical and therapeutic challenges. *Exp. Ther. Med.* **2021**, *21*, 519. [CrossRef] [PubMed]
64. Patel, S.; Parikh, C.; Verma, D.; Sundararajan, R.; Agrawal, U.; Bheemisetty, N.; Akku, R.; Sánchez-Velazco, D.; Waleed, M.S. Bowel ischaemia in COVID-19: A systematic review. *Int. J. Clin. Pract.* **2021**, *75*, e14930. [CrossRef] [PubMed]
65. Yantiss, R.K.; Qin, L.; He, B.; Crawford, C.V.; Seshan, S.; Patel, S.; Wahid, N.; Jessurun, J. Intestinal Abnormalities in Patients With SARS-CoV-2 Infection: Histopathologic Changes Reflect Mechanisms of Disease. *Am. J. Surg. Pathol.* **2021**, *46*, 89–96. [CrossRef] [PubMed]
66. McGonagle, D.; Bridgewood, C.; Ramanan, A.V.; Meaney, J.F.M.; Watad, A. COVID-19 vasculitis and novel vasculitis mimics. *Lancet Rheumatol.* **2021**, *3*, e224–e233. [CrossRef]
67. Huang, C.; Wang, Y.; Li, X. Clinical features of patients infected with 2019 novel coronavirus in Wuhan. *China Lancet* **2020**, *395*, 497–506. [CrossRef]
68. Avila, J.; Long, B.; Holladay, D.; Gottlieb, M. Thrombotic complications of COVID-19. *Am. J. Emerg. Med.* **2021**, *39*, 213–218. [CrossRef]
69. Varga, Z.; Flammer, A.J.; Steiger, P.; Haberecker, M.; Andermatt, R.; Zinkernagel, A.S.; Mehra, M.R.; Schuepbach, R.A.; Ruschitzka, F.; Moch, H. Endothelial cell infection and endotheliitis in COVID-19. *Lancet* **2020**, *395*, 1417–1418. [CrossRef]
70. Maier, C.L.; Truong, A.D.; Auld, S.C.; Polly, D.M.; Tanksley, C.L.; Duncan, A. COVID-19-associated hyperviscosity: A link between inflammation and thrombophilia? *Lancet* **2020**, *395*, 1758–1759. [CrossRef]
71. Miyara, S.J.; Becker, L.B.; Guevara, S.; Kirsch, C.; Metz, C.N.; Shoaib, M.; Grodstein, E.; Nair, V.V.; Jandovitz, N.; McCann-Molmenti, A.; et al. Pneumatosis Intestinalis in the Setting of COVID-19: A Single Center Case Series From New York. *Front. Med.* **2021**, *8*, 638075. [CrossRef] [PubMed]

72. Panigada, M.; Bottino, N.; Tagliabue, P.; Grasselli, G.; Novembrino, C.; Chantarangkul, V.; Pesenti, A.; Peyvandi, F.; Tripodi, A. Hypercoagulability of COVID-19 patients in intensive care unit: A report of thromboelastography findings and other parameters of hemostasis. *J. Thromb. Haemost.* **2020**, *18*, 1738–1742. [CrossRef]
73. Hottz, E.D.; Azevedo-Quintanilha, I.G.; Palhinha, L.; Teixeira, L.; Barreto, E.A.; Pão, C.R.; Righy, C.; Franco, S.; Souza, T.M.; Kurtz, P.; et al. Platelet activation and platelet-monocyte aggregate formation trigger tissue factor expression in patients with severe COVID-19. *Blood J. Am. Soc. Hematol.* **2020**, *136*, 1330–1341. [CrossRef]
74. Stefely, J.A.; Christensen, B.B.; Gogakos, T.; Cone Sullivan, J.K.; Montgomery, G.G.; Barranco, J.P.; Van Cott, E.M. Marked factor V activity elevation in severe COVID-19 is associated with venous thromboembolism. *Am. J. Hematol.* **2020**, *95*, 1522–1530. [CrossRef]
75. Giuffrè, M.; Di Bella, S.; Sambataro, G.; Zerbato, V.; Cavallaro, M.; Occhipinti, A.A.; Palermo, A.; Crescenti, A.; Monica, F.; Luzzati, R.; et al. COVID-19-Induced Thrombosis in Patients without Gastrointestinal Symptoms and Elevated Fecal Calprotectin: Hypothesis Regarding Mechanism of Intestinal Damage Associated with COVID-19. *Trop. Med. Infect. Dis.* **2020**, *5*, 147. [CrossRef] [PubMed]
76. Giuffrè, M.; Vetrugno, L.; Di Bella, S.; Moretti, R.; Berretti, D.; Crocè, L.S. Calprotectin and SARS-CoV-2: A Brief-Report of the Current Literature. *Healthcare* **2021**, *9*, 956. [CrossRef] [PubMed]
77. Buso, G.; Becchetti, C.; Berzigotti, A. Acute splanchnic vein thrombosis in patients with COVID-19: A systematic review. *Dig. Liver Dis.* **2021**, *53*, 937–949. [CrossRef]
78. Thachil, J. The versatile heparin in COVID-19. *J. Thromb. Haemost.* **2020**, *18*, 1020–1022. [CrossRef]
79. Poterucha, T.J.; Libby, P.; Goldhaber, S.Z. More than an anticoagulant: Do heparins have direct anti-inflammatory effects? *Thromb. Haemost.* **2017**, *117*, 437–444. [CrossRef]
80. Wang, M.K.; Yue, H.Y.; Cai, J.; Zhai, Y.J.; Peng, J.H.; Hui, J.F.; Hou, D.Y.; Li, W.P.; Yang, J.S. COVID-19 and the digestive system: A comprehensive review. *World J. Clin. Cases* **2021**, *9*, 3796–3813. [CrossRef]
81. Manolis, A.S.; Manolis, T.A.; Manolis, A.A.; Papatheou, D.; Melita, H. COVID-19 Infection: Viral Macro- and Micro-Vascular Coagulopathy and Thromboembolism/Prophylactic and Therapeutic Management. *J. Cardiovasc. Pharmacol. Ther.* **2021**, *26*, 12–24. [CrossRef] [PubMed]
82. Conti, P.; Caraffa, A.; Gallenga, C.E.; Ross, R.; Kritas, S.K.; Frydas, I.; Younes, A.; Di Emidio, P.; Ronconi, G.; Toniato, E. IL-1 induces throboxane-A2 (TxA2) in COVID-19 causing inflammation and micro-thrombi: Inhibitory effect of the IL-1 receptor antagonist (IL-1Ra). *J. Biol. Regul. Homeost. Agents* **2020**, *34*, 1623–1627. [CrossRef] [PubMed]

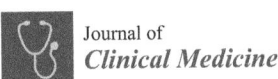

Article

Nationwide COVID-19-EII Study: Incidence, Environmental Risk Factors and Long-Term Follow-Up of Patients with Inflammatory Bowel Disease and COVID-19 of the ENEIDA Registry

Yamile Zabana [1,2,*], Ignacio Marín-Jiménez [3], Iago Rodríguez-Lago [4,5], Isabel Vera [6], María Dolores Martín-Arranz [7], Iván Guerra [8,9], Javier P. Gisbert [2,10,11], Francisco Mesonero [12], Olga Benítez [1], Carlos Taxonera [13,14], Ángel Ponferrada-Díaz [15], Marta Piqueras [16], Alfredo J. Lucendo [2,11,17], Berta Caballol [2,18], Míriam Mañosa [2,19], Pilar Martínez-Montiel [20], Maia Bosca-Watts [21], Jordi Gordillo [22], Luis Bujanda [2,23,24], Noemí Manceñido [25], Teresa Martínez-Pérez [26], Alicia López [27], Cristina Rodríguez-Gutiérrez [28], Santiago García-López [29], Pablo Vega [30], Montserrat Rivero [31], Luigi Melcarne [32], Maria Calvo [33], Marisa Iborra [2,34], Manuel Barreiro-de-Acosta [35], Beatriz Sicilia [36], Jesús Barrio [37], José Lázaro Pérez [38], David Busquets [39], Isabel Pérez-Martínez [40], Mercè Navarro-Llavat [41], Vicent Hernández [42], Federico Argüelles-Arias [43], Fernando Ramírez Esteso [44], Susana Meijide [45], Laura Ramos [46], Fernando Gomollón [2,47], Fernando Muñoz [48], Gerard Suris [49], Jone Ortiz de Zarate [50], José María Huguet [51], Jordina Lláo [52], Mariana Fe García-Sepulcre [53], Mónica Sierra [54], Miguel Durà [55], Sandra Estrecha [56], Ana Fuentes Coronel [57], Esther Hinojosa [58], Lorenzo Olivan [59], Eva Iglesias [60], Ana Gutiérrez [2,61], Pilar Varela [62], Núria Rull [63], Pau Gilabert [64], Alejandro Hernández-Camba [65], Alicia Brotons [66], Daniel Ginard [67], Eva Sesé [68], Daniel Carpio [69], Montserrat Aceituno [1,2], José Luis Cabriada [4,5], Yago González-Lama [6], Laura Jiménez [8,9], María Chaparro [2,10,11], Antonio López-San Román [12], Cristina Alba [13,14], Rocío Plaza-Santos [15], Raquel Mena [16], Sonsoles Tamarit-Sebastián [17], Elena Ricart [2,18], Margalida Calafat [2,19], Sonsoles Olivares [20], Pablo Navarro [21], Federico Bertoletti [22], Horacio Alonso-Galán [23,24], Ramón Pajares [25], Pablo Olcina [26], Pamela Manzano [1], Eugeni Domènech [2,19], Maria Esteve [1,2] and on behalf of the ENEIDA registry of GETECCU [†]

Citation: Zabana, Y.; Marín-Jiménez, I.; Rodríguez-Lago, I.; Vera, I.; Martín-Arranz, M.D.; Guerra, I.; Gisbert, J.P.; Mesonero, F.; Benítez, O.; Taxonera, C.; et al. Nationwide COVID-19-EII Study: Incidence, Environmental Risk Factors and Long-Term Follow-Up of Patients with Inflammatory Bowel Disease and COVID-19 of the ENEIDA Registry. *J. Clin. Med.* 2022, 11, 421. https://doi.org/10.3390/jcm11020421

Academic Editor: Hemant Goyal

Received: 9 December 2021
Accepted: 6 January 2022
Published: 14 January 2022

Publisher's Note: MDPI stays neutral with regard to jurisdictional claims in published maps and institutional affiliations.

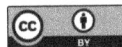

Copyright: © 2022 by the authors. Licensee MDPI, Basel, Switzerland. This article is an open access article distributed under the terms and conditions of the Creative Commons Attribution (CC BY) license (https://creativecommons.org/licenses/by/4.0/).

1   Hospital Universitari Mútua Terrassa, 08221 Terrassa, Spain; olgabl27@gmail.com (O.B.); maceituno1@hotmail.com (M.A.); hermisende@gmail.com (P.M.); mariaesteve@mutuaterrassa.cat (M.E.)
2   Centro de Investigación Biomédica en Red de Enfermedades Hepáticas y Digestivas (CIBEREHD), 28029 Madrid, Spain; javier.p.gisbert@gmail.com (J.P.G.); ajlucendo@hotmail.com (A.J.L.); caballol@clinic.cat (B.C.); mmanosa.germanstrias@gencat.cat (M.M.); luis.bujanda@osakidetza.net (L.B.); marisaiborra@hotmail.com (M.I.); fgomollon@gmail.com (F.G.); gutierrez_anacas@gva.es (A.G.); mariachs2005@gmail.com (M.C.); ericart@clinic.cat (E.R.); margalidasard.calafat@gmail.com (M.C.); eugenidomenech@gmail.com (E.D.)
3   Hospital Gregorio Marañón, 218007 Madrid, Spain; drnachomarin@hotmail.com
4   Gastroenterology Department, Hospital Universitario de Galdakao, 48960 Galdakao, Spain; iago.r.lago@gmail.com (I.R.-L.); jcabriada@gmail.com (J.L.C.)
5   Biocruces Bizkaia Health Research Institute, 48960 Galdakao, Spain
6   Hospital Universitario Puerta de Hierro, 28222 Majadahonda, Spain; isabel.veramendoza@gmail.com (I.V.); ygonzalezlama@gmail.com (Y.G.-L.)
7   Hospital Universitario La Paz, 28046 Madrid, Spain; mmartina.hulp@salud.madrid.org
8   Hospital Universitario de Fuenlabrada, 28942 Fuenlabrada, Spain; ivangm79@gmail.com (I.G.); laujmarquez@gmail.com (L.J.)
9   Instituto de Investigación Hospital Universitario La Paz (IdiPaz), 28046 Madrid, Spain
10 Department of Gastroenterology, Hospital Universitario de La Princesa, Universidad Autónoma de Madrid (UAM), 28049 Madrid, Spain
11 Instituto de Investigación Sanitaria Princesa (IIS-IP), 28006 Madrid, Spain
12 Hospital Universitario Ramón y Cajal, 28034 Madrid, Spain; pacomeso@hotmail.com (F.M.); mibuzon@gmail.com (A.L.-S.R.)

13 Hospital Clínico San Carlos, 28040 Madrid, Spain; ctaxonera.hcsc@salud.madrid.org (C.T.); cristina.alba@telefonica.net (C.A.)
14 Instituto de Investigación del Hospital Clínico San Carlos [IdISSC], 28040 Madrid, Spain
15 Hospital Universitario Infanta Leonor, 28031 Madrid, Spain; angelponmedicina@yahoo.es (Á.P.-D.); rocio_plaza@yahoo.es (R.P.-S.)
16 Consorci Sanitari de Terrassa, 08227 Terrassa, Spain; MPiqueras@cst.cat (M.P.); RMena@cst.cat (R.M.)
17 Hospital General de Tomelloso, 13700 Tomelloso, Spain; sonsolestamarit@hotmail.com
18 Hospital Clínic de Barcelona-IDIBAPS, 08036 Barcelona, Spain
19 Hospital Universitari Germans Trias i Pujol, 08916 Badalona, Spain
20 Fundación Hospital Universitario Doce de Octubre, 28041 Madrid, Spain; pilarmarmon123@telefonica.net (P.M.-M.); sonsolesolivares@hotmail.com (S.O.)
21 Hospital Clinic Universitari de Valencia, 46010 Valencia, Spain; maiabosca@gmail.com (M.B.-W.); pnavarrocortes@gmail.com (P.N.)
22 Hospital de la Santa Creu i Sant Pau, 08041 Barcelona, Spain; jgordillo@santpau.cat (J.G.); fbertoletti@santpau.cat (F.B.)
23 Hospital Universitario Donostia, Instituto Biodonostia, 20014 San Sebastián, Spain; horacio.alonsogalan@osakidetza.eus
24 Universidad del País Vasco (UPV/EHU), 48940 Leioua, Spain
25 Hospital Universitario Infanta Sofía, 28703 San Sebastián de los Reyes, Spain; nmancenido@gmail.com (N.M.); rpajaresvi@gmail.com (R.P.)
26 Hospital Virgen de la Luz, 16002 Cuenca, Spain; terechu.martinez@gmail.com (T.M.-P.); olcinapod@gmail.com (P.O.)
27 Institut Hospital del Mar d'Investigacions Mèdiques (IMIM), Hospital del Mar, 08003 Barcelona, Spain; alicialg84@gmail.com
28 Complejo Hospitalario de Navarra, 31008 Pamplona, Spain; cristina.rodriguez.gutierrez@cfnavarra.es
29 Hospital Universitario Miguel Servet, 50009 Zaragoza, Spain; sgarcia.lopez@gmail.com
30 Complexo Hospitalario Universitario de Ourense, 32005 Ourense, Spain; pablo.vega.villaamil@sergas.es
31 Instituto de Investigación Sanitaria Valdecilla (IDIVAL), Hospital Universitario Marqués de Valdecilla, 39008 Santander, Spain; digrtm@humv.es
32 Hospital Universitari Parc Taulí, 08208 Sabadell, Spain; lmelcarne@tauli.cat
33 Hospital San Pedro-Logroño, 26006 Logroño, Spain; mciniguez@riojasalud.es
34 Hospital Universitario y Politécnico de la Fe de Valencia, 46026 Valencia, Spain
35 Hospital Clínico Universitario de Santiago, 15706 Santiago, Spain; manubarreiro@hotmail.com
36 Hospital Universitario de Burgos, 09006 Burgos, Spain; bsicilia4@gmail.com
37 Hospital Universitario Río Hortega (HURH), 47012 Valladolid, Spain; jbarrioa95@gmail.com
38 Hospital Universitario Fundación de Alcorcón, 28922 Alcorcón, Spain; jlperezc@fhalcorcon.es
39 Hospital Universitari de Girona Doctor Josep Trueta, 17007 Girona, Spain; dbusquets.girona.ics@gencat.cat
40 Instituto de Investigación Sanitaria del Principado de Asturias (ISPA), Hospital Universitario Central de Asturias, 33011 Oviedo, Spain; ipermar_79@hotmail.com
41 Hospital de Sant Joan Despí Moisès Broggi, 08970 Sant Joan Despí, Spain; merce.navarro@sanitatintegral.org
42 Hospital Álvaro Cunqueiro, 36213 Vigo, Spain; vicent.hernandez.ramirez@sergas.es
43 Hospital Universitario Virgen de la Macarena, Universidad de Sevilla, 41009 Sevilla, Spain; farguelles@telefonica.net
44 Hospital General Universitario de Ciudad Real, 13005 Ciudad Real, Spain; fernando.ramirez.est@gmail.com
45 Hospital Universitario de Cruces, 48903 Barakaldo, Spain; susana.meijidedelafuente@osakidetza.eus
46 Hospital Universitario de Canarias, 38320 San Cristobal de la Laguna, Spain; laura7ramos@gmail.com
47 Hospital Clínico Universitario "Lozano Blesa" and IIS Aragón, 50009 Zaragoza, Spain
48 Hospital Universitario de Salamanca, 37007 Salamanca, Spain; jmunozn@gmail.com
49 Hospital Universitari de Bellvitge, 08907 L'Hospitalet de Llobregat, Spain; tsuris@bellvitgehospital.cat
50 Hospital Universitario de Basurto, 48013 Bilbo, Spain; jone.ortizdezaratesagastagoitia@osakidetza.net
51 Consorcio Hospital General Universitario de Valencia, 46014 Valencia, Spain; josemahuguet@gmail.com
52 Althaia Xarxa Assistencial Universitària de Manresa, 08243 Manresa, Spain; jllao@althaia.cat
53 Hospital Universitario de Elche, 03203 Elche, Spain; marifegarciasepulcre@gmail.com
54 Complejo Asistencial Universitario de León, 24071 León, Spain; msierra.ausin@gmail.com
55 Hospital Clínico de Valladolid, 47003 Valladolid, Spain; mdura@saludcastillayleon.es
56 Hospital Universitario Álava, 01009 Gasteiz, Spain; sandra.estrecha@gmail.com
57 Hospital Virgen de la Concha, 49022 Zamora, Spain; amfcoronel@gmail.com
58 Hospital de Manises, 46940 Manises, Spain; hinova200@gmail.com
59 Hospital Universitario San Jorge, 22004 Huesca, Spain; lorenolivan@gmail.com
60 Instituto Maimónides de Investigación Biomédica de Córdoba (IMIBIC), Hospital Universitario Reina Sofía de Córdoba, 14004 Cordoba, Spain; evaiflores@gmail.com
61 Hospital General Universitario de Alicante, 03010 Alicante, Spain
62 Hospital Universitario de Cabueñes, 33394 Gijón, Spain; trastoy@hotmail.com

63 Hospital Universitario Son Llàtzer, 07198 Palma, Spain; nrull@hsll.es
64 Hospital de Viladecans, 08840 Viladecans, Spain; pgilabert.hv@gencat.cat
65 Hospital Universitario Nuestra Señora de Candelaria, 38010 Santa Cruz de Tenerife, Spain; dr.alejandrohc@gmail.com
66 Hospital Vega Baja de Orihuela, 03314 Alicante, Spain; aliciabbrotons@gmail.com
67 Hospital Universitario Son Espases, 07120 Palma, Spain; daniel.ginard@ssib.es
68 Hospital Universitari Arnau de Vilanova de Lleida, 25198 Lleida, Spain; eseseabi@gmail.com
69 Complexo Hospitalario de Pontevedra, 36071 Pontevedra, Spain; daniel.carpio.lopez@sergas.es
* Correspondence: yzabana@gmail.com
† All Co-authors are part of ENEIDA.

Abstract: We aim to describe the incidence and source of contagion of COVID-19 in patients with IBD, as well as the risk factors for a severe course and long-term sequelae. This is a prospective observational study of IBD and COVID-19 included in the ENEIDA registry (53,682 from 73 centres) between March–July 2020 followed-up for 12 months. Results were compared with data of the general population (National Centre of Epidemiology and Catalonia). A total of 482 patients with COVID-19 were identified. Twenty-eight percent were infected in the work environment, and 48% were infected by intrafamilial transmission, despite having good adherence to lockdown. Thirty-five percent required hospitalization, 7.9% had severe COVID-19 and 3.7% died. Similar data were reported in the general population (hospitalisation 19.5%, ICU 2.1% and mortality 4.6%). Factors related to death and severe COVID-19 were being aged ≥ 60 years (OR 7.1, 95% CI: 1.8–27 and 4.5, 95% CI: 1.3–15.9), while having ≥ 2 comorbidities increased mortality (OR 3.9, 95% CI: 1.3–11.6). None of the drugs for IBD were related to severe COVID-19. Immunosuppression was definitively stopped in 1% of patients at 12 months. The prognosis of COVID-19 in IBD, even in immunosuppressed patients, is similar to that in the general population. Thus, there is no need for more strict protection measures in IBD.

Keywords: COVID-19; SARS-CoV-2; inflammatory bowel disease

1. Introduction

The COVID-19 pandemic hit Spain at the end of February 2020 and is far from under complete control. Data on affected cases and mortality are continuously updated [1]. There is evidence that patients suffering from inflammatory bowel disease (IBD) have a greater risk for infections, some of them opportunistic, mainly favoured by immunosuppressive treatment [2–4]. For that reason, experts on IBD, worried by the potential severity of COVID-19 in these patients, recommended, during the initial phases of the pandemic, that whenever possible, starting immunosuppressants should be delayed and treatment deescalated [5–7]. Notwithstanding this information, more than one year after the start of the pandemic, factors related to deleterious prognosis of COVID-19 in patients with IBD are essentially the same as those of the general population (mainly older age and comorbidities), whereas those on immunosuppressants do not appear to have a greater risk for severe COVID-19, except for corticosteroids [8]. In this sense, the international self-reported registry SECURE-IBD (https://covidibd.org (accessed on 24 August 2021)) has provided valuable clinical and therapeutic information [9]. Nevertheless, retrospective studies and registries have important limitations, such as reporting bias, over- or underrepresentation of the more severe cases of COVID-19, and the possibility of including confounding factors that may influence the results.

In addition, some studies have reported a low incidence of COVID-19 in patients with IBD [10], suggesting that IBD and the type of immunosuppressants administered for disease control do not represent risk factors for COVID-19. However, few of these studies are population based and do not address important environmental epidemiological risk factors, such as variability in the incidence of the infection in different regions within the same country. Neither do they address factors that may facilitate the infection, such as occupational risk, or those that may reduce the risk, as they may be specific isolation measures that could be recommended to a particular diseased population [10–16]. Likewise, the impact of COVID-19 on patients with IBD in the long term has not yet been explored.

The present study (COVID-19-EII study) was conducted in the setting of the ENEIDA project, the Spanish registry of patients with IBD, promoted by the Spanish Working Group on Crohn's disease and ulcerative colitis (GETECCU) [17]. The aims of the present study were (1) to describe the incidence of COVID-19 in the ENEIDA registry, the geographical distribution of the infection compared with the distribution in the general Spanish population and exposure factors that may favour or prevent the infection (occupational risk and lockdown measures) during the first wave of the pandemic and (2) to describe the clinical characteristics and the disease course, including a 12-month follow-up after COVID-19.

2. Materials and Methods

2.1. Design

This was an observational prospective cohort study (COVID-19-EII) within the Spanish ENEIDA IBD registry. It included all patients with IBD who had COVID-19 between March and July 2020 (in the first wave) from the participant centres.

2.2. Study Population

The potential population was all patients with IBD registered in ENEIDA. Patients with COVID-19 were identified by an active search from their IBD unit (systematically addressing all the patients with IBD from the unit by email or phone call) or by direct notification from the patient itself, the family physician, the emergency department or the hospitalisation unit.

2.3. Data Collection

A prospective module hosted on the ENEIDA platform was specially designed for this study. Data collected included clinical baseline characteristics such as type of IBD, date of IBD diagnosis and Montreal's classification [18], extraintestinal manifestations, family history of IBD and smoking behaviour at time of infection. The following comorbidities were specifically registered: cirrhosis, chronic renal failure, chronic obstructive pulmonary disease, heart disease, stroke, diabetes mellitus, arterial hypertension, dyslipidaemia, neoplasia, congestive heart failure, dementia, HIV, rheumatological disease or immune-mediated disease. Charlson's index [19] was also calculated. We decided to explore both individual comorbidities and the Charlson comorbidity score, as these two approaches examine different aspects of comorbidity and are complementary. Variables measuring the exposure risk to SARS-CoV-2 included occupational risk (such as health care workers, teachers, basic services as supermarket cashiers, market clerks or pharmacy workers, police and firepersons, workers of closed institutions, veterinaries, animal control workers or conservation and forest technicians), compliance with lockdown measures, social distancing and the route of contagion. At the time of COVID-19 diagnosis, IBD activity was evaluated using the Harvey-Bradshaw index [20] or partial Mayo score [21]. The IBD therapeutic regimen was registered at the time of infection and up to 3 and 12 months before it: systemic steroid treatment, aminosalicylates, immunosuppressants (thiopurines, cyclosporine, methotrexate, tacrolimus and tofacitinib) and biologics (anti-TNF, vedolizumab and ustekinumab). Regarding COVID-19, the data collected included symptoms associated with the infection at the time of diagnosis, diagnostic procedures and specific treatment. The variables registered 3 and 12 months after COVID-19 were IBD activity and COVID-19 sequelae, both physical and psychological. To assess the impact of COVID-19 on IBD treatment, any change in medical therapy, including withdrawal of immunosuppression, both definitive and temporary, was collected during follow-up.

2.4. Definitions

COVID-19 diagnosis was based on a typical clinical picture consisting of fever (>38 °C), respiratory symptoms (cough and/or dyspnoea), anosmia or dysgeusia within the epidemiological setting. COVID-19 was considered confirmed by a positive diagnostic test including polymerase chain reaction (PCR) taken by nasopharyngeal swab or serology (IgM or IgG) for SARS-CoV-2. COVID-19 was considered probable in patients with a typical clinical picture but negative or lacking diagnostic tests. Asymptomatic patients with positive PCR or serology were not included.

It was considered that any patient had a good compliance with the lockdown measures when maintaining social distance by staying at home almost exclusively since 14 March 2020, the date the Spanish government ordered a total lockdown to prevent the spread of SARS-CoV-2.

Sequelae due to COVID-19 were any sign or symptom that the patient and/or physician considered related directly to COVID-19 and that was present at 3 and 12 months after infection.

2.5. Outcomes

To assess the disease course and clinical evolution of COVID-19, the following outcomes were registered and analysed: hospitalisation due to COVID-19, intensive care unit (ICU) admission, sequelae, severe COVID-19 and death. Severe COVID-19 was considered a composite variable that included ICU admission and/or use of active amines and/or respiratory distress and/or invasive oxygen therapy and/or death [22]. Cases with systemic inflammatory response syndrome were also registered. Data on outcomes of our study were compared to those registered on the SECURE-IBD registry (accessed on 24 August 2021) [9], considered the worldwide IBD registry on COVID-19. These outcomes were also compared to those of the general population taking into account data from Catalonia [23].

2.6. Ethical Considerations

The Scientific Committee of ENEIDA approved the study on 16 March 2020. It was also approved by the Ethics Committee of Hospital Universitari Mútua Terrassa (coordinating centre). Informed consent was obtained from all subjects. The patients were not identified by name in the publication, and no one, except the investigators of this study, had access to their local data, in accordance with the local Law of Personal Data Protection.

2.7. Statistical Analysis

Quantitative variables were compared with Student's t test and the Mann–Whitney test, and the results are expressed as the means ($\pm$standard deviation) or median ($\pm$interquartile range (IQR) 25–75 percentiles). Quantitative variables were compared using Student's t test for parametric data and the Mann–Whitney test for nonparametric data, while qualitative variables were compared using the Chi2 test or Fisher's exact test, as appropriate. Univariate and multivariate logistic binary regression analyses were performed to explore the variables related to the need for hospitalisation, ICU admission, severe COVID-19, death and sequelae found at the 3- and 12-month follow-ups. The intensity of the significant associations was measured by calculating the OR and its 95% confidence interval. The multivariate models included significant variables in univariate analysis at the $p < 0.1$ level. In addition, for the outcomes with a small number of events (death and ICU admission), only the 2 most significant covariates in the univariate analysis were included. As the use of aminosalicylates was more frequent in patients with ulcerative colitis (UC) than in Crohn's disease (CD), the model was adjusted to UC diagnosis when this drug was independently associated with a specific outcome.

Due to the great variability in the incidence of COVID-19 between the Spanish territories, the number of cases of both IBD and the general population are shown per province. Data on COVID-19 incidence in the general population as well as the age at COVID-19 diagnosis, age of hospitalized patients (including ICU admission) and age of patients with fatal outcomes were obtained from the National Centre of Epidemiology (CNE) [24,25]. The age- and sex-standardised incidence of every outcome in the IBD cohort was obtained based on all the patients actively followed in each participant centre of ENEIDA.

3. Results

A total of 73 out of the 86 centres adhered to the ENEIDA registry at the time of the study and decided to participate. This registry had, at that moment, 60,512 patients actively followed-up (data as for 15 July 2020), with 53,682 coming from the 73 participating centres (89% of the whole registry). Finally, 482 cases of COVID-19 were reported (251 males (52%); median 52 years (IQR: 42–61); cumulative incidence of 8.97 per 1000 patients with IBD, taking into account the population at risk from the participating centres). Ten centres that agreed to participate did not register any COVID-19 cases during the study period, despite being aware.

3.1. Clinical Baseline Characteristics

Tables 1 and 2 show the most important clinical characteristics of the patients regarding IBD at the time of COVID-19 diagnosis. The activity of the disease and treatment are provided separately for UC and CD (Table 2). Notably, 80% of patients were in remission, and 9% had moderate–severe disease activity. Regarding IBD treatment at the time of the infection, 42% of the patients were on aminosalicylates, 5.4% were receiving systemic steroids, 36% were receiving immunosuppressants, 36% were receiving biologics and 12% were receiving combination therapy. Eleven percent of the patients required steroids within the 3 months before COVID-19 diagnosis.

Table 1. Clinical baseline characteristics regarding inflammatory bowel disease with COVID-19.

Clinical Characteristics	Cases n = 482
Gender	
Male	251 (52)
Female	231 (48)
Age at COVID-19 diagnosis	52 years (IQR 42–61)
IBD duration at COVID-19 diagnosis	12 years (IQR 6–19)
Type of IBD, n (%)	
Crohn's disease	247 (51)
Ulcerative colitis	221 (46)
Unclassified colitis	14 (2.9)
Ulcerative colitis extent (%)	
E1	43 (19)
E2	80 (36)
E3	98 (44)
Crohn's disease location, n (%)	
L1	114 (46)
L2	43 (17)
L3	88 (36)
L4 (isolated)	3 (1.2)
Crohn's disease behaviour, n (%)	
B1	144 (58)
B2	71 (29)
B3	47 (19)
Perianal	59 (24)
B1 + perianal	29 (12)
B2 + perianal	18 (7.3)
B3 + perianal	20 (8.1)

Table 1. *Cont.*

Clinical Characteristics	Cases n = 482
Extraintestinal manifestation, n (%)	125 (26)
Family history of IBD, n (%)	64 (13)
Smoking behaviour, n (%)	
Active	53 (11)
Former smoker	137 (28)
Never smoker	268 (56)

IQR: interquartile rate, IBD: inflammatory bowel disease, L1: ileal, L2: colonic, L3: ileocolonic, L4: upper gastrointestinal tract; B1: inflammatory behaviour, B2: stricturing behaviour, B3: penetrating behaviour.

Table 2. Inflammatory bowel disease activity and treatment at time of COVID-19 diagnosis.

	IBD (Total) n = 482	Crohn's Disease n = 247	Ulcerative Colitis n = 221	p-Value *
	IBD Activity at COVID-19 Diagnosis			
Clinical remission	385 (80)	200 (81)	173 (78)	0.35
Active disease	97 (20)	47 (19)	48 (22)	0.35
Mild	53 (11)	26 (10.5)	26 (12)	
Moderate	42 (8.7)	21 (8.5)	20 (9)	
Severe	2 (0.4)	0	2 (0.9)	
	IBD treatment			
None, n (%)	62 (13)	37 (15)	23 (10.4)	0.15
5-aminosalicylates, n (%)	202 (42)	49 (20)	143 (65)	<0.0001
Oral (oral and topic)	197 (41)	49 (20)	138 (62)	
Topical (exclusive)	5 (1)	0	5 (2.3)	
Monotherapy	131 (27)	31 (12)	91 (41)	
Systemic steroids 3 months before COVID-19 (oral or intravenous), n (%)	53 (11)	30 (12)	21 (9.5)	0.36
Systemic steroids, n (%)	26 (5.4)	16 (6.4)	8 (3.6)	0.37
Immunosuppressants (in monotherapy), n (%)	113 (23)	65 (26)	56 (25)	0.03
Azathioprine	90 (19)	54 (22)	46 (21)	0.04
Mercaptopurine	8 (1.7)	4 (1.6)	2 (0.9)	0.16
Cyclosporine	1 (0.2)	0	1 (0.4)	0.96
Methotrexate	9 (1.9)	6 (2.4)	3 (1.3)	0.06
Tacrolimus	1 (0.2)	1 (0.4)	0	1
Tofacitinib	4 (0.8)	0	4 (1.8)	0.10
Biologics (in monotherapy), n (%)	117 (22)	72 (29)	35 (16)	0.04
Anti-TNF	71 (15)	42 (17)	19 (8.6)	<0.0001
Vedolizumab	25 (5.2)	12 (4.8)	13 (5.9)	0.75
Ustekinumab	21 (4.3)	18 (7.3)	3 (1.3)	0.001
Combotherapy, n (%)	59 (12)	45 (18)	14 (6.3)	0.02
Anti-TNF plus thiopurines	37 (7.7)	28 (11)	9 (4.1)	0.02
Anti-TNF plus methotrexate	9 (1.9)	6 (2.4)	3 (1.3)	0.62
Vedolizumab plus thiopurines	5 (1)	4 (1.6)	1 (0.4)	0.73
Vedolizumab plus methotrexate	1 (0.2)	0	1 (0.4)	0.78
Ustekinumab plus thiopurines	5 (1)	5 (2)	0	0.55
Ustekinumab plus methotrexate	2 (0.4)	2 (0.8)	0	0.98

* Comparison between Crohn's disease and ulcerative colitis. IBD: inflammatory bowel disease; TNF: tumour necrosis factor.

Forty-four percent had at least one comorbidity, and 64% had a Charlson score of one or more. The most frequent comorbidity was arterial hypertension (22% (106/482)), followed by dyslipidaemia (15% (74/482)) and immune-mediated diseases (11% (53/482)) other than IBD (Supplementary Table S1).

3.2. Geografical Distribution of COVID-19 and Epidemiological Risk Factors of Exposure

The geographical distribution of cases is shown in Figure 1A, allowing a comparative approach with the incidence of COVID-19 in the Spanish general population (Figure 1B).

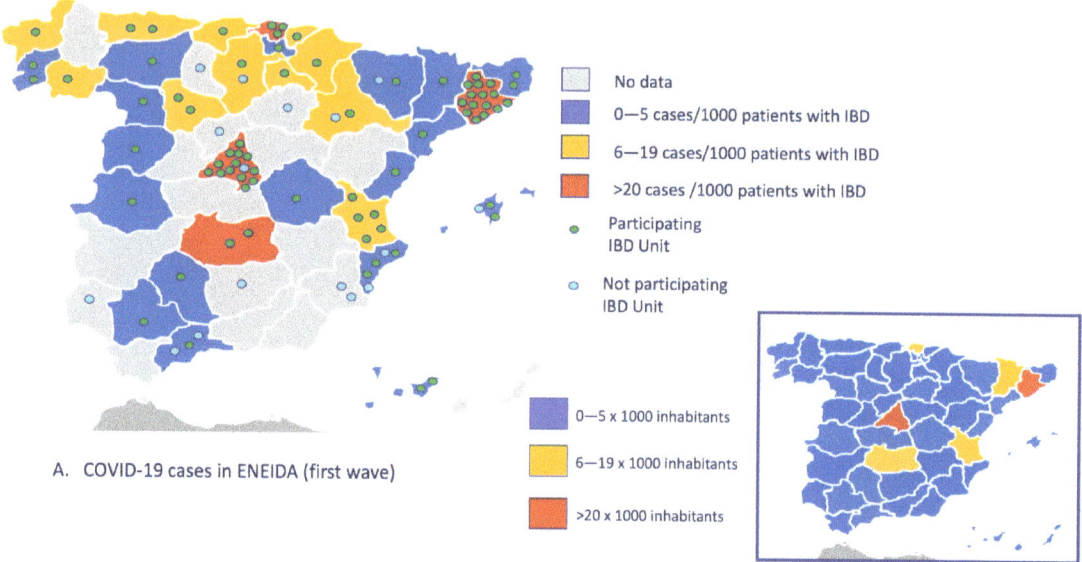

Figure 1. Geographic distribution of COVID-19 cases in the ENEIDA registry and comparison with the general Spanish population in the first wave of the pandemic.

The majority of cases were reported in ENEIDA centres of the communities of Madrid and in those of the metropolitan area of Barcelona (red colour), where there is also the highest proportion of certified IBD units [26]. These two regions have the highest population density in Spain (844 and 743 inhabitants per km^2, respectively, as of January 2021 [27]) and register the highest incidence of COVID-19 in the general population.

Compared to the Spanish population in March 2020 [24], the median age of IBD cases was similar: 52 years old (IQR, 42–61) in patients with IBD vs. 54 years old (IQR, 39–70) in the general population. When considering specific outcomes, a similar trend was observed: the age of hospitalised patients with IBD was 59 years old (IQR, 50–72) vs. 66 years old (IQR, 51–79) in the general population, and the age of ICU/death was 72 years old (IQR, 57–80) in patients with IBD vs. 70 years old (IQR, 59–80 years) in the general population

Regarding risk factors for COVID-19, almost half of the patients declared good adherence to lockdown measures (48% (229/482)). The circumstances that ensured an appropriate domiciliary lockdown were having preventive sick leave (31% (71/229)), being retired (26% (60/229)), doing telecommuting (18% (42/229)) and being unemployed (6.6% (15/229)). Table 3 summarizes the risk for SARS-CoV-2 infection related to occupational risk.

Table 3. Epidemiological factors of SARS-CoV-2 infection and occupational risk.

Route of Contagion, n (%)	
Unknown	242 (50)
Intrafamilial transmission	108 (22)
Occupational	96 (20)
Travel	8 (1.7)
Occupational Risk, n (%)	133 (28)
Healthcare	85 (18)
Basic services (supermarket cashiers, market clerks, pharmacy)	18 (3.7)
Education	15 (3)
Police and fireperson	5 (1)
Closed institutions	2 (0.4)
Veterinary, animal control worker or conservation and forest technician	4 (0.8)

Almost one-third of the patients had a job position considered as posing a high risk of infection, which was the main cause for not having proper adherence to lockdown measures. Health care professions were the most frequent occupational hazard (18% (85/482). Table 4 shows the relationship between infection and occupational risk in patients with and without good adherence to a total lockdown.

Table 4. Relationship between the route of contagion and occupational risk in patients with and without a total lockdown.

Risk Variable	Patients with Total Lockdown (n = 229)	Patients without Total Lockdown (n = 225)	p-Value
Route of contagion, n (%)			
Intrafamilial transmission	70 (31)	38 (17)	0.001
Infection on March 2020	47 (20)	26 (12)	0.007
Infection on April–July 2020	23 (10)	12 (5.3)	0.034
Occupational	19 (8.3)	77 (34)	<0.0001
Infection on March 2020	19 (8.2)	48 (21)	<0.0001
Infection on April–July 2020	0	29 (13)	<0.0001
Travel	3 (1.3)	5 (2.2)	0.69
Infection on March 2020	3 (1.3)	5 (2.2)	0.69
Infection on April–July 2020	-	-	
Unknown	137 (60)	105 (47)	0.005
Infection on March 2020	83 (36)	69 (31)	0.167
Infection on April–July 2020	54 (24)	36 (16)	0.003
Occupational risk, n (%)			
Occupational risk (all)	38 (17)	92 (41)	<0.0001
Healthcare	18 (7.9)	65 (29)	<0.0001

Despite declaring good adherence, patients became infected mainly by intrafamilial transmission, particularly during the first 2 weeks (March 2020) after the Spanish government established lockdown.

3.3. COVID-19 Diagnosis and Treatment

Symptoms of COVID-19 diagnosis can be found in Supplementary Table S2, with fever (69% (336/482)) and cough (63% (305/482)) as the most frequently observed symptoms. Diarrhoea was reported in 26% (126/482) of patients, with no significant differences between patients with active or inactive IBD.

Supplementary Table S3 includes the tests performed for COVID-19 diagnosis. Notably, 90% of IBD patients had a diagnostic test performed, whether PCR (80% (388/482)) or SARS-CoV-2 serology (35% (167/482)). Only 49 patients did not have any diagnostic test performed. It is also important to emphasize that 28% of patients (85/301) had a positive PCR after one or more negative PCRs, with no difference between immunosuppressed and non-immunosuppressed patients (19% vs. 21%, $p = 0.67$).

COVID-19 treatment followed the trend used and recommended by health authorities at that time. It included chloroquine/hydroxychloroquine in 41% (198/482), antibiotics in 38% (182/482), antivirals in 18% (88/482), systemic corticosteroids in 12% (58/482) and biologic therapy in 2.9% (14/482) (tocilizumab in 1.7% (8/482), interferon in 1.2% (6/482) and anakinra in 0.2% (1/482)). Antifungal therapy was used in 1.9% (9/482), vasoactive amines in 1.2% (6/482) and invasive oxygen therapy in 2.9% (14/482) of the patients (one patient received invasive oxygen therapy in a conventional floor due to occupation limitations of the ICU).

3.4. Outcomes

Patients attended their primary care facility in 55% of the cases (266/482), received emergency room assistance in 52% (251/482) and required hospitalisation due to COVID in 35% (167/482). Eleven patients (0.2%) required IBD-related hospitalisation during the study period. Twenty-four patients had respiratory distress (4.9%), 56 (12%) presented with systemic inflammatory response syndrome upon admission and 6.4% (31/482) presented with systemic inflammatory response syndrome during hospitalisation. Thirteen (2.5%) required ICU admission, 38 (7.9%) fulfilled the criteria of severe COVID-19 and 21 patients died during the study. Of those who died, 18 (3.7%) died due to COVID-19 and 3 due to causes other than COVID-19, 2 of them during the first wave of the pandemic (one case with signet-ring cell adenocarcinoma of digestive origin and one case of pulmonary neoplasia) and the third 9 months after COVID-19 infection due to urinary sepsis. Only one death occurred outside the hospital (80-year-old female with inactive ileal CD treated with oral aminosalicylates). Compared to the general population in Spain, the severe outcomes were similar, with a mortality proportion of 4.6% and ICU requirement proportion of 2.1% with a slightly lower proportion of patients requiring hospitalisation (19.5%) [23].

Univariate and multivariate analyses of factors associated with hospitalisation, ICU admission, severe COVID-19 and death are detailed in Supplementary Tables S4–S7. In that case, predictive factors for hospitalisation due to COVID-19 were being 50 years of age or more (OR 2.09, 95% CI 1.3–3.4), having at least one comorbidity (OR 2.28, 95% CI 1.4–3.6) and being treated with steroids for IBD within the 3 months before COVID-19 diagnosis (OR 1.3, 95% CI 1.1–1.6). Predictors for ICU admission were having a Charlson score of at least 2 (OR 5.4, 95% CI 1.5–20.1) and the use of aminosalicylates (OR 4.6, 95% CI 1.2–17). However, when adjusted for diagnosis, the effect of aminosalicylates disappeared (OR 3.6, 95% CI 0.85–15.2, $p = 0.08$). Independent risk factors related to death due to COVID-19 were being 60 years of age or more (OR 7.1, 95% CI 1.8–27.4) and having at least 2 comorbidities (OR 3.9, 95% CI 1.3–11.6). The only predictor for severe COVID-19 was being 60 years of age or more (OR 4.59, 95% CI 1.3–15.9), while having CD with an inflammatory behaviour was protective for this outcome (OR 0.29, 95% CI 0.09–0.89). There were no differences in the proportion of hospitalisation, ICU admission, severe COVID-19 or death between patients found under active search (18% of the centres) vs. those that were found by direct notification from the patient itself, the family physician, the emergency department or the hospitalisation unit (data not shown). The proportion of patients under specific IBD treatment, taking into account each predefined outcome, is shown in Table 5.

Table 5. Outcome of the COVID-19-EII cohort and treatment administered. The results are compared with those reported in the SECURE-IBD cohort (as for 24 August 2021) [9] ¶.

A. Outcomes

Outcome	Hospitalised		ICU Admission		Severe COVID-19		Death	
	COVID-19-EII n = 482	SECURE-IBD n = 6438	COVID-19-EII n = 482	SECURE-IBD n = 6438	COVID-19-EII n = 482	SECURE-IBD n = 6438	COVID-19-EII n = 482	SECURE-IBD n = 6438
	n = 168 (35%)	n = 977 (15%)	n = 13 (2.6%)	n = 184 (2.8%)	n = 38 * (7.8%)	n = 257 ** (3.9%)	n = 18 (3.7%)	n = 104 (1.6%)

B. Treatment taking into account each specific outcome

DRUG	Total		Hospitalised		ICU		Severe COVID-19		Death	
Cohort	COVID-19-EII n = 482	SECURE-IBD n = 6438	COVID-19-EII n = 168	SECURE-IBD n = 977	COVID-19-EII n = 13	SECURE-IBD n = 184	COVID-19-EII * n = 38	SECURE-IBD ** n = 257	COVID-19-EII n = 18	SECURE-IBD n = 104
5-aminosalicylates, Alone	202 (42) 131 (27)	1924 (30) -	79 (47) 52 (31)	411 (42) -	10 (77) 5 (38)	81 (44) -	24 (63) 16 (42)	118 (46) -	9 (50) 6 (33)	53 (51) -
With other IBD drugs	71 (15)	-	27 (16)	-	5 (28)	-	8 (21)	-	3 (17)	-
Systemic steroids	26 (5.4)	414 (6.4)	11 (6.5)	146 (15)	1 (7.7)	41 (22)	4 (10.5)	53 (21)	1 (5.6)	28 (27)
Thiopurines (monotherapy)	108 (22)	551 (8.6)	38 (23)	114 (12)	3 (23)	26 (14)	5 (13)	33 (13)	1 (5.6)	11 (10.6)
Methotrexate (monotherapy)	9 (1.9)	49 (0.8)	4 (2.4)	13 (1.3)	1 (7.7)	1 (0.5)	2 (5.3)	3 (1.2)	1 (5.6)	2 (1.9)
Anti-TNF (monotherapy)	71 (15)	2082 (32)	11 (6.5)	178 (18)	2 (15)	24 (13)	3 (7.9)	31 (12)	2 (11)	10 (9.6)
Anti-TNF in combotherapy	46 (9.5)	636 (9.9)	20 (12)	91 (9.3)	0	17 (9)	2 (5.3)	21 (8.2)	2 (11)	6 (5.8)
Vedolizumab	30 (6.2)	706 (11)	15 (8.9)	94 (9.6)	0	21 (11)	4 (10.5)	28 (10.9)	2 (11)	9 (8.6)
Ustekinumab	28 (5.8)	602 (9)	6 (3.6)	50 (5.1)	1 (7.7)	9 (4.9)	1 (2.6)	11 (4.3)	1 (5.6)	5 (4.8)
Tofacitinib	4 (0.8)	103 (1.6)	2 (1.2)	12 (1.2)	0	4 (2.2)	0	4 (1.5)	0	1 (0.9)

ICU: intensive care unit, TNF: tumour necrosis factor. ¶ Brenner EJ, Ungaro RC, Colombel JF, Kappelman MD. SECURE-IBD Database Public Data, https://covidibd.org/current-data/ accessed on 24 August 2021. * Severe COVID-19 for the COVID-19-EII study: composite of intensive care unit admission and/or use of active amines and/or respiratory distress and/or invasive oxygen therapy and/or death. ** Severe COVID-19 for the SECURE-IBD registry: composite of intensive care unit admission and/or use of ventilator and/or death.

There were no differences in any outcomes between patients with probable or confirmed COVID-19 (data not shown). To compare the results of the present study with those of the SECURE-IBD (accessed on 24 August 2021) [9], the results of the two cohorts are provided in the same table. In Supplementary Table S8, we show the incidence of adverse outcomes of COVID-19 in patients with IBD, taking into account sex and age. Of note, being ≥50 years old increases the incidence of the reported adverse outcomes from 3 to 7, with a greater frequency in males than in females.

3.5. Follow-Up

IBD treatment and the presence of sequelae related to COVID-19 at the 3- and 12-month follow-up are described in Table 6.

Table 6. Sequelae at 3- and 12-months of COVID-19 and the impact of the infection on changes in therapeutic regimens for IBD.

	3 Months Follow-Up (n = 462)	12 Months Follow-Up (n = 451)
COVID-19 sequelae, n (%)	65 (14)	72 (15)
Psychologic sequelae, n (%)	20 (4.3)	15 (3.3)
Physical sequelae, n (%)	55 (12)	67 (15)
Asthenia	21 (4.5)	22 (4.8)
Myalgia/Arthralgia	7 (1.5)	3 (0.7)
Anosmia	4 (0.9)	7 (1.5)
Dyspnoea	4 (0.9)	6 (1.3)
Odynophagia	2 (0.4)	2 (0.4)
Dysgeusia	2 (0.4)	2 (0.4)
Hair loss	1 (0.2)	1 (0.2)
Pulmonary fibrosis	1 (0.2)	3 (0.6)
Bronchial hyperreactivity	1 (0.2)	1 (0.2)
Deep venous thrombosis/pulmonary thrombosis	1 (0.2)	1 (0.2)
Headache	1 (0.2)	6 (1.3)
Obstructive pulmonary disease	1 (0.2)	3 (0.6)
Paraesthesia	1 (0.2)	3 (0.6)
Wegener's vasculitis	-	1 (0.2)
Immunosuppression withdrawal, n (%)	65 (14)	6 (1.3)
Transient	58 (13)	1 (0.2)
Definitive	7 (1.5)	5 (1.1)
De-escalation from combo to monotherapy	13 (2.9)	1 (0.2)
Patients requiring Immunosuppression initiation or modification, n (%)	12 (2.6)	43 * (9.5)
Systemic corticosteroids	1 (0.2)	7 (1.6)
Thiopurines	2 (0.4)	5 (1.1)
Methotrexate	0	1 (0.2)
Anti-TNF	5 (1)	18 (4)
Vedolizumab	1 (0.2)	7 (1.6)
Ustekinumab	2 (0.4)	12 (2.7)
Tofacitinib	1 (0.2)	6 (1.3)

* Some patients required more than one new immunosuppressant (combined or sequential); therefore, this number expresses the total number of patients that required immunosuppression initiation/modification from 3 to 12 months after COVID-19. IBD = inflammatory bowel disease; TNF: tumour necrosis factor.

Only 13% of patients had short-term immunosuppression withdrawal due to COVID-19 (12% partial and 1.4% definitive), and only 1% kept their withdrawal of immunosuppression in the long term.

At the 3-month follow-up, 65 patients (13%) presented COVID-19 sequelae, of which 4% (20/482) were psychological and 11% (55/482) were physical (Table 6). At the 12-month follow-up, 72 patients (15%) were considered to have sequelae, of which 3.1% (15/482) were psychological and 14% (67/482) were physical. The most frequent physical sequelae were asthenia, myalgia/arthralgia and anosmia. The only predictive factor for having physical sequelae at the 3-month follow-up was the use of steroid treatment for IBD within the 3 months before COVID-19 (OR 1.4, 95% CI 1.07–1.7) (Supplementary Table S9). No predictive factor for physical sequelae was found at the long-term follow-up (12 months) (Supplementary Table S10). Only one patient reported SARS-CoV-2 reinfection 6 months after the index diagnosis.

IBD activity both at COVID-19 diagnosis and at 3- and 12-month follow-ups is shown in Figure 2. Two-thirds of patients (68%, 330/482) remained in remission throughout the study period.

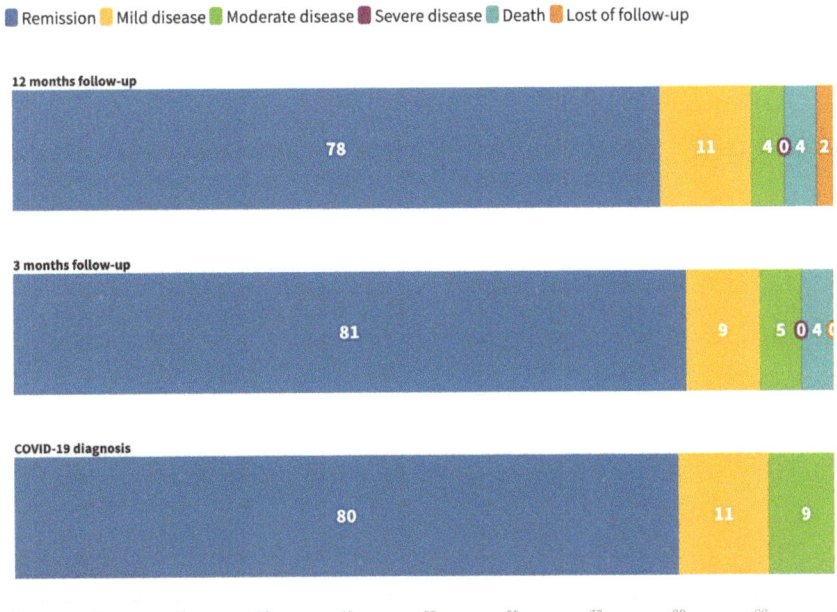

Figure 2. Inflammatory bowel disease activity at COVID-19 diagnosis and 3- and 12-month follow-up.

4. Discussion

We report the largest cohort of patients with IBD and symptomatic COVID-19 prospectively recruited with a one-year follow-up after infection. This is a national, multicentre study that was conducted within the ENEIDA project and included 482 patients with COVID-19 among 53,682 patients with IBD, giving a cumulative incidence of 8.97 per 1000. These data are in the upper limit of the wide range of incidence previously described [10,14,28], ranging from 0.95 [29] to 100 per 1000 [15]. The universal access to health care within the National Health System in Spain (less than 3% of IBD patients with private insurance never use public services [30]) and the adherence of most centres to the nationwide certification programme in IBD [26] provide homogeneity to the cohort, minimizing potential bias in the clinical characteristics. We did not calculate the comparative incidence of COVID-19 between the IBD cohort and data obtained from the general population because the identification of cases did not use the same methodology. However, it is clearly observed in Figure 1 that the number of cases with COVID-19 and IBD is the highest in areas with the highest incidence of infection. The high variability in incidence between relatively close geographical areas was also observed, with a maximum in those areas with the highest population density. We decided to exclude asymptomatic patients, as there was no policy for a universal testing in our patients nor in the general population during the first wave. Therefore data on asymptomatic patients with IBD and positive SARS-CoV-2 test are scarce and can imply a selection bias.

It has been suggested that patients with IBD are at lower risk of having COVID-19, and most studies support this assertion [10,31–35]. However, only a few of these studies performed in Denmark and Sweden were population based [36,37], which is how differences in the incidence of infection between population groups should be addressed. In our cohort, we recorded the influence of occupational risk, lockdown strategies and other risk factors, in addition to IBD treatment, that may have influenced, either increasing or decreasing, the risk of contagion. We observed, for example, that one-third of infected patients received special protection measures such as sick leave simply because they were considered a risk group. However, many patients became infected, perhaps because they were infected early before mandatory lockdown or through close family-infected contact. Lockdown has been demonstrated to be the most effective strategy precluding SARS-CoV-2 expansion [38–40], also in patients with IBD [41]. Thus, the low incidence of COVID-19 in IBD cohorts does not necessarily reflect a lower susceptibility to infection but a higher protection attitude towards IBD patients based on recommendations [6,42] or because they spontaneously adopt more rigorous self-protecting measures [43]. It has been shown that patients under biologic drugs perceive themselves to be at greater risk of SARS-CoV-2 infection, but, despite that, they do not perform more strict social distancing practices than patients with IBD without biologics or in remission [43]. However, in our cohort, only 49% exhibited good adherence to lockdown measures. Currently, data on the exposure environment of noninfected patients are very limited [44]. The study also showed that one-third of IBD patients with COVID-19 had occupational risks, mainly working in health care facilities. It has been reported that health care providers bore a great burden during the pandemic, as shown in data coming from Italy and China [22,45]. Nonetheless, we did not find that occupational risk or failure to meet lockdown measures were predictors for a worse evolution of COVID-19 in patients with IBD.

The reported outcomes of COVID-19 are highly variable [10,28,33,36,46] and may depend on many factors, such as age, comorbidity, ethnicity, socioeconomic status and the quality of health care. In our cohort, as in others, the most important factors influencing outcomes were age and comorbidity. Thirty-five percent of the patients required hospitalisation, 7.9% had severe COVID-19, 2.5% required ICU admission and 3.7% died. These figures are similar to those extracted from the general population in Spain [23] (hospitalisation 19.5%, ICU 2.1% and mortality 4.6%) and are also identical to those reported in the first publication of SECURE-IBD, including the first 525 registered cases [8].

Age is known to be one of the most consistent risk factors for severe COVID-19 and death worldwide [47,48], both in the general population and in patients with IBD [10,49]. We found that patients 50 years old or older were at greater risk for hospitalization, while those 60 years old or older were more prone to severe COVID-19 or death due to COVID-19. Comorbidities have also been considered the other important risk factor for deleterious COVID-19 evolution, both in patients with IBD [16,29,33,36,46] and in the general population [22,50], and we also found consistent results in our cohort. Thus, differences in the percentages of parameters of the severity of COVID-19 between cohorts can be largely explained by these two factors, not only by themselves. The median age of patients in the initial SECURE-IBD cohort was 41 years versus 52 years in our cohort, and the percentage of comorbidities was 36% versus 44%, respectively. Data from SECURE-IBD accessed on 24 August 2021 [9], showed significantly improved outcomes compared to previous outcomes, with a fifty percent reduction in indicators of severity, including hospitalisation, severe COVID-19 and death (more than 70% of the patients were younger than 49 years). Although it can be speculated that improved knowledge of COVID-19 management may account for a better outcome over time, important selection bias accounting for differences in this type of registry cannot be ruled out.

The only protective factor for severe COVID-19 was CD with inflammatory behaviour. As this was found to be independent of IBD activity and treatment, we speculate that this is because this pattern has less disease burden, as it was also related to a shorter duration of the disease (11 years of disease in inflammatory IBD vs. 18 years in stricturing or penetrating disease, $p < 0.0001$).

As stated previously, IBD-related immunosuppression has not been found to be a risk factor for severe COVID-19 or death [28,29,51]. Our cohort confirms that there is no relationship between anti-TNF or any other form of therapeutic immunosuppression and COVID-19 severity. Some authors suggested that the risk of hospitalisation is higher in patients under biologics, but this may reflect a precaution more than COVID-19 severity itself, as overall mortality related to COVID has not been demonstrated to be increased in ours and other previous studies [28,36,46,51,52]. This consistent evidence reinforces the message that biologics can be safely continued in most cases. The use of steroids in this pandemic has been controversial [53,54]. In contrast to SECURE-IBD [8], we did not find that current treatment with systemic steroids was related to a worse COVID-19 evolution, an outcome that we have previously found related to other relevant infections in patients with IBD [3]. This might be due to the small proportion of patients under this treatment (5.4%) or the type of schedule administered. However, the use of steroids three months before COVID-19 diagnosis was an independent risk factor for hospitalisation and physical sequelae (at the 3-month follow-up). This could be indirectly related to a probable active IBD that was challenging to treat and required the use of systemic steroids.

Finally, we describe the evolution of patients at 3 and 12 months after COVID-19. Thirteen percent withdrew IBD medication during COVID-19. This is less than previously reported, ranging between 27% [15] and 34% [55]. This is certainly encouraging, as the first guidelines on the treatment of patients with IBD during the pandemic were very clear in recommending the withdrawal of immunosuppressants and biologics in infected individuals [6]. However, as our experience increased, it was assured that the inappropriate cessation of effective agents for IBD treatment due to unjustified fear of adverse events could lead to IBD relapse and then to the use of steroids or hospitalisation, thus increasing the risk of COVID-19 exposure and infection. The last outcome that we explored was COVID-19 sequelae, present in 13% at 3 months and 15% at 12 months in our cohort. The only predictive factor for having physical sequelae at the 3-month follow-up was the use of steroid treatment for IBD 3 months before COVID-19 (OR 1.4, 95% CI 1.07–1.7). It has been shown that severe sequelae were lower in patients with IBD when matched to non-IBD controls [49], so IBD does not seem to be a disease linked to more sequelae due to COVID-19. In contrast, a recent population-based Danish study has suggested that sequelae are a common phenomenon, affecting almost 44% of patients [56]. It has to be noted that this study accessed sequelae only in 222 of the 516 patients included and that they were self-reported sequalae, limiting the confirmation of a real effect that might be caused by COVID-19. In addition, another study found that patients with IBD, hospitalized due to COVID-19, have a greater risk of severe infections requiring further hospitalisation [57], a situation that has not been found in our cohort.

Our study has several limitations to be aware of. First, only 18% of centres performed an active search of cases (82% of cases were collected by direct notification from the patient itself, the family physician, the emergency department or the hospitalisation unit, as stated in the Methods section). Thus, it is possible that very mild cases did not consult their IBD unit; thus, mild COVID-19 cases might be underrepresented. However, data on hospitalisation, severe COVID-19, ICU admission and death from the general population are similar to our cohort and we did not find differences in specific outcomes between these two searching strategies; therefore, this bias is probably small. On the other hand, the majority of participant centres were certified IBD units that had open access to their outpatient clinics, nurse-led advice lines and/or emails for emergencies as mandatory quality criteria [26]. Second, this study, including only the first wave of an ongoing pandemic, is observational and cannot establish causation or account for unmeasured confounders. Finally, discovering the real number of infected patients remains a global challenge because PCR or serology were not performed universally at the beginning and there is evidence of false negative results. This occurred in 10% of this cohort. Notwithstanding these issues, there are some important strengths. First, it has national coverage with active participation of almost 90% of the IBD units from the ENEIDA registry. However, the main strength relies on prospective data, collecting IBD activity, and other important variables. In addition, although nationwide series on COVID-19 and IBD have been published before [29,33], our study is the largest cohort of patients with IBD and COVID-19 with the longest follow-up after infection.

5. Conclusions

In conclusion, we have shown that occupational risk and intrafamilial transmission are relevant epidemiological risk factors and that a high proportion of patients receive preventive sick leave. We have also demonstrated that IBD does not worsen COVID-19 prognosis, even when immunosuppressants and biological drugs are used. Age and comorbidity are the most important prognostic factors for more severe COVID-19 in patients with IBD and are even more relevant than epidemiological risk factors such as occupational risk. Finally, COVID-19 is not a condition that affects the prognosis of IBD or its treatment, either in the short or the long term and is not a cause of significant sequelae in patients already suffering from IBD. Therefore, there is no need for more strict protection measures than those adopted for the general population.

Supplementary Materials: The following are available online at https://www.mdpi.com/article/10.3390/jcm11020421/s1, Table S1. Comorbidities; Table S2. Symptoms at COVID-19 diagnosis; Table S3. Tests performed for COVID-19 diagnosis; Table S4. Clinical characteristics and treatment for IBD in patients who required hospitalization; Table S5. Clinical characteristics and treatment for IBD in patients who required ICU admission; Table S6. Clinical characteristics and treatment for IBD in patients who died due to COVID-19; Table S7. Clinical characteristics and treatment for IBD in patients with severe COVID-19; Table S8. Incidence of adverse outcomes of COVID-19 patients in the ENEIDA registry; Table S9. Clinical characteristics and treatment for IBD in patients with 3-month physical sequelae; Table S10. Clinical characteristics and treatment for IBD in patients with 12-month physical sequelae.

Author Contributions: Study design: Y.Z., I.M.-J., I.R.-L., M.E.; study conduction: Y.Z., P.M.; data collection: Y.Z., I.M.-J., I.R.-L., I.V., M.D.M.-A., I.G., J.P.G., F.M. (Francisco Mesonero)., O.B., C.T., Á.P.-D., M.P., A.J.L., B.C., M.M., P.M.-M., M.B.-W., J.G., L.B., N.M., T.M.-P., A.L., C.R.-G., S.G.-L., P.V. (Pablo Vega), M.R., L.M., M.C. (Maria Calvo), M.I., M.B.d.-A., B.S., J.B., J.L.P., D.B., I.P.-M., M.N.-L., V.H., F.A.-A., F.R.E., S.M., L.R., F.G., F.M. (Fernando Muñoz), G.S., J.O.d.Z., J.M.H., J.L., M.F.G.-S., M.S., M.D., S.E., A.F.C., E.H., L.O., E.I., A.G., P.V. (Pilar Varela), N.R., P.G., A.H.-C., A.B., D.G., E.S., D.C., M.A., J.L.C., Y.G.-L., L.J., M.C. (María Chaparro), A.L.-S.R., C.A., R.P.-S., R.M., S.T.-S., E.R., M.C. (Margalida Calafat), S.O., P.N., F.B., H.A.-G., R.P., P.O., P.M., E.D., M.E.; data analysis and interpretation: Y.Z., I.M.-J., I.R.-L., M.E.; manuscript drafting: Y.Z., I.M.-J., I.R.-L., M.E. All authors have read and agreed to the published version of the manuscript, including the authorship list.

Funding: This study is funded by the Carlos III Health Institute (COV20/00227: Co-IP Dra. Maria Esteve and Dra. Yamile Zabana), FEDER (Fondo Europeo de Desarrollo Regional) and supported by GETECCU. The ENEIDA Registry of GETECCU is supported by Takeda, Pfizer, Galápagos, AbbVie and Biogen.

Institutional Review Board Statement: The study was conducted according to the guidelines of the Declaration of Helsinki, and approved by the Scientific Committee of ENEIDA on 16 March 2020. It was also approved by the Ethics Committee of Hospital Universitari Mútua Terrassa (coordinating centre).

Informed Consent Statement: Informed consent was obtained from all subjects involved in the study.

Data Availability Statement: The data underlying this article are available in the article and Supplementary Materials.

Acknowledgments: The authors would like to thank the centres that registered no cases during the study period but performed an active search of IBD patients with COVID-19: Hospital Sant Joan de Deu, Hospital Sant Jaume de Calella, Hospital de Castellón, Hospital Materno-Infantil de Málaga, Hospital de Granollers, Hospital Joan XXIII, Hospital Niño Jesús, Hospital de Cáceres, Hospital de Vic, and Complejo Hospitalario La Mancha Centro.

Conflicts of Interest: Y. Zabana has received support for conference attendance, speaker fees, research support and consulting fees from Abbvie, Adacyte, Almirall, Amgen, Dr Falk, FAES Pharma, Ferring, Jannsen, MSD, Otsuka, Pfizer, Shire, Takeda and Tillotts. I. Marín-Jiménez has received financial support for travelling and educational activities from or has served as an advisory board member to MSD, Pfizer, Abbvie, Amgen, Takeda, Janssen, Sandoz, Shire Pharmaceuticals, Ferring, Dr. Falk Pharma, and Otsuka Pharmaceutical. I. Rodríguez-Lago has received financial support for travelling and educational activities from or has served as an advisory board member to MSD, Pfizer, Abbvie, Takeda, Janssen, Tillotts Pharma, Roche, Shire Pharmaceuticals, Ferring, Dr. Falk Pharma, Adacyte and Otsuka Pharmaceutical. MD Martín-Arranz has received fees as a speaker, consultant and advisory member for or has received funding from MSD, AbbVie, Hospira, Pfizer, Takeda, Janssen, Shire Pharmaceuticals, Tillotts Pharma, Faes farma. J. P. Gisbert has served as speaker, consultant, and advisory member for or has received research funding from MSD, Abbvie, Pfizer, Kern Pharma, Biogen, Mylan, Takeda, Janssen, Roche, Sandoz, Celgene, Gilead/Galapagos, Ferring, Faes Farma, Shire Pharmaceuticals, Dr. Falk Pharma, Tillotts Pharma, Chiesi, Casen Fleet, Gebro Pharma, Otsuka Pharmaceutical and Vifor Pharma. F. Mesonero has served as a speaker or has received education funding or advisory fees from MSD, Abbvie, Takeda, Janssen, Pfizer, Kern Pharma, Ferring and Dr. Falk Pharma. O. Benítez has received financial support for travelling and educational activities from Janssen, Biogen and MSD. C. Taxonera has served as a speaker, consultant and advisory board member for or has received research funding from MSD, AbbVie, Pfizer, Taked, Janssen, Ferring, Faes Pharma, Shire Pharmaceuticals, Dr Falk Pharma, Galapagos and Tillotts. M. Piqueras has received financial support or has served as speaker for Takeda, Abbvie and Janssen. N. Manceñido has been a consultant or speaker for Abbvie, Janssen, Takeda, Ferring, Dr. Falk Pharma and Tillotts Pharma. M. Rivero has served as a speaker, consultant and advisory member for Merck Sharp and Dohme, Abbvie, Pfizer, Takeda and Janssen. M. Barreiro has served as a speaker, consultant and advisory member for or has received research funding from MSD, AbbVie, Janssen, Kern Pharma, Celltrion, Takeda, Gillead, Celgene, Pfizer, Sandoz, Biogen, Fresenius, Ferring, Faes Farma, Dr. Falk Pharma, Chiesi, Gebro Pharma, Adacyte and Vifor Pharma. F. Argüelles has received financial support for travelling and educational activities from or has served as an advisory board member to MSD, Pfizer, Abbvie, Amgen, Takeda, Janssen, Sandoz, Shire Pharmaceuticals, Ferring and Dr Falk Pharma. JM. Huguet has participated in educational activities, research projects, scientific meetings or advisory boards sponsored by Merck Sharp Dohme (MSD), Ferring, Abbvie, Janssen, Biogen, Sandoz, Kern Pharma, Faes Farma, Vifor Pharma and Takeda. A. Hernández-Camba has served as speaker, or has received education funding from AbbVie, Takeda, Kern Pharma, Pfizer, Janssen, Adacyte Therapeutics and Ferring. D. Ginard has received support for conference attendance, speaker fees, research support and consulting fees from Abbvie, Adacyte, Janssen, Takeda, Sandoz, Ferring, Pfizer and Biogen. M. Aceituno has received educational grants from Ferring, Pfizer, Janssen and AbbVie. M. Chaparro has served as a speaker and consultant and has received research or education funding from MSD, Abbvie, Hospira, Pfizer, Takeda, Janssen, Ferring, Shire Pharmaceuticals, Dr. Falk Pharma, Tillotts Pharma, Faes Pharma, Biogen and Gilead. H. Alonso-Galán has received financial support for travelling and educational activities from or has served as an advisory board member to Janssen, MSD, Abbvie, Takeda, Ferring, Pfizer and Dr. Falk Pharma. E. Domènech has served as a speaker, or has received research or education funding or advisory fees from AbbVie, Adacyte Therapeutics, Biogen, Celltrion, Gilead, Janssen, Kern Pharma, MSD, Pfizer, Roche, Samsung, Takeda, and Tillotts. M. Esteve: has received support for conference attendance, speaker fees, research support and consulting fees from Abbvie, Ferring, Janssen, MSD, Otsuka, Pfizer, Takeda and Tillotts. I.V. era, I. Guerra, A. Ponferrada-Díaz, A. Lucendo, B. Caballol, M.Mañosa, P. Martínez-Montiel, M. Bosca-Watts, J. Gordillo, L. Bujanda, T. Martínez-Pérez, A. López, C. Rodríguez, S. García-López, P. Vega, L. Melcarne, M. Calvo, M. Iborra, B. Sicilia, J. Barrio, JL. Pérez, D. Busquets, I. Martínez-Pérez, M. Navarro-Llavat, V. Hernández, F. Ramírez Esteso, S. Mejilde, L. Ramos, F.Gomollón, F. Muñoz, G. Suris, J. Ortiz de Zarate, J. Lló, M. García-Sepulcre, M. Sierra, M. Durà. S. Estrecha, A. Fuentes Coronel, E. Hinojosa, L. Olivan, E. Iglesias, A. Gutiérrez, P. Varela, N. Rull, P. Gilabert, A. Brotons, E. Sesé, D. Carpio, JL Cabriada, Y. González-Lama, L. Giménez, A. López-San Román, C. Alba, R. Plaza-Santos, R. Mena, S. Tamarit-Sebastián, E. Ricart, M. Calafat, S. Olivares, P. Navarro, F. Bertoletti,

R. Pajares, P. Olcina and P. Manzano have no conflict of interest. The funders had no role in the design of the study; in the collection, analyses, or interpretation of data; in the writing of the manuscript, or in the decision to publish the results.

References

1. John Hopkins University Coronavirus Resource Center. Coronavirus COVID-19 Global Cases. Available online: https://coronavirus.juy.edu/map.html (accessed on 21 August 2021).
2. Kirchgesner, J.; Lemaitre, M.; Carrat, F.; Zureik, M.; Carbonnel, M.F.; Dray-Spira, R.; Carbonnel, F.; Dray-Spira, R. Risk of Serious and Opportunistic Infections Associated with Treatment of Inflammatory Bowel Diseases. *Gastroenterology* **2018**, *155*, 337–346. [CrossRef] [PubMed]
3. Zabana, Y.; Rodríguez, L.; Lobatón, T.; Gordillo, J.; Montserrat, A.; Mena, R.; Beltrán, B.; Dotti, M.; Benitez, O.; Guardiola, J.; et al. Relevant Infections in Inflammatory Bowel Disease, and Their Relationship with Immunosuppressive Therapy and Their Effects on Disease Mortality. *J. Crohn's Colitis* **2019**, *13*, 828–837. [CrossRef] [PubMed]
4. Tinsley, A.; Navabi, S.; Williams, E.D.; Liu, G.; Kong, L.; Coates, M.D.; Clarke, K. Increased Risk of Influenza and Influenza-Related Complications among 140,480 Patients with Inflammatory Bowel Disease. *Inflamm. Bowel Dis.* **2019**, *25*, 369–376. [CrossRef] [PubMed]
5. Rubin, D.T.; Feuerstein, J.D.; Wang, A.Y.; Cohen, R.D. AGA Clinical Practice Update on Management of Inflammatory Bowel Disease during the COVID-19 Pandemic: Expert Commentary. *Gastroenterology* **2020**, *159*, 350–357. [CrossRef]
6. Kennedy, N.A.; Jones, G.-R.; Lamb, C.A.; Appleby, R.; Arnott, I.; Beattie, R.M.; Bloom, S.; Brooks, A.J.; Cooney, R.; Dart, R.J.; et al. British Society of Gastroenterology guidance for management of inflammatory bowel disease during the COVID-19 pandemic. *Gut* **2020**, *69*, 984–990. [CrossRef] [PubMed]
7. Abreu, C. 1st Interview COVID-19 ECCO Taskforce. 2020. Available online: https://ecco-ibd.eu/images/6_Publication/6_8_Surveys/1st_interview_COVID-19%20ECCOTaskforce_published.pdf (accessed on 2 August 2021).
8. Brenner, E.J.; Ungaro, R.C.; Gearry, R.B.; Kaplan, G.G.; Kissous-hunt, M.; Lewis, J.D.; Ng, S.C.; Rahier, J.; Reinisch, W.; Ruemmele, F.M.; et al. Corticosteroids, but Not TNF Antagonists, Are Associated with Adverse COVID-19 Outcomes in Patients with Inflammatory Bowel Diseases: Results from an International Registry. *Gastroenterology* **2020**, *159*, 481–491. [CrossRef] [PubMed]
9. Brenner, E.; Ungaro, R.; Colombel, J.; Kappelman, M. SECURE-IBD Database Public Data. Available online: https://covidibd.org/current-data/ (accessed on 24 August 2021).
10. Aziz, M.; Fatima, R.; Haghbin, H.; Smith, W.L.; Nawras, A. The incidence and outcomes of COVID-19 in ibd patients: A rapid review and meta-Analysis. *Inflamm. Bowel Dis.* **2020**, *26*, E132–E133. [CrossRef]
11. Mao, R.; Liang, J.; Shen, J.; Ghosh, S.; Zhu, L.-R.; Yang, H.; Wu, K.-C.; Chen, M.-H. Implications of COVID-19 for patients with pre-existing digestive diseases. *Lancet Gastroenterol. Hepatol.* **2020**, *5*, 425–427. [CrossRef]
12. Norsa, L.; Indriolo, A.; Sansotta, N.; Cosimo, P.; Greco, S.; D'Antiga, L. Uneventful course in IBD patients during SARS-CoV-2 outbreak in northern Italy. *Gastroenterology* **2020**, *159*, 371–372. [CrossRef]
13. Allocca, M.; Fiorino, G.; Zallot, C.; Furfaro, F.; Radice, S.; Danese, S.; Peyrin-biroulet, L. Incidence and patterns of COVID-19 among inflammatory bowel disease patients from the Nancy and Milan cohorts. *Clin. Gastroenterol. Hepatol.* **2020**, *18*, 2134–2135. [CrossRef]
14. Taxonera, C.; Sagastagoitia, I.; Alba, C.; Mañas, N.; Olivares, D.; Rey, E. 2019 novel coronavirus disease (COVID-19) in patients with inflammatory bowel diseases. *Aliment. Pharmacol. Ther.* **2020**, *52*, 276–283. [CrossRef]
15. Guerra, I.; Algaba, A.; Jiménez, L.; Aller, M.M.; Garza, D.; Bonillo, D.; Esteban, L.M.M.; Bermejo, F. Incidence, Clinical Characteristics, and Evolution of SARS-CoV-2 Infection in Patients with Inflammatory Bowel Disease: A Single-Center Study in Madrid, Spain. *Inflamm. Bowel Dis.* **2021**, *27*, 25–33. [CrossRef]
16. Rodríguez-Lago, I.; Ramírez de la Piscina, P.; Elorza, A.; Merino, O.; Ortiz de Zárate, J.; Cabriada, J.L. Characteristics and Prognosis of Patients with Inflammatory Bowel Disease during the SARS-CoV-2 Pandemic in the Basque Country (Spain). *Gastroenterology* **2020**, *159*, 781–783. [CrossRef]
17. Zabana, Y.; Panés, J.; Nos, P.; Gomollón, F.; Esteve, M.; García-Sánchez, V.; Gisbert, J.P.; Barreiro-de-Acosta, M.; Domènech, E. The ENEIDA registry (Nationwide study on genetic and environmental determinants of inflammatory bowel disease) by GETECCU: Design, monitoring and functions. *Gastroenterol. Hepatol.* **2020**, *43*, 551–558. [CrossRef]
18. Silverberg, M.S.; Satsangi, J.; Ahmad, T.; Arnott, I.D.; Bernstein, C.N.; Brant, S.R.; Caprilli, R.; Colombel, J.-F.; Gasche, C.; Geboes, K.; et al. Toward an integrated clinical, molecular and serological classification of inflammatory bowel disease: Report of a Working Party of the 2005 Montreal World Congress of Gastroenterology. *Can. J. Gastroenterol.* **2005**, *19* (Suppl. A), 5–36. [CrossRef]
19. Huang, Y.Q.; Gou, R.; Diao, Y.S.; Yin, Q.H.; Fan, W.X.; Liang, Y.P.; Chen, Y.; Wu, M.; Zang, L.; Li, L.; et al. Charlson comorbidity index helps predict the risk of mortality for patients with type 2 diabetic nephropathy. *J. Zhejiang Univ. Sci. B* **2014**, *15*, 58–66. [CrossRef]
20. Harvey, R.F.; Bradshaw, J.M. A simple index of Crohn's-disease activity. *Lancet* **1980**, *1*, 514. [CrossRef]
21. Lewis, J.D.; Chuai, S.; Nessel, L.; Lichtenstein, G.R.; Aberra, F.N.; Ellenberg, J.H. Use of the noninvasive components of the Mayo score to assess clinical response in ulcerative colitis. *Inflamm. Bowel Dis.* **2008**, *14*, 1660–1666. [CrossRef] [PubMed]

22. Guan, W.-J.; Ni, Z.-Y.; Hu, Y.; Liang, W.-H.; Ou, C.-Q.; He, J.-X.; Liu, L.; Shan, H.; Lei, C.-L.; Hui, D.S.C.; et al. Clinical Characteristics of Coronavirus Disease 2019 in China. *N. Engl. J. Med.* **2020**, *382*, 1708–1720. [CrossRef] [PubMed]
23. Alves-Cabratosa, L.; Comas-Cufí, M.; Blanch, J.; Martí-Lluch, R.; Ponjoan, A.; Castro-Guardiola, A.; Hurtado-Ganoza, A.; Pérez-Jaén, A.; Rexach-Fumaña, M.; Faixedas-Brunsoms, D.; et al. Persons with SARS-CoV-2 during the First and Second Waves in Catalonia (Spain): A Retrospective Observational Study Using Daily Updated Data. *JMIR Public Heal. Surveill.* **2021**, *8*, e30006. [CrossRef] [PubMed]
24. ISC; CNE. Informe Sobre la Situación de COVID-19 en España. Informe COVID-19 no12, 20 Marzo, 2020. Available online: https://www.isciii.es/QueHacemos/Servicios/VigilanciaSaludPublicaRENAVE/EnfermedadesTransmisibles/Paginas/-COVID-19.-Informes-previos.aspx (accessed on 2 August 2021).
25. CNE; ISC; ICI. COVID-19 en España. Available online: https://cnecovid.isciii.es/covid19/#provincias (accessed on 2 August 2021).
26. Barreiro-de Acosta, M.; Gutiérrez, A.; Zabana, Y.; Beltrán, B.; Calvet, X.; Chaparro, M.; Domènech, E.; Esteve, M.; Panés, J.; Gisbert, J.P.; et al. Inflammatory bowel disease integral care units: Evaluation of a nationwide quality certification programme. The GETECCU experience. *United Eur. Gastroenterol. J.* **2021**, *9*, 766–772. [CrossRef]
27. Instituto Nacional de Estadística (INE). Población por Provincias y Sexo. 2021. Available online: https://www.ine.es/jaxiT3/Datos.htm?t=2852#!tabs-tabla (accessed on 2 September 2021).
28. Burke, K.E.; Kochar, B.; Allegretti, J.R.; Winter, R.W.; Lochhead, P.; Khalili, H.; Colizzo, F.P.; Hamilton, M.J.; Chan, W.W.; Ananthakrishnan, A.N. Immunosuppressive Therapy and Risk of COVID-19 Infection in Patients with Inflammatory Bowel Diseases. *Inflamm. Bowel Dis.* **2021**, *27*, 155–161. [CrossRef]
29. Khan, N.; Patel, D.; Xie, D.; Lewis, J.; Trivedi, C.; Yang, Y.-X. Impact of Anti-Tumor Necrosis Factor and Thiopurine Medications on the Development of COVID-19 in Patients with Inflammatory Bowel Disease: A Nationwide Veterans Administration Cohort Study. *Gastroenterology* **2020**, *159*, 1545–1546.e1. [CrossRef]
30. Chaparro, M.; Garre, A.; Núñez Ortiz, A.; Diz-Lois Palomares, M.T.; Rodríguez, C.; Riestra, S.; Vela, M.; Benítez, J.M.; Fernández Salgado, E.; Sánchez Rodríguez, E.; et al. Incidence, Clinical Characteristics and Management of Inflammatory Bowel Disease in Spain: Large-Scale Epidemiological Study. *J. Clin. Med.* **2021**, *10*, 2885. [CrossRef] [PubMed]
31. Khan, N.; Mahmud, N.; Trivedi, C.; Reinisch, W.; Lewis, J.D. Risk factors for SARS-CoV-2 infection and course of COVID-19 disease in patients with IBD in the Veterans Affair Healthcare System. *Gut* **2021**, *70*, 1657–1664. [CrossRef]
32. Ardizzone, S.; Ferretti, F.; Monico, M.C.; Carvalhas Gabrielli, A.M.; Carmagnola, S.; Bezzio, C.; Saibeni, S.; Bosani, M.; Caprioli, F.; Mazza, S.; et al. Lower incidence of COVID-19 in patients with inflammatory bowel disease treated with non-gut selective biologic therapy. *J. Gastroenterol. Hepatol.* **2021**, *36*, 3050–3055. [CrossRef]
33. Derikx, L.A.A.P.; Lantinga, M.A.; de Jong, D.J.; van Dop, W.A.; Creemers, R.H.; Römkens, T.E.H.; Jansen, J.M.; Mahmmod, N.; West, R.L.; Tan, A.C.I.T.L.; et al. Clinical Outcomes of Covid-19 in Patients with Inflammatory Bowel Disease: A Nationwide Cohort Study. *J. Crohn's Colitis* **2020**, *15*, 529–539. [CrossRef] [PubMed]
34. Singh, S.; Khan, A.; Chowdhry, M.; Bilal, M.; Kochhar, G.S.; Clarke, K. Risk of Severe Coronavirus Disease 2019 in Patients with Inflammatory Bowel Disease in the United States: A Multicenter Research Network Study. *Gastroenterology* **2020**, *159*, 1575–1578.e4. [CrossRef] [PubMed]
35. Wetwittayakhlang, P.; Albader, F.; Golovics, P.A.; Bessissow, T.; Bitton, A.; Afif, W.; Wild, G.; Lakatos, P.L. Clinical Outcomes of COVID-19 and Impact on Disease Course in Patients with Inflammatory Bowel Disease. *Can. J. Gastroenterol. Hepatol.* **2021**, *2021*, 7591141. [CrossRef]
36. Attauabi, M.; Poulsen, A.; Theede, K.; Pedersen, N.; Larsen, L.; Jess, T.; Rosager Hansen, M.; Verner-Andersen, M.K.; Haderslev, K.V.; Berg Lødrup, A.; et al. Prevalence and Outcomes of COVID-19 Among Patients with Inflammatory Bowel Disease—A Danish Prospective Population-Based Cohort Study. *J. Crohn's Colitis* **2020**, *15*, 540–550. [CrossRef]
37. Ludvigsson, J.F.; Axelrad, J.; Halfvarson, J.; Khalili, H.; Larsson, E.; Lochhead, P.; Roelstraete, B.; Simon, T.G.; Söderling, J.; Olén, O. Inflammatory bowel disease and risk of severe COVID-19: A nationwide population-based cohort study in Sweden. *United Eur. Gastroenterol. J.* **2021**, *9*, 177–192. [CrossRef]
38. Guzzetta, G.; Riccardo, F.; Marziano, V.; Poletti, P.; Trentini, F.; Bella, A.; Andrianou, X.; Del Manso, M.; Fabiani, M.; Bellino, S.; et al. Impact of a Nationwide Lockdown on SARS-CoV-2 Transmissibility, Italy. *Emerg. Infect. Dis.* **2021**, *27*, 267–270. [CrossRef] [PubMed]
39. Pan, A.; Liu, L.; Wang, C.; Guo, H.; Hao, X.; Wang, Q.; Huang, J.; He, N.; Yu, H.; Lin, X.; et al. Association of Public Health Interventions with the Epidemiology of the COVID-19 Outbreak in Wuhan, China. *JAMA* **2020**, *323*, 1915–1923. [CrossRef] [PubMed]
40. Lodyga, M.; Maciejewska, K.; Eder, P.; Waszak, K.; Stawczyk-Eder, K.; Dobrowolska, A.; Kaczka, A.; Gąsiorowska, A.; Stępień-Wrochna, B.; Cicha, M.; et al. Social distancing during COVID-19 pandemic among inflammatory bowel disease patients. *J. Clin. Med.* **2021**, *10*, 3689. [CrossRef] [PubMed]
41. Allocca, M.; Chaparro, M.; Gonzalez, H.A.; Bosca-Watts, M.M.; Palmela, C.; D'Amico, F.; Zacharopoulou, E.; Kopylov, U.; Ellul, P.; Bamias, G.; et al. Patients with Inflammatory Bowel Disease Are Not at Increased Risk of COVID-19: A Large Multinational Cohort Study. *J. Clin. Med.* **2020**, *9*, 3533. [CrossRef] [PubMed]

42. Magro, F.; Rahier, J.F.; Abreu, C.; MacMahon, E.; Hart, A.; van der Woude, C.J.; Gordon, H.; Adamina, M.; Viget, N.; Vavricka, S.; et al. Inflammatory bowel disease management during the COVID-19 outbreak:The ten do's and don'ts from the ECCO-COVID task force. *J. Crohn's Colitis* **2020**, *14*, S798–S806. [CrossRef]
43. Bezzio, C.; Pellegrini, L.; Manes, G.; Arena, I.; Picascia, D.; Della Corte, C.; Devani, M.; Schettino, M.; Saibeni, S. Biologic therapies may reduce the risk of COVID-19 in patients with inflammatory bowel disease. *Inflamm. Bowel Dis.* **2020**, *26*, E107–E109. [CrossRef]
44. Iborra, I.; Puig, M.; Marín, L.; Calafat, M.; Cañete, F.; Quiñones, C.; González-González, L.; Cardona, G.; Mañosa, M.; Domènech, E. Treatment Adherence and Clinical Outcomes of Patients with Inflammatory Bowel Disease on Biological Agents during the SARS-CoV-2 Pandemic. *Dig. Dis. Sci.* **2021**, *66*, 4191–4196. [CrossRef]
45. The Lancet. COVID-19: Protecting health-care workers. *Lancet* **2020**, *395*, 922. [CrossRef]
46. Bezzio, C.; Saibeni, S.; Variola, A.; Allocca, M.; Massari, A.; Gerardi, V.; Casini, V.; Ricci, C.; Zingone, F.; Amato, A.; et al. Outcomes of COVID-19 in 79 patients with IBD in Italy: An IG-IBD study. *Gut* **2020**, *69*, 1213–1217. [CrossRef]
47. Williamson, E.J.; Walker, A.J.; Bhaskaran, K.; Bacon, S.; Bates, C.; Morton, C.E.; Curtis, H.J.; Mehrkar, A.; Evans, D.; Inglesby, P.; et al. Factors associated with COVID-19-related death using OpenSAFELY. *Nature* **2020**, *584*, 430–436. [CrossRef]
48. Nowak, J.K.; Lindstrøm, J.C.; Kalla, R.; Ricanek, P.; Halfvarson, J.; Satsangi, J. Age, Inflammation, and Disease Location Are Critical Determinants of Intestinal Expression of SARS-CoV-2 Receptor ACE2 and TMPRSS2 in Inflammatory Bowel Disease. *Gastroenterology* **2020**, *159*, 1151–1154.e2. [CrossRef]
49. Lukin, D.J.; Kumar, A.; Hajifathalian, K.; Sharaiha, R.Z.; Scherl, E.J.; Longman, R.S. Baseline Disease Activity and Steroid Therapy Stratify Risk of COVID-19 in Patients with Inflammatory Bowel Disease. *Gastroenterology* **2020**, *159*, 1541–1544.e2. [CrossRef] [PubMed]
50. Chan, J.F.-W.; Yuan, S.; Kok, K.-H.; To, K.K.-W.; Chu, H.; Yang, J.; Xing, F.; Liu, J.; Yip, C.C.-Y.; Poon, R.W.-S.; et al. A familial cluster of pneumonia associated with the 2019 novel coronavirus indicating person-to-person transmission: A study of a family cluster. *Lancet* **2020**, *395*, 514–523. [CrossRef]
51. Axelrad, J.E.; Malter, L.; Hong, S.; Chang, S.; Bosworth, B.; Hudesman, D. From the American Epicenter: Coronavirus Disease 2019 in Patients with Inflammatory Bowel Disease in the New York City Metropolitan Area. *Inflamm. Bowel Dis.* **2020**, *27*, 662–666. [CrossRef] [PubMed]
52. Bataille, P.; Amiot, A.; Claudepierre, P.; Paris, N.; Neuraz, A.; Lerner, I.; Garcelon, N.; Rance, B.; Grisel, O.; Moreau, T.; et al. Letter: Severe COVID-19 infection and biologic therapies—A cohort study of 7 808 patients in France. *Aliment. Pharmacol. Ther.* **2020**, *52*, 1245–1248. [PubMed]
53. Shang, L.; Zhao, J.; Hu, Y.; Du, R.; Cao, B. On the use of corticosteroids for 2019-nCoV pneumonia. *Lancet* **2020**, *395*, 683–684. [CrossRef]
54. Zhou, W.; Liu, Y.; Tian, D.; Wang, C.; Wang, S.; Cheng, J.; Hu, M.; Fang, M.; Gao, Y. Potential benefits of precise corticosteroids therapy for severe 2019-nCoV pneumonia. *Signal. Transduct. Target. Ther.* **2020**, *5*, 18. [CrossRef]
55. Agrawal, M.; Brenner, E.J.; Zhang, X.; Colombel, J.-F.; Kappelman, M.D.; Ungaro, R.C.; Gearry, R.B.; Kalpan, G.G.; Kissous-Hunt, M.; Lewis, J.D.; et al. Physician Practice Patterns in Holding Inflammatory Bowel Disease Medications due to COVID-19, in the SECURE-IBD Registry. *J. Crohns. Colitis* **2021**, *15*, 860–863. [CrossRef]
56. Attauabi, M.; Dahlerup, J.F.; Poulsen, A.; Hansen, M.R.; Verner-Andersen, M.K.; Eraslan, S.; Prahm, A.P.; Pedersen, N.; Larsen, L.; Jess, T.; et al. Outcomes and long-term effects of COVID-19 in patients with inflammatory bowel diseases—A Danish prospective population-based cohort study with individual-level data. *J. Crohn's Colitis* **2021**, in press. [CrossRef] [PubMed]
57. Mertz, B.; Dijkstra, F.; Nielsen, J.; Kjeldsen, J. Post COVID-19 hospitalizations in patients with chronic inflammatory diseases—A nationwide cohort study. *J. Autoimmun.* **2021**, *125*, 102739.

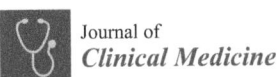

Article

Assessment of Gastrointestinal Symptoms and Dyspnea in Patients Hospitalized due to COVID-19: Contribution to Clinical Course and Mortality

Krzysztof Kaliszewski [1,*], Dorota Diakowska [2], Łukasz Nowak [3], Urszula Tokarczyk [1], Maciej Sroczyński [1], Monika Sępek [1], Agata Dudek [1], Karolina Sutkowska-Stępień [1], Katarzyna Kiliś-Pstrusińska [4], Agnieszka Matera-Witkiewicz [5], Michał Pomorski [6], Marcin Protasiewicz [7], Janusz Sokołowski [8], Barbara Adamik [9], Krzysztof Kujawa [10], Adrian Doroszko [11], Katarzyna Madziarska [12,†] and Ewa Anita Jankowska [13,†]

1. Department of General, Minimally Invasive and Endocrine Surgery, Wroclaw Medical University, Borowska Street 213, 50-556 Wroclaw, Poland; urszula.tokarczyk@student.umw.edu.pl (U.T.); maciej.sroczynski@o2.pl (M.S.); moniasep@wp.pl (M.S.); agatadudek7@gmail.com (A.D.); karolina.sutkowska@onet.pl (K.S.-S.)
2. Department of Basic Science, Faculty of Health Science, Wroclaw Medical University, Bartel Street 5, 51-618 Wroclaw, Poland; dorota.diakowska@umed.wroc.pl
3. Department of Urology and Urological Oncology, Wroclaw Medical University, Borowska Street 213, 50-556 Wroclaw, Poland; lllukasz.nowak@gmail.com
4. Department of Pediatric Nephrology, Wroclaw Medical University, Borowska Street 213, 50-556 Wroclaw, Poland; katarzyna.kilis-pstrusinska@umed.wroc.pl
5. Screening Laboratory of Biological Activity Tests and Collection of Biological Material, Faculty of Pharmacy, Wroclaw Medical University, Borowska Street 211A, 50-556 Wroclaw, Poland; agnieszka.matera-witkiewicz@umed.wroc.pl
6. Department of Gynecology and Obstetrics, Wroclaw Medical University, Borowska Street 213, 50-556 Wroclaw, Poland; michal.pomorski@umed.wroc.pl
7. Department and Clinic of Cardiology, Wroclaw Medical University, Borowska Street 213, 50-556 Wroclaw, Poland; marcin.protasiewicz@umed.wroc.pl
8. Department of Emergency Medicine, Wroclaw Medical University, Borowska Street 213, 50-556 Wroclaw, Poland; janusz.sokolowski@umed.wroc.pl
9. Department of Anaesthesiology and Intensive Therapy, Wroclaw Medical University, Borowska Street 213, 50-556 Wroclaw, Poland; barbara.adamik@umed.wroc.pl
10. Statistical Analysis Center, Wroclaw Medical University, Marcinkowski Street 2-6, 50-368 Wroclaw, Poland; krzysztof.kujawa@umed.wroc.pl
11. Department of Internal Medicine, Hypertension and Clinical Oncology, Wroclaw Medical University, Borowska 213, 50-556 Wroclaw, Poland; adrian.doroszko@umed.wroc.pl
12. Department of Nephrology and Transplantation Medicine, Wroclaw Medical University, Borowska Street 213, 50-556 Wroclaw, Poland; katarzyna.madziarska@umed.wroc.pl
13. Centre for Heart Diseases, Department of Heart Diseases, Wroclaw Medical University, Borowska Street 213, 50-556 Wroclaw, Poland; ewa.jankowska@umed.wroc.pl

* Correspondence: krzysztof.kaliszewski@umed.wroc.pl; Tel./Fax: +48-71-734-3000
† These authors contributed equally to this work.

Abstract: Gastrointestinal manifestations may accompany the respiratory symptoms of COVID-19. Abdominal pain (AP) without nausea and vomiting is one of the most common. To date, its role and prognostic value in patients with COVID-19 is still debated. Therefore, we performed a retrospective analysis of 2184 individuals admitted to hospital due to COVID-19. We divided the patients into four groups according to presented symptoms: dyspnea, $n = 871$ (39.9%); AP, $n = 97$ (4.4%); AP with dyspnea together, $n = 50$ (2.3%); and patients without dyspnea and AP, $n = 1166$ (53.4%). The patients with AP showed tendency to be younger than these with dyspnea, but without AP (63.0 [38.0–70.0] vs. 65.0 [52.0–74.0] years, $p = 0.061$), and they were more often females as compared to patients with dyspnea (57.7% vs. 44.6%, $p = 0.013$, for females). Patients with AP as a separate sign of COVID-19 significantly less often developed pneumonia as compared to individuals with dyspnea or with dyspnea and AP together ($p < 0.0001$). Patients with AP or AP with dyspnea were significantly less frequently intubated or transferred to the intensive care unit ($p = 0.003$ and $p = 0.031$, respectively).

Individuals with AP alone or with dyspnea had significantly lower rate of mortality as compared to patients with dyspnea ($p = 0.003$). AP as a separate symptom and also as a coexisting sign with dyspnea does not predispose the patients with COVID-19 to the worse clinical course and higher mortality.

Keywords: COVID-19; SARS-CoV-2; gastrointestinal manifestations; abdominal pain; dyspnea; clinical course; mortality

1. Introduction

In December 2019, a large number of pneumonia cases of unknown origin were first reported in Wuhan, Hubei Province, China [1]. Next, after several weeks, the new pathological agent was recognized as a novel coronavirus responsible for this severe acute respiratory syndrome (SARS). The virus was named SARS coronavirus 2 (SARS-CoV-2) as a member of the Coronaviridae family [1,2]. This group of viruses is routinely presented among animals and humans, and contains nonsegmented enveloped RNA viruses with a single-strand linear positive-sense RNA (2). Subsequently, the disease caused by SARS-CoV-2 was introduced as coronavirus disease-2019 (COVID-19) [1–3]. The new, unknown virus disease spread rapidly worldwide, and 11 March 2020 was established as the start date of the global pandemic by the World Health Organization (WHO) [3]. Since that time, over 212 million patients with a COVID-19 diagnosis and 4.4 million COVID-19-associated deaths have been observed [4]. The prevalence of COVID-19 is steadily increasing [5].

Initially, according to many studies, COVID-19 was recognized only as a respiratory tract infection. However, later, many authors described COVID-19 as a disease with a wide range spectrum of symptoms due to its involvement of not only the lungs but also other organs [6,7]. Hoffmann et al. [8] revealed that it is caused by the interaction of SARS-CoV-2 with other human organs mediated by angiotensin converting enzyme 2 (ACE 2). ACE 2 is expressed on many anatomical structures on the cell surface. ACE 2 was identified as an integral membrane protein that is recognized as the host cell receptor for SARS-CoV-2. Additionally, Chen et al. [9] observed ACE 2 as the host cell receptor in a large quantity in patients with COVID-19. Varga et al. [10] established that endothelial ACE 2-positive cells obtained from COVID-19 patients present significant morphological changes, such as disruptions of intercellular junctions, cell swelling, and damaged contacts of the basement membrane. Despite the fact that ACE 2 is mostly localized in the alveolar epithelium, some authors have highlighted its presence in the liver and biliary epithelium, enterocytes, or the vascular endothelium [11,12]. Therefore, it can be expected that such pathophysiological reactions may lead to some other clinical manifestations of the extrapulmonary locations.

It was estimated that on 19 January 2020, in Washington (USA), the first COVID-19-positive patient manifested, in addition to respiratory sings, abdominal symptoms such as abdominal pain (AP), nausea, and vomiting [13]. Some authors noticed that several individuals with COVID-19, who presented to the emergency department (ED) had only AP without any typical respiratory signs characteristic of this infection [1]. Others described an interesting situation, that was individually observed in EDs: in patients with severe AP, when radiologists subsequently performed abdominal computed tomography [CT] due to the abdominal symptoms, they recognized the SARS-CoV-2 infection due to the typical findings of peripheral and subpleural ground-glass opacities in the lower lobes of the lung [14–16]. Regarding some observational studies describing connections between COVID-19 and digestive system failure symptoms [17–19], we can ask whether they should be treated as specific signs for SARS-CoV-2 infections, especially in patients without any respiratory symptoms. However, there are also other important issues, which in our opinion stand in contrast to previously mentioned ones. Namely, some authors recognize AP in patients with COVID-19 as a side effect of virus infection treatment and as secondary to systemic inflammation and ischemia [20]. Others say that AP may also occur in patients with basilar pneumonia [12,21]. However, many authors have reported an association between SARS-CoV-2 infections and other abdominal diseases, such as acute pancreatitis, which has been well documented by clinical studies [22–26]. On the other hand, there are analyses that have considered such observations, even well-documented ones, inappropriate [27]. These authors recommend treating the relationship between SARS-CoV-2 infections and, for instance, mentioning acute pancreatitis as a casual association, due to insufficient etiological evaluation.

Due to these observations and many doubts about the COVID-19 disease, we performed a retrospective analysis of 2184 individuals with COVID-19 to determine whether, and how many patients infected by SARS-CoV-2 manifested AP. Second, we checked, whether the patients with COVID-19 disease, who presented with AP, had significantly elevated specific markers for digestive system involvement. Third, we assessed the correlation between respiratory symptoms and AP to establish how often they occur together and separately. Finally, we assessed how AP may influence the clinical course and mortality of patients with COVID-19.

2. Materials and Methods

2.1. Study Population

We retrospectively analyzed 2184 medical records of patients admitted and treated at the university and temporary COVID-19 hospital arranged by the Medical University Hospital in Wroclaw (Poland) between February 2020 and June 2021.

The study protocol was approved by the Institutional Review Board and Ethics Committee of Wroclaw Medical University, Wroclaw, Poland (No: KB-444/2021). All our patients provided informed consent for admission into the study, which stipulated that the results may be used for research purposes. The data were analyzed retrospectively and anonymously from established medical records. The authors did not have access to identifying patient information or direct access to the study participants.

The patients were divided into four groups according to presented symptoms at the time of admission to the hospital: group A—patients without dyspnea and AP, (study control population); group B—patients with dyspnea; group C—patients with AP; and group D—patients with dyspnea and AP. Patients in Group A did not have dyspnea and AP, and they were included to this group as the patients with COVID-19 positive test and other signs of virus infection (except of AP and dyspnea): cough, fever, pain in the chest, standstill, stressed sounds, and whistling sounds heard over the lung fields, diarrhea, vomiting, deterioration of health, weakness, and elevated inflammatory parameters. The patients infected by SARS-CoV-2 in whom we confirmed acute abdominal disease such as appendicitis, cholecystitis, diverticulitis, incarcerated and strangulated abdominal hernia, occlusion of mesenteric artery or aortic aneurysm were excluded from the study (see supplementary materials). They were transported to the department of surgery for potential surgical intervention. They were not admitted to the temporary COVID-19 hospital.

2.2. Statistical Analysis

Descriptive data were presented as number of observation and percent (for categorical variables) or as mean, standard deviation ($\pm$SD), median and interquartile range (Q25–Q75) (for continuous variables). Distribution of continuous variables was tested by Kolmogorov-Smirnoff with Lillefor's correction or Shapiro-Wilk normality tests. Chi-square test and Fisher exact test were used for comparison of qualitative variables. Quantitative variables were tested by ANOVA Kruskal-Wallis analysis with post-hoc Dunn test with Bonferroni correction. A significance level of 0.05 was assumed in the analyzes.

Univariable and multivariable logistic regression analysis was used for the determination of independent clinical and laboratory predictors of patients' death. Results of $p > 0.1$ in univariable logistic analyzes were assumed as exclusion criterion in multivariable analysis. Odds ratios (OR) and confidence intervals ($\pm$95% CI) were calculated. In some cases, it was observed a strong correlation between the variables ($r = 1.0$, $p < 0.0001$), the matrix model was improperly conditioned and the criteria for logistic regression analysis were not met, these variables were removed from the analysis. Clinical and laboratory variables were analyzed separately in multivariable log analysis.

Statistical calculations were performed using Statistica v.13.3 (Tibco Software Inc., Palo Alto, CA, USA).

3. Results

3.1. Patient Characteristics

The study group consisted of 2184 COVID-19 patients. There were 1102 (50.5%) women and 1082 (49.5%) men, with a mean age of 60.1 ± 18.8 years old. Group A consists of 1166 (53.4%) patients, group B contains 871 (39.9%) individuals, group C 97 (4.4%) patients, and group D consists of 50 (2.3%) patients. Groups were different in sex ($p = 0.0001$) and age ($p = 0.001$) parameters (Table 1), therefore subsequent data were analyzed separately according sex. The "age" variable was not significant in selected "women" and "men" groups in post-hoc tests ($p > 0.05$).

Table 1. Baseline characteristics of 2184 patients hospitalized due to COVID-19, divided into four study groups.

Variables	No Dyspnea and No Abdominal Pain $n = 1166$; (Group A)	Dyspnea $n = 871$; (Group B)	Abdominal Pain $n = 97$; (Group C)	Dyspnea and Abdominal Pain $n = 50$; (Group D)	p-Value
Sex:					
- women	629 (54.0)	388 (44.6)	56 (57.7)	29 (58.0)	0.0001
- men	537 (46.0)	483 (55.4)	41 (42.3)	21 (42.0)	
Age (years old)	63.0 (41.0–73.0) [1]	65.0 (52.0–74.0) [1,2]	63.0 (38.0–70.0) [2]	64.0 (40.0–75.0)	0.001

Values for continuous variables were showed as or median (Q25–Q75), and values for categorical variables were presented as number of observation (percent) [1]: A vs. B, $p = 0.002$; [2]: B vs. C, $p = 0.061$ tendency to statistical significance.

Baseline characteristics of patients with COVID-19 according to clinical symptoms reported by patients during admission time to the hospital was presented in Table 1.

The patients with dyspnea (Group B) were significantly older than patients without respiratory sign and AP (Group A) (65.0 [52.0–74.0] vs. 63.0 [41.0–73.0] years, $p = 0.002$), and they showed tendency to be older than patients with AP (Group C) ($p = 0.061$). The patients with dyspnea were more often male as compared to other study groups (55.4% vs. 46.0% or 42.0%, $p < 0.0001$).

3.2. Relationship between Presented Symptoms in Four Study Groups and Other Clinical and Laboratory Parameters Obtained on Admission to Hospital and during Hospitalization

Table 2 showed the prevalence of clinical factors and results of laboratory parameters in COVID-19 patients divided into four study groups in two time periods, namely at the time of admission to the hospital and during hospitalization.

Table 2. Comparison of the clinical and laboratory parameters in four tested groups of patients with COVID-19 at the time of admission to hospital and during hospitalization.

Variables	Control Group $n = 1166$; (Group A)	Dyspnoea $n = 871$; (Group B)	Abdominal Pain $n = 97$; (Group C)	Dyspnoea and Abdominal Pain $n = 50$; (Group D)	p-Value
Parameters Obtained at the Admission to the Hospital					
Saturation (SaO_2) without oxygen therapy (%)	96.0 (94.0–98.0) [1,2]	90.0 (85.0–95.0) [1,3]	97.0 (95.0–98.0) [3,4]	92.4 ± 4.5 [2,4]	<0.0001
PaO_2 [mmHg]	61.5 ± 31.4	54.0 (35.5–73.5)	42.0 (26.0–50.0)	49.8 ± 26.4	0.045

Table 2. Cont.

Variables	Control Group n = 1166; (Group A)	Dyspnoea n = 871; (Group B)	Abdominal Pain n = 97; (Group C)	Dyspnoea and Abdominal Pain n = 50; (Group D)	p-Value
Pain in the chest	50 (4.3)	101 (11.6)	3 (3.1)	9 (18.0)	<0.0001
Cough	171 (14.7)	434 (49.8)	15 (15.5)	28 (56.0)	<0.0001
Standstill heard over the lung fields	109 (9.4)	233 (26.8)	10 (10.3)	15 (30.0)	<0.0001
Stressed sounds heard over the lung fields	108 (9.3)	189 (21.7)	10 (10.3)	12 (24.0)	<0.0001
Whistling sounds heard over the lung fields	63 (5.4)	147 (16.9)	4 (4.1)	5 (10.0)	<0.0001
Diarrhea	35 (3.0)	58 (6.7)	21 (21.7)	13 (26.0)	<0.0001
Vomiting	35 (3.0)	21 (2.4)	30 (30.9)	12 (24.0)	<0.0001
Respiratory support:					
- oxygen mustache cannula	127 (10.9)	277 (31.9)	8 (8.3)	16 (32.0)	
- face mask	34 (2.9)	104 (12.0)	1 (1.0)	5 (10.0)	
- Venturi mask	3 (0.3)	12 (1.4)	2 (2.1)	0 (0.0)	<0.0001
- passive oxygen therapy	33 (2.8)	176 (20.3)	2 (2.1)	5 (10.0)	
- HFNC	1 (0.1)	9 (1.0)	0 (0.0)	0 (0.0)	
- BiPAP/CPAP	1 (0.1)	8 (0.9)	0 (0.0)	0 (0.0)	
- respirator therapy	72 (6.2)	11 (1.3)	0 (0.0)	0 (0.0)	
ASPAT (U/L)	32.0 (21.0–55.0) [5]	43.0 (29.0–69.0) [5,6]	33.0 (22.0–56.0) [6]	42.5 (26.0–59.0)	<0.0001
ALAT (U/L)	25.0 (16.0–45.0) [7]	35.0 (21.0–58.0) [7]	26.0 (17.0–47.0)	32.0 (20.0–46.0)	<0.0001
Total bilirubin (mg/dL)	0.6 (0.5–0.9)	0.6 (0.5–0.8)	0.6 (0.5–1.0)	0.6 (0.5–0.9)	0.365
Amylase in blood (U/L)	50.5 (31.0–75.0)	50.0 (32.0–72.0)	50.5 (31.0–63.0)	55.0 (42.0–60.0)	0.834
Lipase (U/L)	29.0 (16.0–63.0)	31.0 (18.0–56.0)	30.0 (15.0–63.0)	41.0 (22.0–57.0)	0.742
CRP (mg/L)	30.7 (5.2–89.8) [8,9]	74.4 (32.7–144.3) [8,10]	40.7 (11.3–100.8) [10]	71.2 (31.4–128.15) [9]	<0.0001
Procalcitonin (ng/mL)	0.09 (0.04–0.31)	0.09 (0.04–0.30)	0.07 (0.04–0.22)	0.07 (0.04–0.26)	0.351
Parameters obtained during hospitalization					
Deterioration of health—The need for maximum aggressive oxygen therapy	329 (28.2)	371 (42.6)	26 (26.8)	17 (34.0)	<0.0001
The most aggressive respiratory support during hospitalization:					
- HFNC	32 (2.8)	92 (10.6)	3 (3.1)	4 (8.0)	<0.0001
- BiPAP/CPAP	9 (0.8)	32 (3.7)	0 (0.0)	1 (2.0)	
- respirator therapy	112 (9.6)	96 (11.0)	3 (3.1)	1 (2.0)	
Whistling/rattling sounds	274 (23.5)	441 (50.7)	20 (20.6)	28 (56.0)	<0.0001
Pneumonia	397 (34.1)	599 (68.8)	32 (33.0)	33 (66.0)	<0.0001
Hypovolemic shock	19 (1.6)	12 (1.4)	4 (4.1)	0 (0.0)	0.199
Cardiac shock	18 (1.5)	13 (1.5)	1 (1.0)	0 (0.0)	0.643
Septic shock	80 (6.9)	57 (6.5)	4 (4.1)	0 (0.0)	0.046

Table 2. Cont.

Variables	Control Group n = 1166; (Group A)	Dyspnoea n = 871; (Group B)	Abdominal Pain n = 97; (Group C)	Dyspnoea and Abdominal Pain n = 50; (Group D)	p-Value
Digestive tract hemorrhage:					
- upper part	17 (1.5)	12 (1.4)	3 (3.1)	0 (0.0)	0.500
- lower part	4 (0.3)	3 (0.3)	1 (1.0)	1 (2.0)	
Respiratory hemorrhage	14 (1.2)	17 (2.0)	1 (1.0)	2 (4.0)	0.330
The need for intubation	111 (9.5)	100 (11.5)	3 (3.1)	1 (2.0)	0.003
Transfer to the Intensive Care Unit	106 (9.1)	101 (11.6)	5 (5.2)	2 (4.0)	0.031
Ventilation mode:					
- A/C	65 (65.0)	39 (54.9)	1 (50.0)	0 (0.0)	0.507
- CMV	19 (19.0)	12 (16.9)	1 (50.0)	0 (0.0)	
- SIMS	16 (16.0)	20 (28.2)	0 (0.0)	0 (0.0)	
Hospitalization:					
- Discharge home	741 (63.6)	481 (55.2)	65 (67.0)	29 (58.0)	
- Transferred to another hospital for specialist treatment or deterioration of health	129 (11.1)	128 (14.7)	14 (14.4)	9 (18.0)	0.003
- Transferred to another hospital for rehabilitation	143 (12.3)	104 (11.9)	8 (8.3)	7 (14.0)	
- Patient's death	153 (13.1)	158 (18.1)	10 (10.3)	5 (10.0)	
ASPAT (U/L)	29.0 (20.0–48.0) [11]	35.0 (24.0–57.0) [11]	28.0 (21.0–45.0)	34.0 (24.0–58.0)	<0.0001
ALAT (U/L)	28.0 (17.0–53.0) [12]	41.0 (22.0–75.0) [12,13]	28.0 (15.0–48.0) [13]	39.0 (20.0–61.0)	<0.0001
Total bilirubin (mg/dL)	0.6 (0.4–0.8)	0.6 (0.5–0.8)	0.6 (0.4–0.9)	0.6 (0.4–0.9)	0.930
Amylase in blood (U/L)	49.5 (30.0–71.0)	50.0 (34.0–69.0)	45.5 (28.0–65.0)	52.7 ± 15.9	0.805
Lipase (U/L)	30.0 (16.0–65.0)	34.0 (19.0–58.0)	33.0 (15.0–63.0)	41.0 (21.0–54.0)	0.876
CRP (mg/L)	15.6 (3.9–65.6) [14]	19.6 (5.0–94.4) [14]	20.7 (6.6–54.0)	28.9 (7.4–94.7)	0.006
Procalcitonin (ng/mL)	0.06 (0.03–0.30)	0.05 (0.03–0.2)	0.05 (0.03–0.13)	0.06 (0.03–0.14)	0.292

HFNC, high flow nasal cannula; BiPAP/CPAP, bilevel positive airway pressure/continuous positive airway pressure; A/C, assist/control; CMV, continuous mandatory ventilation; SIMV, synchronized intermittent mandatory ventilation; ASPAT, aspartate transaminase; ALAT, alanine aminotransferase; CRP, C-reactive protein. Values for continuous variables were showed as mean ± SD and for variables without normal distribution as median (Q25-Q75), and values for categorical variables were presented as number of observation (percent). [1]: A vs. B, $p < 0.0001$, [2]: A vs. D, $p = 0.0004$; [3]: B vs. C, $p < 0.0001$; [4]: C vs. D, $p < 0.001$; [5]: A vs. B, $p < 0.0001$; [6]: B vs. C, $p = 0.009$; [7]: A vs. B, $p < 0.0001$; [8]: A vs. B, $p < 0.0001$; [9]: A vs. D, $p < 0.001$; [10]: B vs. C, $p < 0.001$; [11]: A vs. B, $p < 0.0001$; [12]: A vs. B, $p < 0.0001$; [13]: B vs. C, $p = 0.003$; [14]: A vs. B, $p = 0.013$.

At the time of admission to the hospital we observed statistically significant correlation between the prevalence of the clinical signs characteristic for analyzed groups. In the groups of patients with dyspnea (Group B) and with dyspnea and AP (Group D), the clinical respiratory signs (cough, standstill, stressed sounds, and whistling sounds heard over the lung fields) were observed significantly more often as compared to the patients without dyspnea (Group A) and to the patients presented only AP (Group C) ($p < 0.0001$ for all) (Table 2). Similarly, the clinical signs characteristic for patients with AP (Group C) and AP with dyspnea (Group D) (diarrhea and vomiting) were significantly more often observed in these groups comparing to the groups without AP (Groups A and

B) (*p* < 0.0001 for all) (Table 2). Saturation (SaO$_2$) without oxygen therapy significantly differed between comparing groups (A vs. B, *p* < 0.0001, A vs. D, *p* = 0.0004; B vs. C, *p* < 0.0001; C vs. D, *p* < 0.001) what correlated with clinical symptoms presented by patients (Table 2). Consequently, respiratory supports (oxygen mustache cannula, face mask, Venturi mask, passive oxygen therapy, High Flow Nasal Cannula (HFNC), Bilevel Positive Airway Pressure/Continuous Positive Airway Pressure (BiPAP/CPAP), and lastly respirator therapy) were significantly more often introduced in patients with dyspnea and with dyspnea and AP (Groups B and D). However, none of the patients with AP and AP with dyspnea did not need HFNC, BiPAP/CPAP, and respirator therapy. What is interesting, we observed significantly higher levels of aspartate transaminaze (ASPAT) and alanine aminotransferaze (ALAT) in the blood of the patients presented dyspnea separately and with AP (Groups B and D) when compared to the patients with AP alone (Group C) (A vs. B, *p* < 0.0001; B vs. C, *p* = 0.009; A vs. B, *p* < 0.0001) (Table 2). We observed the analogous situation with C-reactive protein (CRP) in compared groups (A vs. B, *p* < 0.0001; A vs. D, *p* < 0.001; B vs. C, *p* < 0.001) (Table 2). We did not observe statistically significant correlations in analyzed groups in case of blood levels of total bilirubin, amylase, and procalcitonin.

During hospitalization the patients with dyspnea and with dyspnea and AP (Groups B and D) presented significantly more often deterioration of health what needed maximum aggressive oxygen therapy (*p* < 0.0001) (Table 2). The most aggressive respiratory support during hospitalization (HFNC, BiPAP/CPAP and respirator therapy) was significantly more often introduced in patients with dyspnea (Group B) as compared to the patients with AP or with AP and dyspnea (Groups C and D). Patients with AP (Group C) significantly less frequently developed pneumonia compared to patients with dyspnea and patients with dyspnea and AP (Groups B and D) (*p* < 0.0001) (Table 2). Patients with AP and AP with dyspnea (Groups C and D) were significantly less frequently intubated and transferred to the Intensive Care Unit as compared to the patients with dyspnea (Group B) (*p* = 0.003 and *p* = 0.031, respectively) (Table 2). Patients with AP as a separate sign (Group C) and with AP and dyspnea (Group D) had significantly lower rate of mortality as compared to patients with dyspnea as a separate symptom (Group B) (*p* = 0.003) (Table 2). We observed significantly higher levels of ASPAT and ALAT in the blood of the patients presented dyspnea separately and with AP (Groups B and D) when compared to the patients with AP alone (Group C) (A vs. B, *p* < 0.0001; A vs. B, *p* < 0.0001; B vs. C, *p* = 0.003) (Table 2). During hospitalization we observed significantly higher level of CRP in patients with AP and dyspnea (Group D) (*p* = 0.006) (Table 2).

3.3. Selected Determinants of COVID-19 Patient Death

In order to test the risk of qualifying a COVID-19 patient to a given group on the basis of the presented symptoms at the time of admission to the hospital, we conducted a logistic analysis for three study groups (A, B and C) as predictors of death (Table 3).

Table 3. Logistic regression analysis of membership in selected groups of COVID-19 patients as predictors of patient's death.

Groups	OR (± 95% CI)	*p*-Value
gr. B vs. gr. A (for gr. B)	1.47 (1.15–1.87)	0.002
gr. C vs. gr. A (for gr. C)	0.87 (0.62–1.22)	0.428
gr. B vs. gr. C (for gr. C)	0.52 (0.26–1.02)	0.057

Qualifying the patient to group B, but not to group C, significantly influenced the prevalence of patient's death.

We analyzed numerous risk factors and potential predictors of patient's death. Univariable logistic regression analysis was used for precise assessment of each parameter's influence. Then two multivariable models of selected determinants were obtained for patients with dyspnea (Group B, *n* = 871) and patients with AP (Group C, *n* = 97). A corresponding model for group of patients with dyspnea and AP (Group D, n = 50) was not possible due to the low number of subjects.

In the univariable logistic analysis for patients with dyspnea as a separate symptom (Group B), majority of tested risk factors significantly influenced the prevalence of patients' death (p < 0.05 for all) (Table 4).

Table 4. Univariable and multivariable logistic regression analysis of selected variables as predictors of death in group of patients with dyspnea (Group B; n = 871).

Risk Parameters	Univariable		Multivariable	
	OR (±95% CI)	p-Value	OR (±95% CI)	p-Value
Parameters at the Time of Admission to the Hospital:				
Sex (for men)	1.44 (1.01–2.05)	0.045	1.55 (1.05–2.29)	0.027
Age (for ≥65 years old)	4.13 (2.78–6.15)	<0.0001	3.35 (2.20–5.11)	<0.0001
Pain in the chest	1.13 (0.67–1.90)	0.644		
Cough	0.43 (0.29–0.61)	<0.0001	0.52 (0.35–0.77)	0.001
Standstill heard over the lung fields	2.51 (1.75–3.59)	<0.0001	2.10 (1.41–3.13)	<0.001
Stressed sounds heard over the lung fields	1.77 (1.20–2.61)	0.003	1.35 (0.87–2.10)	0.174
Whistling sounds heard over the lung fields	2.00 (1.32–3.02)	<0.001	1.49 (0.95–2.33)	0.082
Diarrhea	0.93 (0.46–1.90)	0.854		
Vomiting	1.06 (0.35–3.22)	0.913		
Respiratory suport:				
Oxygen mustache	0.48 (0.31–0.73)	<0.001	0.65 (0.40–1.05)	0.081
Face mask	1.24 (0.74–2.05)	0.403		
Venturi mask	3.28 (1.02–10.51)	0.044	3.37 (0.99–11.47)	0.051
Passive oxygen therapy	2.41 (1.64–3.54)	<0.0001	1.91 (1.21–3.01)	0.005
HFNC	5.77 (1.53–21.80)	0.009	6.62 (1.56–27.96)	0.010
BiPAP/CPAP	1.18 (0.92–1.50)	0.171		
Respirator therapy	1.70 (0.44–6.49)	0.437		
Laboratory parameters at admission:				
ASPAT (for: >40 U/L)	1.44 (0.98–2.13)	0.059	1.49 (0.59–3.79)	0.395
ALAT (for: >40 U/L)	0.65 (0.44–0.96)	0.031	0.67 (0.29–1.68)	0.419
Total bilirubin (for: >1.1 mg/dL)	2.80 (1.57–4.98)	<0.0001	1.93 (0.71–5.23)	0.194
Amylase in blood (for: >160 U/L)	19.78 (2.38–163.90)	0.005	10.47 (1.05–104.63)	0.044
Lipase (for >150 U/L)	1.20 (0.34–4.09)	0.772		
CRP (for: >5 mg/L)	2.22 (0.78–6.32)	0.134		
Procalcitonin (for: > 0.1 ng/mL)	5.23 (3.41–8.03)	<0.0001	6.13 (2.49–15.06)	<0.0001
Parameters during hospitalization:				
The most aggressive respiratory support during hospitalization:				
HFNC	3.45 (2.17–5.48)	<0.0001	16.38 (6.71–39.93)	<0.0001
BiPAP/CPAP	6.41 (3.11–13.20)	<0.0001	46.04 (15.55–136.23)	<0.0001
Respirator therapy	6.70 (4.27–10.51)	<0.0001	1.41 (0.10–19.31)	0.792
Whistling/rattling sounds	0.34 (0.23–0.49)	<0.0001	2.63 (1.14–6.07)	0.022

Table 4. Cont.

Risk Parameters	Univariable		Multivariable	
	OR (±95% CI)	p-Value	OR (±95% CI)	p-Value
Pneumonia	2.19 (1.42–3.36)	0.0003	1.01 (0.68–1.48)	0.963
Hypovolemic shock	6.56 (2.1–20.99)	0.001	2.54 (0.37–17.26)	0.338
Cardiac shock	26.50 (5.82–121.54)	<0.0001	14.34 (2.32–88.46)	0.004
Septic shock	26.21 (13.16–52.17)	<0.0001	10.45 (2.54–43.01)	0.001
Digestive tract hemorrhage:				
- upper part	3.29 (1.03–10.54)	0.044	2.51 (0.57–11.07)	0.221
- lower part	2.26 (0.20–25.21)	0.505		
Respiratory hemorrhage	4.17 (1.58–11.00)	0.004	1.59 (0.42–5.99)	0.491
Transferred to the Intensive Care Unit	5.17 (3.32–8.02)	<0.0001	5.06 (3.01–8.28)	<0.001
The need for intubation	7.53 (4.82–11.74)	<0.0001	46.95 (5.09–432.87)	<0.001
Ventilation mode:				
- A/C	0.96 (0.36–2.55)	0.933		
- CMV	2.06 (0.49–8.60)	0.314		
- SIMV	0.67 (0.22–1.94)	0.449		
Laboratory parameters during hospitalization:				
ASPAT (for: >40 U/L)	2.89 (1.96–4.27)	<0.0001	2.27 (1.26–4.08)	0.006
ALAT (for: >40 U/L)	0.85 (0.58–1.23)	0.385		
Total bilirubin (for: >1.1 mg/dL)	5.33 (3.08–9.22)	<0.0001	4.99 (1.91–13.08)	0.001
Amylase in blood (for: >160 U/L)	1 ref.	-		
Lipase (for >150 U/L)	0.88 (0.22–3.41)	0.852		
CRP (for: >5 mg/L)	66.67 (9.24–481.12)	<0.0001	23.84 (3.06–185.30)	0.002
Procalcitonin (for: > 0.1 ng/mL)	30.64 (17.66–53.18)	<0.0001	22.56 (11.86–42.91)	<0.0001

HFNC, high flow nasal cannula; BiPAP/CPAP, bilevel positive airway pressure/continuous positive airway pressure; A/C, assist/control; CMV, continuous mandatory ventilation; SIMV, synchronized intermittent mandatory ventilation; ASPAT, aspartate transaminase; ALAT, alanine aminotransferase; CRP, C-reactive protein; OR, odds ratio; ±95%CI, 95% confidence intervals.

Model of multivariable analysis presented for patients with dyspnea alone (Group B) (Table 4) revealed, that an increase in age above 65 years old, male gender, standstill heard over the lung fields, passive oxygen therapy, HFNC therapy, and also levels of amylase in blood above 160 U/L (normal range: 20–160 U/L) and procalcitonin above 0.1 ng/mL (normal range <0.1 ng/mL) at the time of admission to the hospital were connected with significantly higher risk of death ($p < 0.05$ for all). Predictors of patients' death in patients with dyspnea without AP (Group B) during hospitalization were HFNC, BiPAP/CPAP, cardiac and septic shock, the need for intubation, transfer to the intensive care unit, ASPAT above 40 U/L (normal range: 0–40 U/L), total bilirubin above 1.1 mg/dL (normal range: 0.3–1.1 mg/dL), CRP above 5 mg/L (normal range: 3.0–5.0 mg/L), and elevated procalcitonin above 0.1 ng/mL ($p < 0.05$ for all) (Table 4).

In the univariable logistic regression analysis for patients with AP as a separate symptom (Group C), respirator therapy, pneumonia, hypovolemic shock, septic shock, transfer to the intensive care unit, procalcitonin level above 0.1 ng/mL at the time of admission to the hospital, and during hospitalization were predictors of patient's death ($p < 0.05$). Model of multivariable analysis constructed for patients with AP (Group C) (Table 5) revealed that increase of procalcitonin level above 0.1 ng/mL at the time of admission to the hospital and during hospitalization was the only risk factor of patients' death ($p < 0.05$) (Table 5).

Table 5. Univariable and multivariable logistic regression analysis of selected variables as predictors of death in group of patients with abdominal pain ($n = 97$).

Risk Parameters	Univariable		Multivariable	
	OR (±95% CI)	p-Value	OR (±95% CI)	p-Value
Parameters at the Admission to the Hospital:				
Sex (for men)	0.90 (0.23–3.48)	0.878		
Age (for ≥65 years old)	2.34 (0.60–9.05)	0.213		
Pain in the chest	4.72 (0.38–59.22)	0.223		
Cough	1 ref.	-		
Standstill heard over the lung fields	2.46 (0.43–13.97)	0.300		
Stressed sounds heard over the lung fields	0.96 (0.11–8.79)	0.972		
Whistling sounds heard over the lung fields	3.11 (0.28–34.14)	0.346		
Diarrhea	0.37 (0.04–3.20)	0.362		
Vomiting	0.95 (0.22–4.04)	0.946		
Respiratory suport:				
Oxygen mustache cannula	3.38 (0.56–20.01)	0.175		
Face mask	1 ref.	-		
Venturi mask	9.55 (0.53–172.35)	0.121		
Passive oxygen therapy	1 ref.	-		
HFNC	1 ref.	-		
BiPAP/CPAP	1 ref.	-		
Respiratory therapy	1 ref.	-		
Laboratory parameters at admission:				
ASPAT (for: >40 U/L)	1.83 (0.42–7.91)	0.406		
ALAT (for: >40 U/L)	2.14 (0.51–9.05)	0.290		
Total bilirubin (for: >1.1 mg/dL)	0.86 (0.09–8.01)	0.890		
Amylase in blood (for: >160 U/L)	1 ref.	-		
Lipase (for >150 U/L)	1 ref.	-		
CRP (for: >5 mg/L)	1 ref.	-		
Procalcitonin (for: > 0.1 ng/mL)	8.00 (1.41–45.21)	0.016	8.00 (1.41–45.21)	0.016
Parameters during hospitalization:				
The most aggressive respiratory support during hospitalization:				
Whistling/rattling sounds	1.76 (0.40–7.68)	0.443		
HFNC	1 ref.	-		
BiPAP/CPAP	1 ref.	-		
Respirator therapy	21.50 (1.69–272.56)	0.016	0.085 (0.00–15.35)	0.346
Pneumonia	5.78 (1.35–24.63)	0.016	6.20 (0.92–41.74)	0.057
Hypovolemic shock	10.62 (1.27–88.22)	0.027	1.84 (0.02–138.23)	0.779
Cardiac shock	1 ref.	-		
Septic shock	36.85 (3.27–415.19)	0.003	1.31 (0.04–47.73)	0.882

Table 5. Cont.

Risk Parameters	Univariable		Multivariable	
	OR (±95% CI)	p-Value	OR (±95% CI)	p-Value
Digestive tract hemorrhage:- upper part- lower part	4.72 (0.37–59.22)1 ref.	0.223-		
Respiratory hemorrhage	1 ref.	-		
Transferred to the Intensive Care Unit	18.21 (2.52–131.04)	0.003	10.35 (0.13–848.87)	0.292
Laboratory parameters during hospitalization:				
ASPAT (for: >40 U/L)	0.65 (0.11–3.60)	0.620		
ALAT (for: >40 U/L)	0.62 (0.11–3.33)	0.574		
Total bilirubin (for: >1.1 mg/dL)	2.26 (0.38–13.32)	0.360		
Amylase in blood (for: >160 U/L)	1 ref.	-		
Lipase (for >150 U/L)	1 ref.	-		
CRP (for: >5 mg/L)	1 ref.	-		
Procalcitonin (for: > 0.1 ng/mL)	16.62 (2.78–99.32)	0.002	16.62 (2.78–99.32)	0.002

HFNC, high flow nasal cannula; BiPAP/CPAP, bilevel positive airway pressure/continuous positive airway pressure; ASPAT, aspartate transaminase; ALAT, alanine aminotransferase; CRP, C-reactive protein; OR, odds ratio; ±95% CI, 95% confidence intervals.

4. Discussion

Since the COVID-19 pandemic is ongoing, it was estimated, that although respiratory signs are predominant, extrapulmonary manifestations are also present. Clinical observations revealed, that almost all organs and systems can be involved in SARS-CoV-2 infections [28]. Guan et al. [15] suggests, that among many others, AP may occur as an isolated clinical finding in patients with COVID-19. Digestive symptoms such as nausea, vomiting, and diarrhea may accompany respiratory symptoms. In our study group, we estimated that patients with dyspnea without AP presented diarrhea and vomiting in 6.7% and 2.4% of cases, respectively. In patients with AP and dyspnea, digestive symptoms were presented more often (i.e., diarrhea in 26.0% of the patients and vomiting in 24.0%). A similar situation was observed in patients presenting only AP without dyspnea. In this group we observed diarrhea in 21.7% and vomiting in 30.9% of the patients.

Sanku et al. [29] noticed, that gastrointestinal bleeding is a rare and unusual finding since patients with COVID-19 are often hypercoagulable, so they are more likely to clot than to bleed. In our study, we noticed digestive tract hemorrhage from the upper part in 1.4% of the patients presenting dyspnea. Interestingly, we did not observe this symptom in patients with dyspnea and AP and only observed digestive tract hemorrhage from the upper part in 3.1% of the patients with AP but without dyspnea. Bleeding from the lower part of the digestive tract was only observed in 0.3% of the patients presenting dyspnea at admission, in 2.0% of the patients with AP, and dyspnea in 1.0% of the patients, who presented only AP as an isolated symptom. We also observed hemorrhage from the respiratory tract, especially in patients, who presented only dyspnea as a main clinical symptom of COVID-19. In this group we observed respiratory tract hemorrhage in 17 (2.0%) individuals.

In addition to respiratory parameters, liver, biliary tract, and pancreatic laboratory tests are routinely ordered in patients with SARS-CoV-2 infections, especially in those presenting with abdominal complaints. In our study we did not perform the analysis of the imaging tests of the abdominal cavity (CT, ultrasonography, endoscopy) due to low number of the completed examinations. Despite good evidence of a correlation between elevated pancreatic enzymes, liver and biliary injury markers, and diseases of these organs, there is still a lack of data regarding these observations during SARS-CoV-2 infections and the course of the disease. Generally, in our analysis we did not observe any significant correlation of elevated pancreatic and hepatic enzymes, and abdominal complaints. In the analyzed groups of patients with dyspnea (Group B), AP (Group C), and dyspnea with AP together (Group D) were investigated for women and men at the time of admission and during hospitalization, and we noticed only two significant differences. Interestingly, in contrast to other studies, we noticed that the blood level of aspartate transaminase (ASPAT) was significantly higher in the groups of patients with dyspnea as a main clinical symptom and with AP (Groups B and D), but not in patients with AP (Group C). This significant difference was also seen during hospitalization. At the time of admission and during hospitalization we observed, that the blood level of alanine aminotransferase (ALAT) was significantly higher in the groups of patients with dyspnea and AP with dyspnea (Group B and D), but not in the group with AP alone (Group C vs. A and B). Revzin et al. [30] estimated that liver failure in patients with COVID-19 is rather mild and transient, but severe liver injury might be diagnosed in the case of sepsis and coagulopathy with microthrombosis. In our study, we confirmed a higher rate of sepsis in the group with dyspnea. Bhayana et al. [31] established that bowel injury in patients with SARS-CoV-2 infection is most likely caused by direct virus spreading into the gut epithelium or by small vessel thrombosis with subsequent ischemia. However, Balaban et al. [12] noticed, that other pathologies are also observed, such as hemorrhagic complications leading to hematomas in the gut walls. Some authors have established potential proposals for the mechanisms of digestive system involvement in patients infected with SARS-CoV-2 [20,32,33]. It might be the explanation for our observations, that in the groups of patients, who complained of AP as a separate symptom or with dyspnea (Groups C and D), vomiting, and diarrhea were observed significantly more often. For hepatobiliary injury, some authors proposed direct viral cytopathic damage, congestive hepatopathy, drug-induced liver injury, systemic inflammatory response and exacerbation of preexisting chronic liver disease. For pancreas failure, some authors proposed direct viral cytopathic injury, systemic inflammation, and dehydration. In the end, gastrointestinal tract damage, according to these authors, is mainly caused by virus cytopathic injury, systemic inflammation, thrombosis, and adverse effects of COVID-19-related drugs [12,20,32,33]. Additionally, some other authors state that the presence of SARS-CoV-2 within endothelial cells, in addition to direct viral effects, also produces perivascular inflammation [10]. Han et al. [17] assessed that 57% of COVID-19-positive patients with a low severity of disease manifested AP alone or in combination with respiratory symptoms. In our study, there was definitely a lower number of patients with AP alone or with dyspnea, at 6.7%. Liu et al. [34] revealed that clinically observed AP in patients with COVID-19 infection usually comes from involvement of the gastrointestinal tract and hepatobiliary-pancreatic system, whereas urinary tract failure and spleen involvement were not commonly observed. In our study, we did not observe any symptoms from a spleen or urinary tract injury, so we did not note any details in our clinical base.

Jutzeler et al. [35] noticed that men are more commonly affected by SARS-CoV-2 infections, and their hospital mortality rate is significantly higher than that of women infected with SARS-CoV-2. In our study we confirmed, that men were significantly more often observed in the group of patients with dyspnea as a separate sign (Group B). However, they more rarely complained of AP than women. The mortality rate was also higher in the group of patients, who complained of dyspnea alone during hospitalization than in the other groups. What is interesting, regarding the patients, who complained of AP (separately or with dyspnea), the mortality rate was at the same level (18.1 vs. 10.3 and 10.0). Han et al. [17] noticed, that patients with abdominal symptoms, compared to those presenting with only respiratory difficulties, had a longer time between the onset of the disease symptoms and viral clearance. They also observed, that patients with digestive components were referred later to medical care units than those with pulmonary symptoms caused by SARS-CoV-2. The delay might be due to these nonspecific manifestations of COVID-19. The authors also identified SARS-CoV-2 in stool samples in a proportion of COVID-19-positive individuals [17]. Hung et al. [36] identified replication of SARS-CoV-2 in the wall of the small and large intestines. Varga et al. [10] analyzed the small intestine of two infected patients and confirmed endotheliitis of the submucosa vessels with mononuclear cell infiltrates within the intima along the lumen of the vessels. They also noticed direct virus presence in endothelial cells. Effenberger et al. [37] confirmed elevated fecal calprotectin concentrations as the result of the inflammatory response in the intestines of patients with SARS-CoV-2 infections, who presented with diarrhea. Elevated concentrations were not observed in the individuals without diarrhea. Goldberg-Stein et al. [38] performed a retrospective analysis of 141 patients with COVID-19 and revealed, that the most common gastrointestinal symptom in these patients was AP. It was observed in 73.8% of the individuals with negative abdominal CT scans and in 53.8% of the patients with positive abdominal CT findings [38]. The authors noticed that 64% of COVID-19-positive patients without any pathological signs in abdominal CT scans had characteristic changes for SARS-CoV-2 infections at the lung bases [38]. Thus, some other authors suggest, that patients with COVID-19 disease without any pathological signs of the abdominal organs may present AP and may have secondary pleural inflammation [39]. Durmus et al. [40] noticed that during the COVID-19 pandemic, it is important to consider a diagnosis of COVID-19 disease in patients with non-severe flank pain if no urological pathology is evident on abdominal CT scans. In our study, a large majority of the patients did not have any imaging tests performed, what we included in the limitations of the study.

The gastrointestinal lesions produced by COVID-19 pose a major challenge in meeting individuals' nutritional needs. Szefel et al. [41] noticed that the lack of nutrients for the intestinal mucosa may produce atrophy of the lymphoid tissue and subsequently cause immune system deficiency and intestinal bacterial translocation. According to some authors' observations, diarrhea was the first symptom of COVID-19, before respiratory involvement, and sometimes might even be the only sign of the disease [42,43]. In our study, diarrhea was observed in 5.8% of all patients.

In the end, it is worth emphasizing that the liver was estimated to be the second most injured organ following the lungs in patients infected by the SARS-CoV-2 virus [44]. ACE 2 receptors are widely expressed, especially on cholangiocytes, and even more expressed on cholangiocytes than on hepatocytes [4,45]. Zhao et al. [46] described the virus's damaging effects on the bile acid barrier in cholangiocytes and the disruption of genes, which destroy cell connections and bile acid transport. According to some authors, the immune-mediated cytokine storm is often included in liver damage [1]. The authors observed elevated plasma levels of C-reactive protein, lymphocytes, neutrophils, and some cytokines, especially interleukin-6. Nardo et al. [47] suggested that the effort to stop cytokine dysregulation at the very beginning of COVID-19 disease may decrease the progression of liver injury. All pathological events with respiratory-induced liver hypoxia and drug-induced liver toxicity produce coagulopathy and consequently, cause damaging changes in microcirculation with microthrombosis within the liver sinusoids [15]. According to Han et al. [17], 14.0% of patients with COVID-19 present elevated serum ASPAT, ALAT, and total bilirubin (TBIL), what is evidence of liver injury. Zhang et al. [6] noticed that 50% of SARS-CoV-2-infected patients presented elevated plasma levels of gamma-glutamyl transferase (GGT). Individuals with elevated liver laboratory tests were at higher risk of severe disease progression, which becomes more noticeable within the first two weeks of hospitalization [4]. ALAT, ASPAT, TBIL, and GGT levels can be elevated to more than three times the upper limit of the normal range [48]. Additionally, some authors state that patients with severe liver injury have a higher rate of intubation and dializotherapy than patients with mild, moderate or no liver injury during the course of COVID-19 disease [1]. According to an analysis presented by the Institute of the American Society of Gastroenterology, more than 60% of patients with COVID-19 have mild liver injury [21]. Of course, the liver condition of patients during SARS-CoV-2 infections depends on the hepatic disease history and the liver function before COVID-19 disease, such as chronic hepatitis or steatosis. Some authors estimated the undisputed impact of pre-existing liver diseases in patients with COVID-19 and its course [49]. They noticed that the risk of hospitalization and death in such individuals was significantly higher.

AP caused by pancreatic involvement in patients with SARS-CoV-2 infections has also been reported [50]. Although, the pathogenetic mechanisms are not as well described for pancreatic involvement as for liver injury, the most likely reasons are the cytopathic effect of the virus and immune-mediated storm. Liu et al. [50] estimated that 17.9% and 16.4% of patients with COVID-19 had elevated plasma amylase and lipase levels, respectively. Others highlighted elevated blood glucose levels as the next marker of pancreatic injury during a COVID-19 infection [51].

In addition to this fact, that we did not observe such lesions, according to some authors, the spleen is the next abdominal organ involved in SARS-CoV-2 infections [52]. In their opinion, ACE 2 receptors are also localized on red pulp and vascular endothelial cell surfaces. Xu et al. [52] stated, that the virus may directly influence macrophages and dendritic cells. These authors reported splenic parenchyma congestion, hemorrhage and lymphatic vesicle absence with spleen parenchyma atrophy, which were noticed during the autopsies of patients, who died of COVID-19. AP originating from splenic injury is caused by splenomegaly and solitary or multifocal splenic infarcts [52].

The outcomes of COVID-19 patients reported by many authors suggest an association between the presence of AP and important clinical observations such as delay in presentation, disease severity and mortality [53]. In summary, we can say that gastrointestinal and respiratory involvement in COVID-19 often occur together. This is probably why Zhou et al. [54] started to promote the concept of the "gut-lung axis". They suggested that stimulation on one side triggers a response on the other side in patients infected by SARS-CoV-2 [54]. However, in our opinion, there is still too few evidence and completed pathophysiological studies to promote such concept.

Our work has some limitations. First, it was a retrospective study, and access to some necessary specific details was limited. Second, this study was observational, which makes it difficult to control for all potential confounding factors, including age, sex, smoking or vaccination status. Third, there was selection bias since patients included in this study were admitted to the hospital, which indicates that the patients were not representative of the whole population. Fourth, the analyzed data came from a single medical center, so the possibility of selection bias cannot be ruled out. Fifth, we performed our study and made conclusions after an analysis of clinical and biochemical parameters, which only indirectly indicated their pragmatic value in disease prognosis. The large majority of patients did not have imaging tests of the abdominal cavity performed, so we did not decide to include the analysis of them in our study. Many parameters of COVID-19 patients did not show any significant correlation with the clinical course of the disease. This might be since our study included a relatively small number of individuals.

To conclude, AP as a separate symptom and also as a coexisting sign with dyspnea does not predispose the patients with COVID-19 to the worse clinical course and higher mortality. COVID-19 is a systemic disease involving not only the lungs but also the abdominal organs. Thus, the clinical symptoms might be variable.

Supplementary Materials: The following supporting information can be downloaded at: https://www.mdpi.com/article/10.3390/jcm11071821/s1.

Author Contributions: Conceptualization: K.K. (Krzysztof Kaliszewski); Data acquisition: K.K. (Krzysztof Kaliszewski), D.D., Ł.N. and K.K. (Krzysztof Kujawa); Formal analysis: K.K. (Krzysztof Kaliszewski); Investigation: K.K. (Krzysztof Kaliszewski), D.D. and K.K. (Krzysztof Kujawa), Methodology: K.K. (Krzysztof Kaliszewski), D.D. and K.K. (Krzysztof Kujawa); Project administration: K.K. (Krzysztof Kaliszewski); Resources: K.K. (Krzysztof Kaliszewski), Ł.N., U.T., M.S. (Maciej Sroczyński), M.S. (Monika Sępek), A.D. (Agata Dudek), K.S.-S., K.K.-P., A.M.-W., M.P. (Michał Pomorski), M.P. (Marcin Protasiewicz), J.S., and B.A.; Supervision: K.K. (Krzysztof Kaliszewski), A.D. (Adrian Doroszko), K.M. and E.A.J.; Validation: K.K. (Krzysztof Kaliszewski) and D.D. Writing the original draft: K.K. (Krzysztof Kaliszewski) and D.D.; Writing: K.K. (Krzysztof Kaliszewski); Reviewing and editing: K.K. (Krzysztof Kaliszewski) and D.D. All authors reviewed the manuscript. All authors agreed to submit the article to the current journal. All authors also gave final approval of the version to be published and decided to be accountable for all aspects of the work. All authors have read and agreed to the published version of the manuscript.

Funding: This study was not supported by any funds.

Institutional Review Board Statement: The study was conducted according to the guidelines of the Declaration of Helsinki and approved by the Bioethics Committee of Wroclaw Medical University, Wroclaw, Poland (Signature number: KB-444/2021).

Informed Consent Statement: The routine data were collected retrospectively; therefore, writteninformed consent to participate in the study was not required. The Bioethics Committee approvedthe publication of anonymized data.

Data Availability Statement: The datasets used and/or analyzed during the current study are available from the corresponding author upon reasonable request.

Acknowledgments: The authors are grateful to all of the staff and the patients at the study center who contributed to this work.

Conflicts of Interest: The authors declare no conflict of interest.

Abbreviations

COVID-19	Coronavirus Disease-2019
AP	Abdominal pain
SARS	Severe acute respiratory syndrome
SARS-CoV-2	SARS coronavirus 2
WHO	World Health Organization
ACE 2	Angiotensin converting enzyme 2
ED	Emergency department
CT	Computed tomography
HFNC	High Flow Nasal Cannula
BiPAP	Bilevel Positive Airway Pressure
CPAP	Continuous Positive Airway Pressure
A/C	Assist/Control
CMV	Continuous Mandatory Ventilation
SIMV	Synchronized Intermittent Mandatory Ventilation
ASPAT	Aspartate transaminase
ALAT	Alanine aminotransferase
CRP	C-reactive protein

References

1. Boraschi, P.; Giugliano, L.; Mercogliano, G.; Donati, F.; Romano, S.; Neri, E. Abdominal and gastrointestinal manifestations in COVID-19 patients: Is imaging useful? *World J. Gastroenterol.* **2021**, *27*, 4143–4159. [CrossRef] [PubMed]
2. Mahajan, A.; Hirsch, J.A. Novel coronavirus: What neuroradiologists as citizens of the world need to know. *AJNR Am. J. Neuroradiol.* **2020**, *41*, 552–554. [CrossRef] [PubMed]
3. World Health Organization. WHO Director-General's Opening Remarks at the Media Briefing on COVID-19. Available online: https://www.who.int/dg/speeches/detail/who-director-general-s-opening-remarks-at-the-media-briefing-on-covid-19 (accessed on 11 March 2020).
4. Shah, M.D.; Sumeh, A.S.; Sheraz, M.; Kavitha, M.S.; Venmathi Maran, B.A.; Rodrigues, K.F. A mini-review on the impact of COVID 19 on vital organs. *Biomed. Pharmacother.* **2021**, *143*, 112158. [CrossRef] [PubMed]
5. Kallem, V.R.; Sharma, D. COVID-19 in neonates. *J. Matern. Fetal Neonatal Med.* **2020**, *35*, 1610–1618. [CrossRef]
6. Zhang, C.; Shi, L.; Wang, F.S. Liver injury in COVID-19: Management and challenges. *Lancet Gastroenterol. Hepatol.* **2020**, *5*, 428–430. [CrossRef]
7. Consiglio, C.R.; Cotugno, N.; Sardh, F.; Pou, C.; Amodio, D.; Rodriguez, L.; Tan, Z.; Zicari, S.; Ruggiero, A.; Pascucci, G.R.; et al. The immunology of multisystem inflammatory syndrome in children with COVID-19. *Cell* **2020**, *183*, 968–981.e7. [CrossRef]
8. Hoffmann, M.; Kleine-Weber, H.; Schroeder, S.; Krüger, N.; Herrler, T.; Erichsen, S.; Schiergens, T.S.; Herrler, G.; Wu, N.H.; Nitsche, A.; et al. SARS-CoV-2 cell entry depends on ACE2 and TMPRSS2 and is blocked by a clinically proven protease inhibitor. *Cell* **2020**, *181*, 271–280.e8. [CrossRef]
9. Chen, J.; Jiang, Q.; Xia, X.; Liu, K.; Yu, Z.; Tao, W.; Gong, W.; Han, J.J. Individual variation of the SARS-CoV-2 receptor ACE2 gene expression and regulation. *Aging Cell* **2020**, *19*, e13168. [CrossRef]
10. Varga, Z.; Flammer, A.J.; Steiger, P.; Haberecker, M.; Andermatt, R.; Zinkernagel, A.S.; Mehra, M.R.; Schuepbach, R.A.; Ruschitzka, F.; Moch, H. Endothelial cell infection and endotheliitis in COVID-19. *Lancet* **2020**, *395*, 1417–1418. [CrossRef]

11. Hamming, I.; Timens, W.; Bulthuis, M.L.; Lely, A.T.; Navis, G.; Van Goor, H. Tissue distribution of ACE2 protein, the functional receptor for SARS coronavirus. A first step in understanding SARS pathogenesis. *J. Pathol.* **2004**, *203*, 631–637. [CrossRef]
12. Balaban, D.V.; Baston, O.M.; Jinga, M. Abdominal imaging in COVID-19. *World J. Radiol.* **2021**, *13*, 227–232. [CrossRef] [PubMed]
13. Holshue, M.L.; DeBolt, C.; Lindquist, S.; Lofy, K.H.; Wiesman, J.; Bruce, H.; Spitters, C.; Ericson, K.; Wilkerson, S.; Tural, A.; et al. First case of 2019 novel coronavirus in the United States. *N. Engl. J. Med.* **2020**, *382*, 929–936. [CrossRef] [PubMed]
14. Luo, S.; Zhang, X.; Xu, H. Don't overlook digestive symptoms in patients with 2019 novel coronavirus disease (COVID-19). *Clin. Gastroenterol. Hepatol.* **2020**, *18*, 1636–1637. [CrossRef] [PubMed]
15. Guan, W.J.; Ni, Z.Y.; Hu, Y.; Liang, W.H.; Ou, C.Q.; He, J.X.; Liu, L.; Shan, H.; Lei, C.L.; Hui, D.S.C.; et al. Clinical characteristics of coronavirus disease 2019 in China. *N. Engl. J. Med.* **2020**, *382*, 1708–1720. [CrossRef]
16. Siegel, A.; Chang, P.J.; Jarou, Z.J.; Paushter, D.M.; Harmath, C.B.; Arevalo, J.B.; Dachman, A. Lung base findings of coronavirus disease (COVID-19) on abdominal CT in patients with predominant gastrointestinal symptoms. *AJR Am. J. Roentgenol.* **2020**, *215*, 607–609. [CrossRef]
17. Han, C.; Duan, C.; Zhang, S.; Spiegel, B.; Shi, H.; Wang, W.; Zhang, L.; Lin, R.; Liu, J.; Ding, Z.; et al. Digestive symptoms in COVID-19 patients with mild disease severity: Clinical presentation, stool viral RNA testing, and outcomes. *Am. J. Gastroenterol.* **2020**, *115*, 916–923. [CrossRef]
18. Tariq, R.; Saha, S.; Furqan, F.; Hassett, L.; Pardi, D.; Khanna, S. Prevalence and mortality of COVID-19 patients with gastrointestinal symptoms: A systematic review and meta-analysis. *Mayo Clin. Proc.* **2020**, *95*, 1632–1648. [CrossRef]
19. Cheung, K.S.; Hung, I.F.N.; Chan, P.P.Y.; Lung, K.C.; Tso, E.; Liu, R.; Ng, Y.Y.; Chu, M.Y.; Chung, T.W.H.; Tam, A.R.; et al. Gastrointestinal manifestations of SARS-CoV-2 infection and virus load in fecal samples from a Hong Kong cohort: Systematic review and meta-analysis. *Gastroenterology* **2020**, *159*, 81–95. [CrossRef]
20. Pasha, S.B.; Swi, A.; Hammoud, G.M. Gastrointestinal and hepatic manifestations of COVID-19 infection: Lessons for practitioners. *World J. Meta Anal.* **2020**, *8*, 348–374. [CrossRef]
21. Sultan, S.; Altayar, O.; Siddique, S.M.; Davitkov, P.; Feuerstein, J.D.; Lim, J.K.; Falck-Ytter, Y.; El-Serag, H.B. AGA institute rapid review of the gastrointestinal and liver manifestations of COVID-19, meta-analysis of international data, and recommendations for the consultative management of patients with COVID-19. *Gastroenterology* **2020**, *159*, 320–334.e27. [CrossRef]
22. De-Madaria, E.; Siau, K.; Cárdenas-Jaén, K. Increased amylase and lipase in patients with COVID-19 pneumonia: Don't blame the pancreas just yet! *Gastroenterology* **2021**, *160*, 1871. [CrossRef]
23. De-Madaria, E.; Capurso, G. COVID-19 and acute pancreatitis: Examining the causality. *Nat. Rev. Gastroenterol. Hepatol.* **2021**, *18*, 3–4. [CrossRef] [PubMed]
24. Aloysius, M.M.; Thatti, A.; Gupta, A.; Sharma, N.; Bansal, P.; Goyal, H. COVID-19 presenting as acute pancreatitis. *Pancreatology* **2020**, *20*, 1026–1027. [CrossRef] [PubMed]
25. McNabb-Baltar, J.; Jin, D.X.; Grover, A.S.; Redd, W.D.; Zhou, J.C.; Hathorn, K.E.; McCarty, T.R.; Bazarbashi, A.N.; Shen, L.; Chan, W.W. Lipase elevation in patients with COVID-19. *Am. J. Gastroenterol.* **2020**, *115*, 1286–1288. [CrossRef] [PubMed]
26. Szatmary, P.; Arora, A.; Raraty, M.G.T.; Dunne, D.F.J.; Baron, R.D.; Halloran, C.M. Emerging phenotype of severe acute respiratory syndrome-Coronavirus 2-associated pancreatitis. *Gastroenterology* **2020**, *159*, 1551–1554. [CrossRef]
27. Juhász, M.F.; Ocskay, K.; Kiss, S.; Hegyi, P.; Párniczky, A. Insufficient etiological workup of COVID-19-associated acute pancreatitis: A systematic review. *World J. Gastroenterol.* **2020**, *26*, 6270–6278. [CrossRef]
28. Cascella, M.; Del Gaudio, A.; Vittori, A.; Bimonte, S.; Del Prete, P.; Forte, C.A.; Cuomo, A.; De Blasio, E. COVID-pain: Acute and late-onset painful clinical manifestations in COVID-19-molecular mechanisms and research perspectives. *J. Pain Res.* **2021**, *14*, 2403–2412. [CrossRef]
29. Sanku, K.; Siddiqui, A.H.; Paul, V.; Ali, M. An unusual case of gastrointestinal bleeding in a patient with COVID-19. *Cureus* **2021**, *13*, e13901. [CrossRef]
30. Revzin, M.V.; Raza, S.; Srivastava, N.C.; Warshawsky, R.; D'Agostino, C.; Malhotra, A.; Bader, A.S.; Patel, R.D.; Chen, K.; Kyriakakos, C.; et al. Multisystem imaging manifestations of COVID-19, part 2: From cardiac complications to pediatric manifestations. *Radiographics* **2020**, *40*, 1866–1892. [CrossRef]
31. Bhayana, R.; Som, A.; Li, M.D.; Carey, D.E.; Anderson, M.A.; Blake, M.A.; Catalano, O.; Gee, M.S.; Hahn, P.F.; Harisinghani, M.; et al. Abdominal imaging findings in COVID-19: Preliminary observations. *Radiology* **2020**, *297*, E207–E215. [CrossRef]
32. Bruno, G.; Fabrizio, C.; Santoro, C.R.; Buccoliero, G.B. Pancreatic injury in the course of coronavirus disease 2019: A not-so-rare occurrence. *J. Med. Virol.* **2021**, *93*, 74–75. [CrossRef] [PubMed]
33. Schaefer, E.A.K.; Arvind, A.; Bloom, P.P.; Chung, R.T. Interrelationship between coronavirus infection and liver disease. *Clin. Liver Dis.* **2020**, *15*, 175–180. [CrossRef] [PubMed]
34. Liu, P.P.; Blet, A.; Smyth, D.; Li, H. The science underlying COVID-19: Implications for the cardiovascular system. *Circulation* **2020**, *142*, 68–78. [CrossRef] [PubMed]
35. Jutzeler, C.R.; Bourguignon, L.; Weis, C.V.; Tong, B.; Wong, C.; Rieck, B.; Pargger, H.; Tschudin-Sutter, S.; Egli, A.; Borgwardt, K.; et al. Comorbidities, clinical signs and symptoms, laboratory findings, imaging features, treatment strategies, and outcomes in adult and pediatric patients with COVID-19: A systematic review and meta-analysis. *Travel Med. Infect. Dis.* **2020**, *37*, 101825. [CrossRef]
36. Hung, I.F.; Lau, S.K.; Woo, P.C.; Yuen, K.Y. Viral loads in clinical specimens and SARS manifestations. *Hong Kong Med. J.* **2009**, *15* (Suppl. 9), 20–22. [CrossRef]

37. Effenberger, M.; Grabherr, F.; Mayr, L.; Schwaerzler, J.; Nairz, M.; Seifert, M.; Hilbe, R.; Seiwald, S.; Scholl-Buergi, S.; Fritsche, G.; et al. Faecal calprotectin indicates intestinal inflammation in COVID-19. *Gut* **2020**, *69*, 1543–1544. [CrossRef]
38. Goldberg-Stein, S.; Fink, A.; Paroder, V.; Kobi, M.; Yee, J.; Chernyak, V. Abdominopelvic CT findings in patients with novel coronavirus disease 2019 (COVID-19). *Abdom. Radiol.* **2020**, *45*, 2613–2623. [CrossRef]
39. Grief, S.N.; Loza, J.K. Guidelines for the evaluation and treatment of pneumonia. *Prim. Care* **2018**, *45*, 485–503. [CrossRef]
40. Durmus, E.; Ok, F.; Erdogan, Ö.; Saglik, S. Could flank pain be an indicator of COVID-19 infection? *Malawi Med. J.* **2020**, *32*, 192–196. [CrossRef]
41. Szefel, J.; Kruszewski, W.J.; Buczek, T. Enteral feeding and its impact on the gut immune system and intestinal mucosal barrier. *Prz. Gastroenterol.* **2015**, *10*, 71–77. [CrossRef]
42. Pan, L.; Mu, M.; Yang, P.; Sun, Y.; Wang, R.; Yan, J.; Li, P.; Hu, B.; Wang, J.; Hu, C.; et al. Clinical characteristics of COVID-19 patients with digestive symptoms in Hubei, China: A descriptive, cross-sectional, multicenter study. *Am. J. Gastroenterol.* **2020**, *115*, 766–773. [CrossRef] [PubMed]
43. Lee, I.C.; Huo, T.I.; Huang, Y.H. Gastrointestinal and liver manifestations in patients with COVID-19. *J. Chin. Med. Assoc.* **2020**, *83*, 521–523. [CrossRef] [PubMed]
44. Xu, L.; Liu, J.; Lu, M.; Yang, D.; Zheng, X. Liver injury during highly pathogenic human coronavirus infections. *Liver Int.* **2020**, *40*, 998–1004. [CrossRef] [PubMed]
45. Li, H.; Liu, S.M.; Yu, X.H.; Tang, S.L.; Tang, C.K. Coronavirus disease 2019 (COVID-19): Current status and future perspectives. *Int. J. Antimicrob. Agents* **2020**, *55*, 105951. [CrossRef] [PubMed]
46. Zhao, B.; Ni, C.; Gao, R.; Wang, Y.; Yang, L.; Wei, J.; Lv, T.; Liang, J.; Zhang, Q.; Xu, W.; et al. Recapitulation of SARS-CoV-2 infection and cholangiocyte damage with human liver ductal organoids. *Protein Cell* **2020**, *11*, 771–775. [CrossRef]
47. Nardo, A.D.; Schneeweiss-Gleixner, M.; Bakail, M.; Dixon, E.D.; Lax, S.F.; Trauner, M. Pathophysiological mechanisms of liver injury in COVID-19. *Liver Int.* **2021**, *41*, 20–32. [CrossRef]
48. Cai, Q.; Huang, D.; Yu, H.; Zhu, Z.; Xia, Z.; Su, Y.; Li, Z.; Zhou, G.; Gou, J.; Qu, J.; et al. COVID-19: Abnormal liver function tests. *J. Hepatol.* **2020**, *73*, 566–574. [CrossRef]
49. Singh, S.; Khan, A. Clinical characteristics and outcomes of coronavirus disease 2019 among patients with preexisting liver disease in the United States: A multicenter research network study. *Gastroenterology* **2020**, *159*, 768–771.e3. [CrossRef]
50. Liu, F.; Long, X.; Zhang, B.; Zhang, W.; Chen, X.; Zhang, Z. ACE2 expression in pancreas may cause pancreatic damage after SARS-CoV-2 infection. *Clin. Gastroenterol. Hepatol.* **2020**, *18*, 2128–2130.e2. [CrossRef]
51. Wang, F.; Wang, H.; Fan, J.; Zhang, Y.; Wang, H.; Zhao, Q. Pancreatic injury patterns in patients with coronavirus disease 19 pneumonia. *Gastroenterology* **2020**, *159*, 367–370. [CrossRef]
52. Xu, X.; Chang, X.N.; Pan, H.X.; Su, H.; Huang, B.; Yang, M.; Luo, D.J.; Weng, M.X.; Ma, L.; Nie, X. Pathological changes of the spleen in ten patients with coronavirus disease 2019 (COVID-19) by postmortem needle autopsy. *Zhonghua Bing Li Xue Za Zhi* **2020**, *49*, 576–582. [CrossRef] [PubMed]
53. Joshi, T.; Ahmed, A.; Cholankeril, G. Gastrointestinal manifestations of coronavirus disease 2019. *Curr. Opin. Infect. Dis.* **2021**, *34*, 471–476. [CrossRef] [PubMed]
54. Zhou, D.; Wang, Q.; Liu, H. Coronavirus disease-19 and the gut-lung axis. *Int. J. Infect. Dis.* **2021**, *113*, 300–307. [CrossRef] [PubMed]

Article

The Effects of COVID-19 on Clinical Outcomes of Non-COVID-19 Patients Hospitalized for Upper Gastrointestinal Bleeding during the Pandemic

Nonthalee Pausawasdi [1,2], Ekawat Manomaiwong [2], Uayporn Kaosombatwattana [1,2], Khemajira Karaketklang [2] and Phunchai Charatcharoenwitthaya [1,2,*]

[1] Siriraj GI Endoscopy Center, Faculty of Medicine Siriraj Hospital, Mahidol University, Bangkok 10700, Thailand; nonthaleep7@gmail.com (N.P.); koigi214@gmail.com (U.K.)
[2] Division of Gastroenterology, Department of Medicine, Faculty of Medicine Siriraj Hospital, Mahidol University, Bangkok 10700, Thailand; e_manomaiwong@hotmail.com (E.M.); oy.kemajira@gmail.com (K.K.)
* Correspondence: phunchai@yahoo.com; Tel.: +66-2-419-7282; Fax: +66-2-411-5013

Abstract: This study aims to investigate the effects of COVID-19 on clinical outcomes of non-COVID-19 patients hospitalized for upper gastrointestinal bleeding (UGIB) during the pandemic. A retrospective review is conducted. We recruited patients with UGIB admitted during the pandemic's first wave (April 2020 to June 2020), and the year before the pandemic. The outcomes between the two groups were compared using propensity score matching (PSM). In total, 60 patients (pandemic group) and 460 patients (prepandemic group) are included. Patients admitted during the pandemic (mean age of 67 ± 14 years) had a mean Glasgow–Blatchford score of 10.8 ± 3.9. They were older ($p = 0.045$) with more underlying malignancies ($p = 0.028$), had less history of NSAID use ($p = 0.010$), had a lower platelet count ($p = 0.007$), and had lower serum albumin levels ($p = 0.047$) compared to those admitted before the pandemic. Esophagogastroduodenoscopy (EGD) was performed less frequently during the pandemic (43.3% vs. 95.4%, $p < 0.001$). Furthermore, the procedure was less likely to be performed within 24 h after admission ($p < 0.001$). After PSM, admissions during the pandemic were significantly associated with decreased chances of receiving an endoscopy (adjusted odds Ratio (OR), 0.02; 95% CI, 0.003–0.06, $p < 0.001$) and longer hospital stay (adjusted OR, 2.17; 95% CI, 1.13–3.20, $p < 0.001$). Additionally, there was a slight increase in 30-day mortality without statistical significance (adjusted OR, 1.92; 95% CI, 0.71–5.19, $p = 0.199$) and a marginally higher rebleeding rate (adjusted OR, 1.34; 95% CI, 0.44–4.03, $p = 0.605$). During the pandemic, the number of EGDs performed in non-COVID-19 patients with UGIB decreased with a subsequent prolonged hospitalization and potentially increased 30-day mortality and rebleeding rate.

Keywords: upper gastrointestinal bleeding; COVID-19; pandemic; endoscopy; outcomes

1. Introduction

Coronavirus disease 2019 (COVID-19), caused by severe acute respiratory syndrome coronavirus 2 (SARS-CoV-2), has significantly impacted public health worldwide. The COVID-19 pandemic has had a disruptive effect on the workflow and safety of healthcare personnel and patients [1]. An endoscopy is considered a high-risk procedure for COVID-19 transmission due to the aerosol-generating nature of the technique despite no evidence of SARS-CoV-2 transmission by endoscopy [2–4]. Operational reorganization has been undertaken to limit viral spreading since the pandemic started. Nonemergent procedures can be postponed during the pandemic; however, the evaluation of gastrointestinal (GI) bleeding is often urgent and cannot be deferred. International guidelines recommend an early endoscopy within 24 h of clinical stabilization as the first-line diagnostic and therapeutic modality for upper GI bleeding (UGIB) [5–7].

Several international GI societies have issued recommendations for performing an endoscopy in the COVID-19 era to reduce transmission risk in resource-limited settings, lacking personal protective equipment (PPE), infrastructures, and staff [8–11]. Endoscopic procedures, mostly therapeutic interventions, should be reserved for patients with urgent or life-threatening conditions [12]. However, the need for PPE, COVID-19 testing, a negative pressure room, the particular method for room disinfection, and the personnel shortage during the initial COVID-19 outbreak all may have caused deferred endoscopies. Delays in identifying the cause of UGIB and performing endoscopic interventions may result in poor outcomes and possibly decreased overall survival. This study aims to evaluate the impact of the COVID-19 pandemic on clinical outcomes of non-COVID-19 patients hospitalized with acute UGIB.

2. Materials and Methods

2.1. Patient Population

This retrospective study was conducted at Siriraj Hospital, a large referral center serving the Bangkok metropolitan area and surrounding communities. The study conformed to the ethical guidelines of the Helsinki Declaration and was approved by the Institutional review board. The COVID-19 pandemic cohort comprised all consecutive non-COVID-19 persons aged $\geq$ 18 years who were hospitalized for the treatment of acute UGIB from 1 April 2020 to 30 June 2020. The pre-COVID-19 pandemic cohort included patients hospitalized with acute UGIB in the year preceding 1 April 2020. Patients who developed UGIB during their hospitalization for other indications were excluded.

2.2. Management of Upper Gastrointestinal Bleeding

Initial resuscitation and risk stratification using Glasgow–Blatchford score (GBS) were performed in all patients. All patients were given nothing by mouth. Intravenous fluid administration and packed red blood cells transfusions were administered as indicated. Patients with clinical suspicion of nonvariceal bleeding received intravenous proton pump inhibitor (PPI), whereas those with suspected variceal bleeding were given intravenous somatostatin or its long-acting analogues prior to endoscopic assessment. Patients with GBS > 1 were evaluated with esophagogastroduodenoscopy (EGD) within 24–72 h unless contraindicated otherwise, and endoscopic hemostasis was applied as indicated. In patients who required endoscopic intervention for peptic ulcer disease with stigmata of active or recent bleeding, high-dose PPIs were administered through infusion for 72 h following the procedure. Band ligation and cyanoacrylate injection were used to treat bleeding esophageal and gastric varices, respectively, in addition to vasoactive medications and intravenous antibiotics. The intravenous somatostatin or its long-acting analogues was continued for 2–5 days after endoscopic treatment.

During the COVID-19 pandemic, aerosol-generating procedures were restricted because of the following: (1) the risk of spreading COVID-19, (2) the limited availability of PPE, (3) the need for preprocedural COVID-19 testing with Reverse Transcription-Polymerase Chain Reaction (RT-PCR), and (4) negative-pressure rooms. Therefore, the timing of EGDs could have deviated from the routine protocol, but the pre-endoscopic management was carried out as usual. EGD was promptly performed if patients had either one or more of the following: hemodynamic instability, ongoing or recurrent GI bleeding after previous hemodynamic stability, or suspected variceal hemorrhage. In cases of delayed or postponed endoscopic evaluation, additional treatments such as intravenous PPI, somatostatin, or its long-acting analogues, were administered until endoscopic evaluation was performed, or bleeding ceased.

2.3. Clinical, Laboratory, and Endoscopic Data

Patient demographics, clinical manifestations, concomitant disorders, laboratory tests, drugs administered during hospitalization, and endoscopic findings were extracted from electronic medical records. The 30-day mortality, the need for endoscopy, rebleeding, the amount of blood transfusion, and the length of hospital stay were reviewed. Rebleeding was defined as the reoccurrence of hematemesis or melena with signs of hemodynamic instability or decrease in hemoglobin level >2 g/dL in a previously stable case. The presence of hemodynamic instability was defined as systolic blood pressure <100 mmHg with heart rate > 100 beats/min or orthostatic changes with a >10% decrease in systolic blood pressure and a >10% increase in heart rate between supine and seated positions. The primary outcome was 30-day mortality, while secondary outcomes included endoscopic performance, transfusions during hospitalization, and length of stay.

2.4. Statistical Analysis

Continuous variables were described as mean ± standard deviation (SD) or median (interquartile range (IQR)) and were analyzed using the Student's *t*-test. Categorical variables were reported as numbers (percentage) and were analyzed using the χ^2 or Fisher exact tests. Multivariate logistic and linear regression models were used to estimate adjusted odds ratios (OR) or differences of means for the study outcomes. Baseline variables with a standardized difference in absolute values greater than 0.15 were considered for multivariate analysis. In the primary analysis, we examined whether admissions during the pandemic had a different risk of 30-day mortality, endoscopy, blood transfusions, and length of stay compared to admissions before the pandemic.

As a secondary analysis, study outcomes were compared in propensity score (PS)-matched patients. Propensity scores were estimated using a logistic regression model for the COVID-19 versus the pre-COVID-19 pandemic cohorts that included demographic characteristics (age, sex), comorbidities (cirrhosis, chronic kidney disease, cardiovascular disease, cerebrovascular accident, malignancy, Charlson comorbidity index), bleeding severity (GBS), use of nonsteroidal anti-inflammatory drugs (NSAIDs), and laboratory tests (albumin, platelet count). Patients hospitalized during the COVID-19 pandemic were matched one-to-three with a caliper of 0.15 to UGIB patients who were managed before the pandemic using PS matching. Statistical analyses were performed using STATA version 14.0 (StataCorp LP, College Station, TX, USA). A two-sided *p*-value of below 0.05 was considered statistically significant.

3. Results

3.1. Characteristics of the Population

A total of 520 patients with UGIB were recruited, out of which 60 patients were admitted during the first wave of the COVID-19 pandemic in Thailand, while the remaining 460 patients were admitted a year before the pandemic. All patients admitted during the pandemic tested negative for SARS-CoV-2 infection. Clinical characteristics and laboratory data of the two cohorts are shown in Table 1. Patients admitted with acute UGIB during the pandemic (mean age of 67 ± 14 years, 61.7% male) had a mean GBS of 10.8 ± 3.9. Patients admitted during the pandemic were older ($p = 0.045$) and had a higher Charlson comorbidity index ($p = 0.039$), especially coexisting with solid organ malignancies ($p = 0.028$), less history of NSAID use ($p = 0.01$), lower serum albumin levels ($p = 0.047$) and platelet count ($p = 0.007$) compared to those hospitalized before the pandemic. Otherwise, there were no differences in terms of sex, underlying liver cirrhosis, chronic kidney disease, atherosclerotic disease, use of antiplatelet or anticoagulants, clinical manifestations, and GBS between both groups.

Table 2 shows the baseline characteristics of the matched populations after the PS matching. In total, 46 patients admitted during the pandemic were matched with 138 patients admitted before the pandemic. The standardized difference for each characteristic of patients admitted during and before the pandemic was comparable.

Table 1. Baseline characteristics of the overall population.

Characteristics	COVID-19 Pandemic (n = 60)	Pre-COVID-19 Pandemic (n = 460)	p Value	Standardized Difference
Male gender, n (%)	37 (61.7)	300 (65.2)	0.588	0.074
Age, mean (SD), year	67.0 (14.3)	62.8 (15.5)	0.045	0.285
Cirrhosis, n (%)	21 (35.0)	151 (32.8)	0.737	0.046
Chronic kidney disease, n (%)	17 (28.3)	95 (20.7)	0.174	0.179
Cardiovascular disease, n (%)	15 (25.0)	83 (18.0)	0.195	0.170
Cerebrovascular disease, n (%)	6 (10.0)	35 (7.6)	0.518	0.085
Malignancy, n (%)	18 (30.0)	83 (18.0)	0.028	0.283
Charlson comorbidity index, mean (SD)	5.1 (3.0)	4.4 (2.7)	0.039	0.273
Presenting symptom, n (%)				
Hematemesis	19 (31.7)	145 (31.5)	0.982	0.003
Coffee-ground emesis	20 (33.3)	166 (36.1)	0.676	0.058
Melena	38 (63.3)	300 (65.2)	0.774	0.039
Hematochezia	1 (1.7)	11 (2.4)	1.000	0.051
Maroon stool	2 (3.3)	24 (5.2)	0.756	0.093
Hemodynamic instability, n (%)	9 (15.0)	83 (18.0)	0.561	0.082
Medication, n (%)				
NSAIDs	6 (10.0)	115 (25.0)		0.403
Aspirin	12 (20.0)	107 (23.3)	0.010	0.079
Warfarin	6 (10.0)	49 (10.7)	0.572	0.021
Direct oral anticoagulant	0 (0)	1 (0.2)	0.877	0.069
Laboratory values on admission, median (IQR)				
Hemoglobin, g/dL				
Platelet, 10^3/μL	7.5 (6.0–9.8)	8.1 (6.3–10.0)	0.320	−0.106
INR	160 (107–243)	198 (139–271)	0.007	−0.331
BUN, mg/dL	1.37 (1.25–3.03)	1.29 (1.09–2.74)	0.262	−0.045
Creatinine, mg/dL	38.1 (26.3–58.4)	32.1 (20.3–48.3)	0.059	0.233
Albumin, g/dL	1.09 (0.82–2.00)	1.06 (0.78–1.48)	0.330	0.146
Laboratory values on admission, median (IQR)	3.00 (2.58–3.50)	3.20 (2.80–3.70)	0.047	−0.295
Glasgow–Blatchford score, mean (SD)	10.8 (3.9)	10.7 (4.0)	0.834	0.041

BUN, blood urea nitrogen; INR, international normalized ratio; IQR, interquartile range; NSAIDs, nonsteroidal anti-inflammatory drugs; SD, standard deviation.

Table 2. Baseline characteristics of the matched population.

Characteristics	COVID-19 Pandemic (n = 46)	Pre-COVID-19 Pandemic (n = 138)	p Value	Standardized Difference
Male gender, n (%)	29 (63.0)	89 (64.5)	0.859	0.030
Age, mean (SD), year	65.7 (14.9)	63.3 (14.7)	0.337	0.163
Cirrhosis, n (%)	18 (39.1)	56 (40.6)	0.862	0.029
Chronic kidney failure, n (%)	9 (19.6)	28 (20.3)	0.915	0.018
Cardiovascular disease, n (%)	9 (19.6)	22 (15.9)	0.570	0.095
Cerebrovascular disease, n (%)	4 (8.7)	12 (8.7)	1.000	0.001
Malignancy, n (%)	12 (26.1)	32 (23.2)	0.690	0.067
Charlson comorbidity index, mean (SD)	4.8 (2.8)	4.6 (2.5)	0.614	0.084
Presenting symptom, n (%)				
Hematemesis	18 (39.1)	41 (29.7)	0.236	0.199
Coffee-ground emesis	13 (28.3)	54 (39.1)	0.185	0.232

Table 2. Cont.

Characteristics	COVID-19 Pandemic (n = 46)	Pre-COVID-19 Pandemic (n = 138)	p Value	Standardized Difference
Melena	31 (67.4)	89 (64.5)	0.721	0.061
Hematochezia	1 (2.2)	0 (0.0)	0.250	0.211
Maroon stool	1 (2.2)	9 (6.5)	0.455	0.214
Hemodynamic instability, n (%)	8 (17.4)	35 (25.4)	0.269	0.195
Medication, n (%)				
NSAID	6 (13.0)	17 (12.3)	0.898	0.022
Aspirin	8 (17.4)	35 (25.4)	0.269	0.195
Warfarin	4 (8.7)	14 (10.1)	1.000	0.050
Direct oral anticoagulant	4 (8.7)	17 (12.3)	0.503	0.118
Laboratory values on admission, median (IQR)				
Hemoglobin, g/dL	7.7 (6.0–10.0)	8.3 (6.3–10.3)	0.565	−0.041
Platelet, $10^3/\mu L$	167 (107–237)	181 (120–263)	0.421	−0.100
INR	1.4 (1.3–2.5)	1.3 (1.1–3.9)	0.664	−0.323
BUN, mg/dL	34.5 (18.4–53.7)	31.2 (2.2–49.2)	0.532	0.103
Creatinine, mg/dL	1.0 (0.8–1.4)	1.1 (0.8–1.7)	0.400	−0.083
Albumin, g/dL	3.1 (2.7–3.5)	3.1 (2.6–3.6)	0.893	0.032
Glasgow–Blatchford score, mean (SD)	10.5 (4.2)	10.8 (3.9)	0.700	−0.040

BUN, blood urea nitrogen; INR, international normalized ratio; IQR, interquartile range; NSAIDs, nonsteroidal anti-inflammatory drugs; SD, standard deviation.

3.2. Primary Outcomes

Overall, 11 patients admitted during the pandemic died, but only one (1.7%) death was associated with bleeding. Of these, six patients died from their underlying malignancies. During the prepandemic period, 41 deaths were reported, and 12 (2.6%) of them were related to bleeding. The causes of deaths are shown in Table 3.

Table 3. Causes of death among the overall population before and during the COVID-19 pandemic.

Cause of Death	COVID-19 Pandemic (n = 60)	Pre-COVID-19 Pandemic (n = 460)
Bleeding-related death	1 (1.7%)	12 (2.6%)
Nonbleeding-related death	10 (16.7%)	29 (6.3%)
Cardiovascular disease	1 (1.7%)	2 (0.4%)
Infection	3 (5.0%)	14 (3.0%)
Extra-gastrointestinal malignancy	6 (10.0%)	13 (2.8%)

Note. Data are presented as the number (percentage) of a condition.

Treatment outcomes of the overall and matched populations are shown in Table 4. In the univariate analysis, the admissions during the pandemic were associated with a higher 30-day mortality than those before the pandemic (unadjusted OR, 2.29; 95%CI, 1.11–4.75, $p = 0.025$). After adjusting for demographics, comorbidities, bleeding severity, and antiplatelet/anticoagulant usage, an increase in the 30-day mortality was still observed during the pandemic, but it did not reach statistical significance (adjusted OR, 1.33; 95% CI, 0.52–3.39, $p = 0.550$). Once the patient population was matched using PS, eight patients (17.4%) died within 30 days of hospitalization during the pandemic, compared to sixteen cases (11.6%) admitted before the pandemic ($p = 0.315$). Despite the increased odds of 30-day mortality among the admissions during the COVID-19 outbreak, the difference was not statistically significant in the multivariable analysis when adjusting for potential residual confounders (adjusted OR, 1.92; 95% CI, 0.71–5.19, $p = 0.199$).

Table 4. Treatment outcomes for the overall and matched populations.

Variable	Overall Population					Matched Population				
	COVID-19 Pandemic (n = 60)	Pre-COVID-19 Pandemic (n = 460)	Unadjusted OR/Difference (95% CI) *	p Value *	Adjusted OR/Difference (95% CI) †	p Value †	COVID-19 Pandemic (n = 46)	Pre-COVID-19 Pandemic (n = 138)	Unadjusted OR/Difference (95% CI) *	p Value *	Adjusted OR/Difference (95% CI) ψ	p Value ψ
30-day mortality, n (%)	11 (18.3)	41 (8.9)	2.29 (1.11–4.75)	0.025	1.33 (0.52–3.39)	0.550	8 (17.4)	16 (11.6)	1.61 (0.64–4.04)	0.315	1.92 (0.71–5.19)	0.199
Endoscopy, n (%)	26 (43.3)	439 (95.4)	0.04 (0.02–0.07)	<0.001	0.01 (0.003–0.03)	<0.001	19 (41.3)	135 (97.8)	0.02 (0.004–0.06)	<0.001	0.02 (0.003–0.06)	<0.001
Endoscopy within 24 h, n (%)	4 (6.7)	208 (45.2)	0.09 (0.03–0.24)	<0.001	0.06 (0.02–0.22)	<0.001	3 (6.5)	68 (49.3)	0.07 (0.02–0.24)	<0.001	0.07 (0.02–0.24)	<0.001
Rebleeding, n (%)	8 (13.3)	41 (8.9)	1.68 (0.74–3.79)	0.212	1.16 (0.44–3.03)	0.764	6 (14.0)	16 (11.9)	1.21 (0.44–3.31)	0.716	1.34 (0.44–4.03)	0.605
Blood transfusion, median (IQR), unit	3 (1–6)	2 (1–3)	2.38 (1.78–2.99)	<0.001	1.18 (0.60–1.75)	0.051	3 (1–5)	2 (1–3)	1.04 (0.51–1.56)	0.153	1.08 (0.54–1.63)	0.144
Length of stay, median (IQR), day	5 (4–12)	2 (1–3)	4.17 (2.14–6.19)	<0.001	2.21 (0.11–4.31)	0.198	5 (3–9)	4 (2–6)	2.0 (1.02–2.98)	0.045	2.17 (1.13–3.20)	<0.001

Abbreviations: OR, odds ratio; CI, confidence interval; IQR, interquartile range. * The p values for mortality, endoscopy, and rebleeding rates were determined using logistic regression analysis. The p values for blood transfusion and length of stay were determined using the linear regression analysis. † Adjusted for variables with standard difference >0.15 among the overall population, including age, chronic kidney disease, cardiovascular disease, malignancies, Charlson comorbidity index, use of nonsteroidal anti-inflammatory drugs, serum levels of albumin, blood urea nitrogen, and platelet count. ψ Adjusted for variables with standard difference >0.15 among the matched population, including age, hematemesis, coffee-ground emesis, hematochezia, maroon stool, hemodynamic instability, use of aspirin, and international normalized ratio.

3.3. Secondary Outcomes

Table 5 shows the number of the overall population requiring in-hospital interventions according to the GBS. During the pandemic, none of the patients with a GBS of ≤3 underwent EGD, received blood transfusion, or died within 30 days. EGD was performed in 26 patients (43.3%) who had hemodynamic instability ($n = 2$), rebleeding after medical treatment ($n = 8$), or a suspicion of variceal bleeding ($n = 16$). In contrast, 439 patients (95.4%) admitted before the pandemic underwent EGD (adjusted OR, 0.01; 95% CI, 0.003–0.03, $p < 0.001$). The median duration from presentation to EGD (70 h, IQR 48–111) during the pandemic was much longer than in the pre-COVID-19 era (25 h, IQR 16–48). EGD was performed within 24 h in only four patients (6.7%) during the pandemic, compared to 208 (45.2%) patients admitted before the pandemic (adjusted OR, 0.06; 95% CI, 0.02–0.22, $p < 0.001$). The distribution of the types of lesions observed among patients undergoing EGD was comparable across patients admitted during and before the pandemic (Table 6). Peptic ulcer was the most common identified lesion, followed by varices. After adjusting for confounders, increased OR was observed for blood transfusion (adjusted OR, 1.18; 95% CI, 0.60–1.75, $p = 0.051$) and length of stay (adjusted OR, 2.21; 95% CI, 0.11–4.31, $p < 0.198$), but the differences did not reach statistical significance. There was no significant difference in the rebleeding rate (adjusted OR, 1.16; 95% CI, 0.44–3.03, $p = 0.764$).

Table 5. The need for endoscopy and blood transfusion among the overall population according to the Glasgow–Blatchford score.

The Glasgow–Blatchford Score	COVID-19 Pandemic ($n = 60$)			Pre-COVID-19 Pandemic ($n = 460$)		
	No. of Patients	In-Hospital Endoscopy	Blood Transfusion	No. of Patients	In-Hospital Endoscopy	Blood Transfusion
0	1	0	0	7	6	1
1	2	0	0	8	6	1
2	0	0	0	12	8	2
3	0	0	0	11	10	3
4	3	1	1	3	3	1
5	2	1	1	6	5	1
6	0	0	0	17	16	7
7	3	1	3	30	27	23
8	2	2	1	31	29	19
9	3	2	2	23	22	19
≥10	44	19	41	312	307	283

Table 6. Endoscopic findings among the overall and matched populations.

Endoscopic Finding	Overall Population				Matched Population			
	COVID-19 Pandemic ($n = 26$) *	Pre-COVID-19 Pandemic ($n = 439$) *	p Value	Standardized Difference	COVID-19 Pandemic ($n = 19$) *	Pre-COVID-19 Pandemic ($n = 135$) *	p Value	Standardized Difference
Peptic ulcer disease, n (%)	10 (38.5)	240 (54.7)	0.107	0.329	8 (42.1)	72 (53.3)	0.359	0.226
Active bleeding	1 (3.8)	19 (4.3)			1 (5.3)	3 (2.2)		
Nonbleeding visible vessel	0 (0.0)	31 (7.1)			0 (0.0)	12 (8.9)		
Clot with underlying vessel	0 (0.0)	19 (4.3)			0 (0.0)	9 (6.7)		
Pigmented spot/clean base	9 (34.6)	199 (45.3)			7 (36.8)	57 (42.2)		
Varices, n (%)	10 (38.5)	128 (29.2)	0.313	0.198	7 (36.8)	48 (35.6)	0.913	0.028
Others, n (%)	7 (26.9)	98 (22.3)	0.586	0.107	5 (26.3)	25 (18.5)	0.535	0.188

* Some patients presented with more than one endoscopic finding.

After PS matching, patients having undergone endoscopies during the pandemic remained considerably lower than those admitted before the pandemic (adjusted OR, 0.02; 95% CI, 0.003–0.06, $p < 0.001$). However, endoscopic findings of peptic ulcer disease, varices, and other lesions were observed similarly. Additionally, admissions during the pandemic had a longer length of stay (adjusted OR, 2.17; 95% CI, 1.13–3.20, $p < 0.001$). The odds of rebleeding were slightly increased during the pandemic but not statistically significant (adjusted OR, 1.34; 95% CI, 0.44–4.03, $p = 0.605$) compared to prepandemic. The units of blood transfusion were similar between the two periods.

4. Discussion

This study exhibited the impact of the COVID-19 pandemic in the management and treatment outcomes of non-COVID-19 patients presenting with UGIB. The results demonstrated that patients admitted during the pandemic were older with more underlying malignancies, had more history of NSAID use, and had more concerning laboratory results. They were less likely to undergo EGD; furthermore, only 6.7% had EGD performed within 24 h. Overall, we found an increased 30-day mortality, blood transfusion, and length of stay. However, the impact of the pandemic on mortality and blood transfusion became insignificant after adjusting for confounding factors and PS matching. Nonetheless, prolonged hospitalization remained associated with admissions during the pandemic after PS matching. The difference in the rebleeding rate was not statistically significant between the two periods.

Patients with UGIB admitted during the pandemic were sicker with more abnormal laboratory results. These observations may be indicative of the patients' unwillingness to present to the hospital during the pandemic unless they had serious underlying diseases with severe symptoms or a higher threshold of hospital admission. Similar findings were observed in a study conducted in the United States [13], underscoring the global impact of COVID-19 on patients' concerns about hospital visits and admission criteria during the pandemic.

Generally, GBS has been recommended by international guidelines for risk stratification for patients presenting with UGIB [14,15]. Patients with GBS ≤ 1 are considered low-risk and can be managed as outpatients, without the necessity for an in-hospital endoscopy. Due to the strain on the healthcare system, and a lack of PPE during the pandemic, new extended low-risk GBS thresholds were proposed and clinical outcomes were assessed. The data from a large international multicenter study involving 3012 consecutive patients with UGIB showed that using GBS ≤ 3 as the threshold to avoid hospitalization resulted in avoidance of admission and an inpatient endoscopy in 32% of patients [16]. In low-risk individuals, the percentage of patients requiring endoscopic treatment (4.1%) and dying within 30 days (1.7%) might be an acceptable number in countries at risk for healthcare system collapse from COVID-19. In our study's population, only three patients (5%) admitted during the pandemic had GBS ≤ 3, suggesting the limited use of this proposed threshold for identifying low-risk patients.

The study by Ilagan-Ying et al. showed that patients admitted during the first wave of the pandemic (1 March–31 May 2020), who required inpatient endoscopic procedures, were sicker with higher ICU admissions and had higher 30-day mortality rates. The indications for endoscopy included volvulus, obstruction, foreign body, food impaction, biliary tract obstruction, acute cholangitis, and GI bleeding. The diagnosis of COVID-19, an age over 65, and ICU admissions were shown to be associated with increased mortality for admissions during the pandemic [17]. However, Kim et al. reported that patients with GI bleeding admitted during the pandemic were more likely to have concerning laboratory results, received blood transfusions, and had a prolonged hospital stay, but the inpatient mortality rate was comparable to those admitted before the pandemic [13]. Our study found an increased 30-day mortality in patients admitted during the pandemic. However, the difference in the mortality rate was not statistically significant between the two periods after PS matching and adjusting for potential confounders, suggesting that patients' coexisting conditions may have had an impact on mortality rather than the GI bleeding itself.

The results also showed that patients admitted during the pandemic tended to have a higher number of blood transfusions; however, the effect was less significant after adjusting for confounders and PS matching. These findings may imply that the number of blood transfusions among patients admitted during the COVID-19 outbreak might be attributable to comorbidities rather than bleeding severity. Furthermore, the volume of EGD in UGIB was less, and there were more delayed endoscopies during the pandemic compared to the year before in the overall and matched population. In addition, the length of hospital stay increased significantly for admissions during COVID-19. This may reflect the physicians' concern for early rebleeding or delayed adverse events.

This study had some limitations. First, the retrospective design of this study had several drawbacks, which raised the possibility of selection bias. Herein, we employed PS matching to overcome the effects of potential confounding factors. Second, this was a single-center study with small numbers. Thus, multicenter prospective research with a larger sample size is required to extend the findings to other populations. Third, the pre-COVID-19 cohort included more patients with stigmata of recent bleeding, raising the possibility of bias. This finding might be attributed to the influence of intensive PPI regimen usage on the resolution of peptic ulcer disease, resulting in a low incidence of high-risk stigmata on the endoscopic assessment during the pandemic. Finally, the assessment of rebleeding can be challenging, because only 43% of the patients admitted during the pandemic underwent EGD.

5. Conclusions

This study suggested that the disruptive effects on the healthcare system during the first wave of the COVID-19 outbreak led to the restriction of endoscopy services, including the performance of urgent procedures. As a result, clinical outcomes of non-COVID-19 patients who required the endoscopic management of UGIB were compromised. The number of performed EGDs decreased, whereas the length of hospitalization and 30-day mortality tended to increase. Thus, healthcare centers with endoscopy services should consider the potential lethal clinical outcomes of patients requiring an endoscopic evaluation when adapting policy to cope with the ongoing COVID-19 pandemic.

Author Contributions: Conceptualization, N.P. and P.C.; Data curation, E.M. and U.K.; Formal analysis, N.P., E.M., K.K. and P.C.; Methodology, N.P. and P.C.; Software, K.K.; Supervision, P.C.; Writing—original draft, N.P., E.M. and P.C.; Writing—review and editing, N.P. and P.C. All authors have read and agreed to the published version of the manuscript.

Funding: This research received no external funding.

Institutional Review Board Statement: The study was conducted according to the guidelines of the Declaration of Helsinki and approved by the Siriraj Institutional Review Board (code no.350/2563).

Informed Consent Statement: Informed consent was obtained from all subjects involved in the study.

Data Availability Statement: All the data are included in the manuscript.

Conflicts of Interest: The authors declare no conflict of interest.

References

1. Antonelli, G.; Karsensten, J.G.; Bhat, P.; Ijoma, U.; Osuagwu, C.; Desalegn, H.; Abera, H.; Guy, C.; Vilmann, P.; Dinis-Ribeiro, M.; et al. Resuming endoscopy during COVID-19 pandemic: ESGE, WEO and WGO joint cascade guideline for resource limited settings. *Endosc. Int. Open* **2021**, *9*, E543–E551. [PubMed]
2. Noorimotlagh, Z.; Jaafarzadeh, N.; Martinez, S.S.; Mirzaee, S.A. A systematic review of possible airborne transmission of the COVID-19 virus (SARS-CoV-2) in the indoor air environment. *Environ. Res.* **2021**, *193*, 110612. [CrossRef] [PubMed]
3. Xiao, F.; Tang, M.; Zheng, X.; Liu, Y.; Li, X.; Shan, H. Evidence for gastrointestinal infection of SARS-CoV-2. *Gastroenterology* **2020**, *158*, 1831–1833. [CrossRef] [PubMed]

4. Lui, R.N.; Wong, S.H.; Sanchez-Luna, S.A.; Pellino, G.; Bollipo, S.; Wong, M.Y.; Chiu, P.W.Y.; Sung, J.J.Y. Overview of guidance for endoscopy during the coronavirus disease 2019 pandemic. *J. Gastroenterol. Hepatol.* **2020**, *35*, 749–759. [CrossRef] [PubMed]
5. Sung, J.J.; Chiu, P.W.; Chan, F.K.L.; Lau, J.Y.; Goh, K.L.; Ho, L.H.; Jung, H.Y.; Sollano, J.D.; Gotoda, T.; Reddy, N.; et al. Asia-Pacific working group consensus on non-variceal upper gastrointestinal bleeding: An update 2018. *Gut* **2018**, *67*, 1757–1768. [CrossRef] [PubMed]
6. Gralnek, I.M.; Stanley, A.J.; Morris, A.J.; Camus, M.; Lau, J.; Lanas, A.; Laursen, S.B.; Radaelli, F.; Papanikolaou, I.S.; Goncalves, T.C.; et al. Endoscopic diagnosis and management of nonvariceal upper gastrointestinal hemorrhage (NVUGIH): European society of gastrointestinal endoscopy (ESGE) guideline—Update 2021. *Endoscopy* **2021**, *53*, 300–332. [CrossRef] [PubMed]
7. Tripathi, D.; Stanley, A.J.; Hayes, P.C.; Patch, D.; Millson, C.; Mehrzad, H.; Austin, A.; Ferguson, J.W.; Olliff, S.P.; Hudson, M.; et al. UK guidelines on the management of variceal haemorrhage in cirrhotic patients. *Gut* **2015**, *64*, 1680–1704. [CrossRef] [PubMed]
8. Gralnek, I.M.; Hassan, C.; Ebigbo, A.; Fuchs, A.; Beilenhoff, U.; Antonelli, G.; Bisschops, R.; Arvanitakis, M.; Bhandari, P.; Bretthauer, M.; et al. ESGE and ESGENA position statement on gastrointestinal endoscopy and COVID-19: Updated guidance for the era of vaccines and viral variants. *Endoscopy* **2022**, *54*, 211–216. [CrossRef] [PubMed]
9. Gralnek, I.M.; Hassan, C.; Beilenhoff, U.; Antonelli, G.; Ebigbo, A.; Pellise, M.; Arvanitakis, M.; Bhandari, P.; Bisschops, R.; Van Hooft, J.E.; et al. ESGE and ESGENA position statement on gastrointestinal endoscopy and COVID-19: An update on guidance during the post-lockdown phase and selected results from a membership survey. *Endoscopy* **2020**, *52*, 891–898. [CrossRef] [PubMed]
10. Sawhney, M.S.; Bilal, M.; Pohl, H.; Kushnir, V.M.; Khashab, M.A.; Schulman, A.R.; Berzin, T.M.; Chahal, P.; Muthusamy, V.R.; Varadarajulu, S.; et al. Triaging advanced GI endoscopy procedures during the COVID-19 pandemic: Consensus recommendations using the Delphi method. *Gastrointest. Endosc.* **2020**, *92*, 535–542. [CrossRef] [PubMed]
11. Rees, C.J.; East, J.E.; Oppong, K.; Veitch, A.; McAlindon, M.; Anderson, J.; Hayee, B.; Edwards, C.; McKinlay, A.; Penman, I. Restarting gastrointestinal endoscopy in the deceleration and early recovery phases of COVID-19 pandemic: Guidance from the British society of gastroenterology. *Clin. Med.* **2020**, *20*, 352–358. [CrossRef] [PubMed]
12. Sethi, A.; Swaminath, A.; Latorre, M.; Behin, D.S.; Jodorkovsky, D.; Calo, D.; Aroniadis, O.; Mone, A.; Mendelsohn, R.B.; Sharaiha, R.Z.; et al. Donning a new approach to the practice of gastroenterology: Perspectives from the COVID-19 pandemic epicenter. *Clin. Gastroenterol. Hepatol.* **2020**, *18*, 1673–1681. [CrossRef] [PubMed]
13. Kim, J.; Doyle, J.B.; Blackett, J.W.; May, B.; Hur, C.; Lebwohl, B.; HIRE Study Group. Effect of the coronavirus 2019 pandemic on outcomes for patients admitted with gastrointestinal bleeding in New York city. *Gastroenterology* **2020**, *159*, 1155–1157. [CrossRef] [PubMed]
14. Barkun, A.N.; Almadi, M.; Kuipers, E.J.; Laine, L.; Sung, J.; Tse, F.; Leontiadis, G.I.; Abraham, N.S.; Calvet, X.; Chan, F.K.L.; et al. Management of nonvariceal upper gastrointestinal bleeding: Guideline recommendations from the international consensus group. *Ann. Intern. Med.* **2019**, *171*, 805–822. [CrossRef] [PubMed]
15. Gralnek, I.M.; Dumonceau, J.M.; Kuipers, E.J.; Lanas, A.; Sanders, D.S.; Kurien, M.; Rotondano, G.; Hucl, T.; Dinis-Ribeiro, M.; Marmo, R.; et al. Diagnosis and management of nonvariceal upper gastrointestinal hemorrhage: European society of gastrointestinal endoscopy (ESGE) guideline. *Endoscopy* **2015**, *47*, a1–a46. [CrossRef] [PubMed]
16. Laursen, S.B.; Gralnek, I.M.; Stanley, A.J. Raising the threshold for hospital admission and endoscopy in upper gastrointestinal bleeding during the COVID-19 pandemic. *Endoscopy* **2020**, *52*, 930–931. [CrossRef] [PubMed]
17. Ilagan-Ying, Y.C.; Almeida, M.N.; Kahler-Quesada, A.; Ying, L.; Hughes, M.L.; Do, A.; Hung, K.W. Increased mortality in patients undergoing inpatient endoscopy during the early COVID-19 pandemic. *Dig. Dis. Sci.* **2022**, 1–10. [CrossRef] [PubMed]

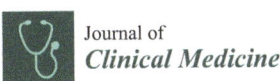

Article

Psychological Effects and Medication Adherence among Korean Patients with Inflammatory Bowel Disease during the Coronavirus Disease 2019 Pandemic: A Single-Center Survey

Ji Eun Ryu [1], Sung-Goo Kang [2], Sung Hoon Jung [3], Shin Hee Lee [1] and Sang-Bum Kang [1,*]

[1] Division of Gastroenterology, Department of Internal Medicine, Daejeon St. Mary's Hospital, College of Medicine, The Catholic University of Korea, Daejeon 34943, Korea; 22101260@cmcnu.or.kr (J.E.R.); shleedjsm@cmcnu.or.kr (S.H.L.)

[2] Department of Family Medicine, St. Vincent Hospital, College of Medicine, The Catholic University of Korea, Suwon 16247, Korea; 10001951@cmcnu.or.kr

[3] Division of Gastroenterology, Department of Internal Medicine, Eunpyeong St. Mary's Hospital, College of Medicine, The Catholic University of Korea, Seoul 03312, Korea; 10002060@cmcnu.or.kr

* Correspondence: sangucsd@gmail.com; Tel.: +82-42-220-7501; Fax: +82-42-252-6807

Abstract: Background and Aim. This study evaluated the impact of coronavirus disease 2019 (COVID-19) on the mental health of inflammatory bowel disease (IBD) patients. We quantified anxiety, depression, and medication adherence among IBD patients through a single-center survey in South Korea during the COVID-19 pandemic. Methods. An electronic survey was made available to patients at the IBD clinic in Daejeon St. Mary's hospital from July 2021 to September 2021. The validated Hospital Anxiety and Depression Scale (HADS) was used to assess depression and anxiety. The Korean version of the Medication Adherence Rating Scale (KMARS) questionnaire was used to assess medication adherence. Results. In total, 407 patients (56.5%; ulcerative colitis, 43.5%; Crohn's disease) participated in the survey. Among the respondents, 14.5% showed significant anxiety and 26.3% showed significant depression. Female sex, presence of mental disease, unvaccinated status, and the presence of Crohn's disease were associated with greater risks of anxiety and depression. Among medications, immunomodulators were associated with a greater risk of anxiety. In terms of KMARS, patients reported favorable medication adherence despite the psychological burden of the pandemic. The KMARS score was 7.3 ± 1.5 (mean ± SD) of 10.0 points. High anxiety and depression were associated with a slight decrease in medication adherence. Conclusions. COVID-19 has increased anxiety and depression among IBD patients, whose medication adherence has nevertheless remained good. Furthermore, anxiety and depression were found to have a negative correlation with adherence. Our results provide insights concerning psychological response and medication adherence among IBD patients in South Korea during the COVID-19 pandemic.

Keywords: COVID-19; inflammatory bowel disease; anxiety; depression; medication adherence

1. Introduction

The coronavirus disease 2019 (COVID-19) pandemic has influenced multiple aspects of life, including social interactions. High rates of anxiety and depression have been reported [1,2]. The risks of anxiety and depression are significantly higher in inflammatory bowel disease (IBD) patients than in the general population [3]. Factors such as disease severity, treatment noncompliance, and socioeconomic deprivation are associated with increased anxiety and depression [4]. In addition, IBD-related disability negatively affects quality of life. [5] However, good drug adherence can result in lower disability and higher quality of life [6].

During the pandemic, data concerning COVID-19 cases and vaccination are frequently updated. IBD patients are susceptible to psychological problems and reduced medication

Citation: Ryu, J.E.; Kang, S.-G.; Jung, S.H.; Lee, S.H.; Kang, S.-B. Psychological Effects and Medication Adherence among Korean Patients with Inflammatory Bowel Disease during the Coronavirus Disease 2019 Pandemic: A Single-Center Survey. *J. Clin. Med.* **2022**, *11*, 3034. https://doi.org/10.3390/jcm11113034

Academic Editor: Angelo Viscido

Received: 24 April 2022
Accepted: 26 May 2022
Published: 27 May 2022

Publisher's Note: MDPI stays neutral with regard to jurisdictional claims in published maps and institutional affiliations.

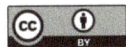

Copyright: © 2022 by the authors. Licensee MDPI, Basel, Switzerland. This article is an open access article distributed under the terms and conditions of the Creative Commons Attribution (CC BY) license (https://creativecommons.org/licenses/by/4.0/).

adherence. Lack of awareness concerning vaccine necessity or existence is a commonly cited reason for not remaining unvaccinated against COVID-19 [7]. Additionally, the number of IBD patients in South Korea has increased in the prior decade, and psychological issues are important among such patients [8]. Compared with non-IBD patients, IBD patients have a higher level of fear concerning the potential for contracting COVID-19 [9,10]. According to a survey conducted by the Korean Association for the Study of intestinal diseases (KASID) in 2021, more than half of IBD patients in South Korea showed a high level of fear of COVID-19 [11].

We evaluated the impact of COVID-19 on the mental well-being and behavior of South Korean patients with IBD. We quantified anxiety, depression, and medication adherence among IBD patients through a single-center survey. We also investigated predictors of increased anxiety and depression. To our knowledge, this is the first study of mental status and medication adherence among IBD patients in South Korea.

2. Materials and Methods

2.1. Study Design and Patients

From July to September 2021, 407 outpatients from the IBD clinic in Daejeon St. Mary's Hospital participated in the survey. Respondents with an underlying diagnosis of IBD and age > 17 years and treatment period more than 6 months were all included. The application of the evaluation battery was in situ. Patients responded to questions related to epidemiologic features, diseases, COVID-19 screening, vaccination, and mental well-being with the provided electronic device after outpatient treatment. To improve the completeness of the survey, clinical research coordinators were assigned to find out blank questions as to outcomes and incomplete questionnaires were excluded from the study. The validated Hospital Anxiety and Depression Scale (HADS) was used to assess anxiety (HADS-A) and depression (HADS-D). The HADS is a 14-item scale with 7 items each for anxiety and depression subscales [12]. Each item is scored from 0 to 3; a total score of >8 indicates significant anxiety or depression. The Korean version of the Medication Adherence Rating Scale (KMARS) was used to assess medication adherence. The parent Medication Adherence Rating Scale was developed by Thompson et al. in 2000 [13,14]. The KMARS is composed of 10 questions, each of which is scored 0 or 1. The total score ranges from 0 to 10; a higher score indicates greater medication adherence. We regarded a KMARS score of >7 as indicative of good adherence. Additionally, a nine-item self-developed questionnaire was used to evaluate behavioral changes during the COVID-19 pandemic. Clinical data were obtained from electronic medical records at the time of survey completion. Surveys were conducted using an electronic device after the provision of informed consent. Information on the COVID-19 situation in Korea was obtained from the following websites; http://ncov.mohw.go.kr (accessed on 20 December 2021), https://ourworldindata.org (accessed on 20 January 2022), https://www.kdca.go.kr (accessed on 10 January 2022).

2.2. Data Analysis

Statistical analysis was conducted using Statistical Analysis Software v. 9.4 (SAS Institute, Cary, NC, USA). Continuous variables are shown as means ± standard deviations (SDs); categorical variables are shown as numbers and proportions (%). Between-group comparisons were carried out by independent sample t-tests for continuous variables and the χ^2 test with or without Fisher's exact test for categorical variables. Univariate and multivariate logistic regression analyses were performed to identify associations of patient characteristics and KMARS score with depression and anxiety. The results are expressed as odds ratios with 95% confidence intervals. p-values < 0.05 were considered indicative of statistical significance.

3. Results

3.1. Patient Characteristics

In total, 407 patients participated in the survey (Table 1). The mean ± SD age of respondents was 41.8 ± 16.4 years, and 68.3% were men. The mean age at IBD diagnosis was 35.3 ± 15.5 years. More than half of the patients had ulcerative colitis (56.5%), and 43.5% of the patients had Crohn's disease. The patients were undergoing treatment with mesalamine (78.4%), immunomodulators (46.0%), and biologics (39.6%). Only 2.5% of the patients were undergoing treatment with steroids during the study period. Most patients were in remission (94.6%) and 5.4% were experiencing disease flares. Approximately half of the patients (54.3%) were married and 74.8% were employed at the time of the survey. Only 6.2% of the patients had a pre-existing diagnosis of depression or anxiety. During the study period, 47.2% of the patients had undergone COVID-19 testing; 2.1% reported positive results. Among the 45.7% of patients who had been vaccinated against COVID-19, only 46.0% were fully vaccinated.

Table 1. Characteristics of patients with IBD responding to the questionnaire.

Characteristic	All (N = 407)
Age (mean ± SD)	41.82 ± 16.35
Gender, n (%)	
Male	278 (68.30)
Female	129 (31.70)
Subtype of IBD, n (%)	
UC	230 (56.51)
CD	177 (43.49)
PO medication, n (%)	
Mesalamine	319 (78.38)
Steroid	10 (2.46)
Immunomodulator	187 (45.95)
Biologics	161 (39.56)
Disease status, n (%)	
Remission	385 (94.59)
Flare	22 (5.41)
Age at IBD diagnosis, mean ± SD	35.25 ± 15.54
Marriage status, n (%)	
Married	221 (54.30)
Unmarried	186 (45.70)
Job status, n (%)	
Employed	303 (74.81)
Unemployed	102 (25.19)
Presence of mental disease, n (%)	
Yes	25 (6.16)
No	381 (93.84)
COVID-19 screening test, n (%)	
Yes	192 (47.17)
No	215 (52.83)
COVID-19 screening result, n (%)	
Positive	5 (2.05)
Negative	239 (97.95)
Vaccination, n (%)	
Yes	189 (45.68)
No	220 (54.32)
Vaccination dose, n (%)	
1st	102 (53.97)
2nd	87 (46.03)
HADS total score, mean ± SD	9.52 ± 6.70
KMARS total score, mean ± SD	7.28 ± 1.49
Smoking, n (%)	
Ex-smoker	109 (29.70)

Table 1. Cont.

Characteristic	All (N = 407)
Never	206 (56.13)
Current smoker	52 (14.17)
Drinking, n (%)	
Never	148 (40.22)
Regular drinking	35 (9.51)
Occasional drinking	185 (50.27)

SD, standard deviation; IBD, inflammatory bowel disease; UC, ulcerative colitis; CD, Crohn's disease; PO, per oral; HADS, hospital anxiety and depression scale; KMARS, Korean version of the medication adherence rating scale.

3.2. Mental Well-Being

The HADS score among the patients was 9.5 ± 6.7 (mean ± SD) (Table 1). Anxiety and depression characteristics are summarized in Table 2. Female sex, unmarried status, unemployed status, presence of mental disease, presence of Crohn's disease, high disease activity, and unvaccinated status were associated with a high HADS score. COVID-19 testing did not strongly influence the level of anxiety or depression. Female sex, presence of mental disease, and unvaccinated status were associated with significant increases in anxiety and depression. Univariate and multivariate analyses were performed to assess predictors of depression and anxiety (Table 3). Among the respondents, 14.5% showed significant anxiety and 26.3% showed significant depression; 11.8% showed both significant anxiety and depression. Multivariate analysis indicated that female sex, presence of mental disease, unvaccinated status, and presence of Crohn's disease were associated with greater risks of anxiety and depression. Among oral medications, immunomodulators were associated with a greater risk of anxiety and steroids were associated with a lower risk of depression. Among ulcerative colitis patients, the medications used were (in decreasing order): mesalamine (92.2%), immunomodulators (22.6%), biologics (20.0%), and steroids (2.2%). Among Crohn's patients, the medications used were immunomodulators (72.9%), biologics (60.5%), mesalamine (57.1%), and steroids (1.7%).

Table 2. Average scores of HADS and KMARS among respondents according to variables.

Variables	HADS Score	p-Value	CohenD	HADS Anxiety	p-Value	CohenD	HADS Depression	p-Value	CohenD	KMARS Score	p-Value	CohenD
Gender		0.01	−0.29		<0.001	−0.41		0.18	−0.54		0.73	0.04
Male	8.90 ± 6.50			3.72 ± 3.24			5.18 ± 3.74			7.29 ± 1.54		
Female	10.84 ± 6.97			5.12 ± 3.76			5.73 ± 3.83			7.24 ± 1.39		
Marital status		0.07	−0.18		0.16	−0.14		0.06	−0.19		0.40	0.08
Married	8.97 ± 6.57			3.94 ± 3.50			5.04 ± 3.57			7.33 ± 1.56		
Unmarried	10.16 ± 6.82			4.42 ± 3.42			5.74 ± 3.97			7.21 ± 1.41		
Job status		0.25	−0.15		0.70	−0.04		0.09	−0.22		0.06	−0.22
Employed	9.25 ± 6.30			4.12 ± 3.38			5.13 ± 3.50			7.21 ± 1.50		
Unemployed	10.24 ± 7.79			4.27 ± 3.77			5.96 ± 4.44			7.53 ± 1.39		
Presence of mental disease		<0.001	1.49		<0.001	1.35		<0.001	1.37		0.14	−0.35
Yes	18.32 ± 8.59			8.36 ± 5.21			9.96 ± 4.06			6.80 ± 1.68		
No	8.93 ± 6.15			3.88 ± 3.15			5.04 ± 3.55			7.32 ± 1.46		
IBD subtype		0.06	−0.19		0.22	−0.12		0.03	−0.22		0.05	0.20
Ulcerative colitis	8.97 ± 6.43			3.97 ± 3.42			5.00 ± 3.59			7.40 ± 1.42		
Crohn's disease	10.23 ± 6.99			4.40 ± 3.53			5.82 ± 3.96			7.11 ± 1.57		
Disease activity		0.18	−0.29		0.31	−0.30		0.27	−0.24		0.55	0.13
Remission	9.41 ± 6.60			4.10 ± 3.40			5.31 ± 3.74			7.29 ± 1.49		
Flare	11.36 ± 8.32			5.14 ± 4.60			6.23 ± 4.28			7.09 ± 1.63		
COVID-19 screening test		0.33	0.10		0.19	0.13		0.61	0.05		0.41	−0.08
Yes	9.86 ± 6.81			4.40 ± 3.63			5.46 ± 3.66			7.21 ± 1.44		
No	9.21 ± 6.61			3.94 ± 3.32			5.27 ± 3.88			7.33 ± 1.54		
Vaccination		0.01	−0.28		0.01	−0.26		0.01	−0.25		0.07	0.18
Yes	8.48 ± 6.17			3.64 ± 3.36			4.83 ± 3.39			7.43 ± 1.47		
No	10.32 ± 7.01			4.55 ± 3.49			5.77 ± 4.03			7.16 ± 1.49		

All values are mean ± SD. p-values were calculated by the t-test. CohenD is Cohen's D.

Table 3. Predictors for moderate depression and anxiety.

Characteristics	Anxiety				Depression			
	Univariate Analysis OR (95% CI)	p-Value	Multivariate Analysis OR (95% CI)	p-Value	Univariate Analysis OR (95% CI)	p-Value	Multivariate Analysis OR (95% CI)	p-Value
Age	1 (0.98, 1.02)	0.928	1.03 (0.98, 1.08)	0.318	1 (0.98, 1.01)	0.694	1 (0.96, 1.05)	0.936
Gender (male vs. female)	0.42 (0.24, 0.73)	0.002	0.38 (0.2, 0.71)	0.003	0.67 (0.42, 1.06)	0.087	0.57 (0.34, 0.95)	0.032
Marital status (married vs. unmarried)	1.08 (0.62, 1.88)	0.786	0.97 (0.43, 2.19)	0.941	0.77 (0.5, 1.2)	0.250	0.65 (0.34, 1.24)	0.188
Job status (employed vs. unemployed)	0.81 (0.44, 1.49)	0.488	1.12 (0.55, 2.26)	0.760	0.84 (0.51, 1.39)	0.505	1.16 (0.65, 2.05)	0.616
Presence of mental disease (yes vs. no)	7.89 (3.4, 18.33)	<0.0001	9.39 (3.74, 23.57)	<0.0001	10.69 (4.14, 27.61)	<0.0001	12.77 (4.67, 34.95)	<0.0001
Age at IBD diagnosis	0.99 (0.98, 1.01)	0.523	0.98 (0.94, 1.03)	0.471	1 (0.98, 1.01)	0.809	1.02 (0.97, 1.06)	0.461
COVID-19 screening test (yes vs. no)	1.01 (0.58, 1.76)	0.962	0.94 (0.51, 1.73)	0.844	1.03 (0.66, 1.6)	0.906	0.95 (0.58, 1.54)	0.823
Vaccination (yes vs. no)	0.63 (0.36, 1.13)	0.120	0.4 (0.19, 0.84)	0.016	0.68 (0.43, 1.07)	0.093	0.5 (0.28, 0.89)	0.019
Subtype of IBD		0.344		0.050		0.055		0.034
Ulcerative colitis	0.77 (0.44, 1.33)		0.44 (0.2, 1)		0.65 (0.42, 1.01)		0.5 (0.27, 0.95)	
Crohn's disease	Index		Index		Index	0.055	Index	
PO medication								
Mesalamine (yes vs. no)	1.15 (0.6, 2.21)	0.671	1.12 (0.47, 2.64)	0.800	1.07 (0.63, 1.81)	0.813	0.7 (0.36, 1.37)	0.293
Steroid (yes vs. no)	1.54 (0.19, 12.38)	0.685	2.88 (0.28, 29.31)	0.371	0.23 (0.06, 0.82)	0.024	0.23 (0.06, 0.92)	0.038
Immunomodulator (yes vs. no)	1.4 (0.79, 2.45)	0.247	2.35 (1.08, 5.12)	0.031	1.01 (0.65, 1.57)	0.971	1.49 (0.81, 2.74)	0.205
Biologics (yes vs. no)	1.59 (0.88, 2.88)	0.127	1.62 (0.77, 3.4)	0.206	0.97 (0.62, 1.51)	0.877	0.86 (0.49, 1.51)	0.595

OR, odds ratio; CI, confidence interval.

3.3. Medication Adherence

The mean ± SD medication adherence score was 7.3 ± 1.5. Approximately 72.5% of the respondents had a KMARS score of >7 points. In a univariate analysis of the association between the KMARS score and variables, for each 1-point increase in HADS-A score, the KMARS score decreased by 0.102 points; this relationship was statistically significant. With respect to HADS-D, the KMARS score decreased by 0.078 points for each 1-point increase in HADS-D; this relationship was statistically significant. Therefore, greater anxiety or depression were associated with a slight decrease in medication adherence. In addition, for each 1-year increase in the age at diagnosis of IBD, the KMARS score increased by 0.010 points; this relationship was statistically significant. In the multivariate analysis, for each 1-point increase in HADS-A score, the KMARS score decreased by 0.074 points; this relationship was statistically significant. Furthermore, each 1-point increase in HADS-D score resulted in a 0.021-point decrease in KMARS score; however, this relationship was not statistically significant. The KMARS score decreased by 0.352 points in employed patients (Table 4).

Table 4. Association between variables and Korean version of Medication Adherence Rating Scale (KMARS).

	Univariate Analysis			Multivariate Analysis		
	β	95% CI	p-Value	β	95% CI	p-Value
HADS Anxiety	−0.102	−0.142 to −0.061	<0.0001	−0.074	−0.135 to −0.013	0.018
HADS Depression	−0.078	−0.116 to −0.040	<0.0001	−0.021	−0.076 to 0.035	0.466
Gender (male vs. female)	0.055	−0.258 to 0.368	0.732	0.006	−0.312 to 0.324	0.972
Marital status (married vs. unmarried)	0.125	−0.167 to 0.417	0.400	−0.045	−0.403 to 0.313	0.804
Job status (employed vs. unemployed)	−0.318	−0.650 to 0.014	0.060	−0.352	−0.695 to −0.010	0.044
Presence of mental disease (yes vs. no)	−0.520	−1.120 to 0.078	0.089	−0.069	−0.702 to 0.564	0.830
Age at IBD diagnosis	0.010	0.001 to 0.020	0.031	0.003	−0.010 to 0.016	0.678
COVID−19 screening test (yes vs. no)	−0.121	−0.413 to 0.170	0.414	−0.043	−0.330 to 0.244	0.768
Vaccination (yes vs. no)	0.269	−0.022 to 0.560	0.070	0.137	−0.188 to 0.461	0.409
Subtype of IBD (Ulcerative colitis vs. Crohn's disease)	0.291	−0.001 to 0.584	0.051	0.181	−0.199 to 0.561	0.350
PO medication						
Mesalamine (yes vs. no)	0.238	−0.115 to 0.591	0.186	0.071	−0.328 to 0.471	0.726
Steroid (yes vs. no)	0.023	−0.918 to 0.964	0.962	0.032	−0.889 to 0.952	0.946
Immunomodulator (yes vs. no)	−0.256	−0.548 to 0.035	0.084	−0.153	−0.508 to 0.202	0.398
Biologics (yes vs. no)	0.034	−0.264 to 0.332	0.823	0.203	−0.134 to 0.540	0.236

3.4. Behavioral Changes

The patients reported that the COVID-19 pandemic reduced their time with friends (76.8%), increased their communication with others concerning health (65.5%), caused them to delay tasks (44.6%) and shop for certain types of food (42.9%), reduced their time with family (37.5%), and increased their efforts to access health care (30.4%) and to obtain medication (18.5%) (Table 5). Fewer than 10% of the patients reported increased smoking (8.9%) and alcohol consumption (7.1%).

Table 5. Impact of COVID-19 on behaviors among patients with inflammatory bowel disease.

Variables	n * (%)
Reduced time with friends	129 (76.8)
More communication with people about health	110 (65.5)
Delay tasks to do	75 (44.6)
Shopping for certain types of food	72 (42.9)
Reduced time with family	63 (37.5)
Increased efforts to access health care service	51 (30.4)
Increased efforts to obtain medication	31 (18.5)
Increased frequency to smoke	15 (8.9)
Increased frequency to drink alcohol	12 (7.1)

* Participants who reported "Yes" to each question.

4. Discussion

According to National Health Insurance Service statistics, the number of IBD patients in South Korea increased from 2010 to 2019. Indeed, KASID reported that the number of IBD patients has increased more than twofold during the past decade, thereby necessitating investigations into changes in disease burden and behavioral patterns [8,15]. The psychological burden of the COVID-19 pandemic has been increased by frequent changes in policies, the introduction of vaccination, and reports of adverse events. The negative effect of disease on mental health in IBD patients has been reported. IBD patients are at least threefold and twofold more likely to develop anxiety and depressive disorders, respectively; treatment of such psychological problems can improve the long-term outcomes [16,17].

As of 7 July 2021, 185.55 million cases of COVID-19 had been reported worldwide, with over 4 million confirmed deaths. In South Korea, these figures were 164,028 cases and 2034 deaths [18]. The South Korean government introduced social distancing rules to slow the spread of COVID-19 in March 2020 and implemented a COVID-19 vaccination program on 26 February 2021 [19,20].

At the beginning of this study, the COVID-19 vaccination rate (at least one dose) in South Korea was higher (30.1%) than the global rate (24.9%). However, other countries have higher vaccination rates, including the United Arab Emirates (74.0%), Canada (68.7%), the United Kingdom (66.9%), and the United States (55.8%). In terms of full vaccination, the United Arab Emirates ranks first (64.1%), followed by the United Kingdom (50.1%), and the United States (48.8%); in South Korea, the rate of full vaccination is 11.1%. During the study period, the South Korean government frequently changed the social distancing rules according to the number of domestic confirmed cases, which was updated daily. At the time the survey began, the highest level (level 4) of social distancing rules was in force. Private gatherings of up to three people were prohibited after 18:00 and restaurants were permitted to offer only take-out and delivery after 22:00. Comprehensive social distancing rules affected all areas of daily life including work, education, and sports activities [18,21].

Data concerning the incidences of anxiety and depression during the COVID-19 pandemic among IBD patients in South Korea are scarce. The patients in this study had higher rates of anxiety (14.5%) and depression (26.3%) than patients in a pre-COVID-19 nationwide study (anxiety, 12.2%; depression, 8.0%) [3]. According to previous studies conducted in Portugal and Italy during the COVID-19 pandemic, more than 50% of respondents showed moderate or severe levels of anxiety. [2,22] Our results reported a lower percentage of anxiety and depression. However, unlike previous studies, this study was conducted one year after the outbreak of the COVID-19 pandemic.

In this study, 6.2% of patients had a previous diagnosis of mental disease. Most of the patients with significant anxiety or depression did not have such a prior diagnosis. The development of such diagnoses could be related to the COVID-19 pandemic, although some patients may have had undiagnosed mental disease before the pandemic.

Multivariate analysis of predictors of significant anxiety or depression can provide insights concerning interventions needed to reduce the mental health burden during the COVID-19 pandemic. Female sex, the presence of mental disease, and the presence of Crohn's disease were associated with greater risks of anxiety and depression. Our results are different from those of Trindade et al., which showed no differences between Crohn's disease and ulcerative colitis patients. [22] With respect to COVID-19 vaccination, unvaccinated patients had greater risks of anxiety and depression, presumably because IBD patients were more likely to take any recommended precautions. A meta-analysis reported a lower incidence of COVID-19 infection among IBD patients than among the general population [23]. Uncertainty concerning the benefits and risks of vaccination may make IBD patients more prone to anxiety and depression.

Immunomodulators were associated with a greater risk of anxiety. In South Korea, some IBD patients regard immunomodulators as suppressants. This could cause fear, despite the unclear relationship between immunomodulators and anxiety. Although previous findings reported reduced medication adherence in IBD patients using steroids, our results for steroids cannot inform conclusions because a small proportion of IBD patients used steroids. [24] Therefore, the mental well-being of patients should be considered when making recommendations concerning the cessation of immunomodulators or biologics among IBD patients during the pandemic.

Medication adherence can considerably affect the quality of life and disease control in IBD patients. A four-item version of the Medicine Adherence Report Scale was previously used to assess medication adherence in IBD patients [25,26]. The Medicine Adherence Report Scale total score ranges from 5 to 20, with each statement scored on a 5-point Likert scale, ranging from always [1] to never [5]. Scores of 17 to 20 are considered good adherence [27]. However, we used the KMARS to assess adherence, which comprises more than four questions. Furthermore, respondents answer each question yes or no. However, a reliable KMARS cut-off score for good adherence has not yet been established. Based on a systematic review before the pandemic, the nonadherence rate among IBD patients is 7% to 72%; most studies reported 30% to 45% [28]. Although it is difficult to compare adherence rates before and after the COVID-19 pandemic, our findings indicate that IBD patients showed good medication adherence despite the psychological effects of the COVID-19 pandemic. Several studies in Asia reported medication nonadherence rates among IBD patients of 20% to 30%, similar to our results [29]. Results of the present study also correspond with those of earlier European studies, which reported COVID-19 prevalence did not affect medication adherence in IBD patients [22,30].

The above findings may be explained as follows. First, the KASID educational materials and campaigns could have promoted medication adherence among South Korean IBD patients. The KASID distributed vaccination guidelines for South Korean IBD patients according to their medications [31,32]. Second, the "Band" social media platform (run by the medical team at our IBD Center) provided patients with comprehensive information. This 24 h online platform enabled communication and question–answer interactions between physicians and patients. Because open communication with healthcare providers is important to maintain control of psychological stress, such social media interventions can reduce the psychological burden of patients and improve their medication adherence [33].

This study had several limitations. First, it was a single-center, cross-sectional study. However, we enrolled 407 outpatients, a considerable number from a single center. A larger multicenter study involving a larger number of outpatients and hospitalized patients is needed to verify the results. Second, we cannot assume that COVID-19 directly affected the mental well-being of IBD patients. Several factors may have affected the results because this was a self-reported survey study. Third, the possibility of unavoidable bias may exist due to uncontrolled factors. The percentage of having previous mental illness was too low and comparisons were not made with this variable. In addition, the survey was conducted for 14 weeks and the frequent changes in restrictions on public activity promulgated by the South Korean government during that period may have affected the responses.

Nonetheless, this study had several strengths. First, it was a timely study. During the study period, COVID-19 vaccination was in the pipeline in South Korea. Our results provide insights concerning how IBD patients reacted to COVID-19 and the effect (if any) of vaccination. Second, this was the first South Korean study of both mental well-being and medication adherence. Third, we evaluated behavioral changes using a self-developed, albeit unvalidated, questionnaire. The high rates of anxiety and depression in IBD patients indicate the need for the development of effective interventions.

5. Conclusions

The COVID-19 pandemic has increased anxiety and depression among IBD patients, whose medication adherence has nevertheless remained good. Furthermore, anxiety and depression were negatively associated with medication adherence. Our results provide insights concerning psychological response and medication adherence among IBD patients in South Korea during the COVID-19 pandemic.

Author Contributions: J.E.R. and S.-B.K. designed the study, reviewed the literature, and contributed to drafting the manuscript; S.-G.K., S.H.J., S.H.L. and S.-B.K. was responsible for revising the manuscript for important intellectual content. All authors have read and agreed to the published version of the manuscript.

Funding: This research received no external funding.

Institutional Review Board Statement: The study was conducted in accordance with the Declaration of Helsinki. Prior to study initiation, the Institutional Review Board at Daejeon St. Mary's Hospital approved the study protocol (DC21QASI0045).

Informed Consent Statement: Written informed consent has been obtained from the patients to publish this paper.

Data Availability Statement: Data can be made available from the corresponding author upon request.

Acknowledgments: We thank the clinical research coordinator, Kyeonghee Hwang, Jian Lee and HyunJoo Kweon, for conducting the survey.

Conflicts of Interest: The authors declare no conflict of interest.

References

1. Cheema, M.; Mitrev, N.; Hall, L. Depression, anxiety and stress among patients with inflammatory bowel disease during the COVID-19 pandemic: Australian national survey. *BMJ Open Gastroenterol.* **2021**, *8*, e000581. [CrossRef] [PubMed]
2. Spagnuolo, R.; Larussa, T.; Iannelli, C. COVID-19 and Inflammatory Bowel Disease: Patient Knowledge and Perceptions in a Single Center Survey. *Medicina* **2020**, *56*, 407. [CrossRef] [PubMed]
3. Choi, K.; Chun, J.; Han, K. Risk of Anxiety and Depression in Patients with Inflammatory Bowel Disease: A Nationwide, Population-Based Study. *J. Clin. Med.* **2019**, *8*, 654. [CrossRef] [PubMed]
4. Nahon, S.; Lahmek, P.; Durance, C. Risk factors of anxiety and depression in inflammatory bowel disease. *Inflamm. Bowel Dis.* **2012**, *18*, 2086–2091. [CrossRef]
5. Ronald, K.; Nazar, M.; Laura, F. Quality of life in inflammatory bowel diseases: It is not all about the bowel. *Intest. Res.* **2021**, *19*, 45–52. [CrossRef]
6. Yoon, J.Y.; Shin, J.E.; Park, S.H. Disability due to Inflammatory Bowel Disease is Correlated with Drug Adherence, Disease Activity, and Quality of Life. *Gut Liver* **2017**, *11*, 370–376. [CrossRef]
7. Yun, H.S.; Min, Y.W.; Chang, D.K. Factors associated with vaccination among inflammatory bowel disease patients in Korea. *Korean J. Gastroenterol.* **2013**, *61*, 203–208. [CrossRef]
8. 2020 Inflammatory Bowel Disease Fact Sheet in Korea. Available online: http://m.kasid.org/file/IBD%20fact%20sheet_1217.pdf (accessed on 23 January 2022).

9. Lee, Y.J.; Kim, K.O.; Kim, M.C. Perceptions and Behaviors of Patients with Inflammatory Bowel Disease during the COVID-19 Crisis. *Gut Liver* **2022**, *16*, 81–91. [CrossRef]
10. Shah, R.; Dua, A.; Naliboff, B.D. Fear of Covid-19, Along with Stress, Anxiety, and Depression, is Associated with Biologic Usage in Patients with Inflammatory Bowel Disease. *Gastroenterology* **2021**, *160*, S335. [CrossRef]
11. Korean Association for the Study for Intestinal Disease (KASID). Available online: https://www.kasid.org/board/list.html?num=1680&start=0&sort=top%20desc,num%20desc&code=m_bbs&key=&keyword=&cate=54 (accessed on 25 January 2022).
12. Zigmond, A.S.; Snaith, P.R. The Hospital Anxiety and Depression Scale. *Acta Psychiatr. Scand.* **1983**, *67*, 361–370. [CrossRef]
13. Thompson, K.; Kulkarni, J.; Sergejew, A.A. Reliability and validity of a new Medication Adherence Rating Scale (MARS) for the psychoses. *Schizophr. Res.* **2000**, *42*, 241–247. [CrossRef]
14. Chang, J.G.; No, D.Y.; Kim, C.Y. The reliability and validity of the Korean version of Medication Adherence Rating Scale (KMARS). *Korean J. Psychopharmacol.* **2015**, *26*, 43–49. [CrossRef]
15. Kwak, M.S.; Cha, J.M.; Lee, H.H. Emerging trends of inflammatory bowel disease in South Korea: A nationwide population-based study. *J. Gastroenterol. Hepatol.* **2019**, *34*, 1018–1026. [CrossRef] [PubMed]
16. Walker, J.R.; Ediger, J.P.; Graff, L.A. The Manitoba IBD cohort study: A population-based study of the prevalence of lifetime and 12-month anxiety and mood disorders. *Am. J. Gastroenterol.* **2008**, *103*, 1989–1997. [CrossRef] [PubMed]
17. Askar, S.; Sakr, M.A.; Alaty, W.H.A. The psychological impact of inflammatory bowel disease as regards anxiety and depression: A single-center study. *Middle East Curr. Psychiatry* **2021**, *28*, 73. [CrossRef]
18. Coronavirus (COVID-19) Vaccinations. Our World in Data. Available online: https://ourworldindata.org/covid-vaccinations (accessed on 20 January 2022).
19. Korea Disease Control and Prevention Agency. Available online: https://www.kdca.go.kr/gallery.es?mid=a20503020000&bid=0003&act=view&list_no=144977 (accessed on 10 January 2022).
20. Ministry of Health and Welfare. Available online: http://www.mohw.go.kr/react/al/sal0301vw.jsp?PAR_MENU_ID=04&MENU_ID=0403&page=184&CONT_SEQ=354112 (accessed on 20 December 2021).
21. Central Disaster Management Headquarters. Overview of Social Distancing System. Available online: http://ncov.mohw.go.kr/en/socdisBoardView.do?brdId=19&brdGubun=191&dataGubun=191&ncvContSeq=&contSeq=&board_id= (accessed on 20 January 2022).
22. Trindade, I.A.; Ferreira, N.B. COVID-19 Pandemic's Effects on Disease and Psychological Outcomes of People with Inflammatory Bowel Disease in Portugal: A Preliminary Research. *Inflamm. Bowel Dis.* **2020**, *27*, 1224–1229. [CrossRef]
23. Aziz, M.; Fatima, R.; Haghbin, H. The incidence and outcomes of COVID-19 in IBD patients: A rapid review and meta-analysis. *Inflamm. Bowel Dis.* **2020**, *26*, e132–e133. [CrossRef]
24. Barnes, A.; Andrews, J.; Spizzo, P. Medication adherence and complementary therapy usage in inflammatory bowel disease patients during the coronavirus disease 2019 pandemic. *JGH Open* **2021**, *29*, 585–589. [CrossRef]
25. Horne, R.; Weinman, J. Self-regulation and self-management in asthma: Exploring the role of illness perceptions and treatment beliefs in explaining non-adherence to preventer medication. *Psychol. Health* **2002**, *17*, 17–32. [CrossRef]
26. Ediger, J.P.; Walker, J.R.; Graff, L. Predictors of medication adherence in inflammatory bowel disease. *Am. J. Gastroenterol.* **2007**, *102*, 1417–1426. [CrossRef]
27. Horne, R.; Parham, R.; Driscoll, R. Patients' attitudes to medicines and adherence to maintenance treatment in inflammatory bowel disease. *Inflamm. Bowel Dis.* **2009**, *15*, 837–844. [CrossRef] [PubMed]
28. Jackson, C.A.; Clatworthy, J.; Robinson, A. Factors associated with non-adherence to oral medication for inflammatory bowel disease: A systematic review. *Am. J. Gastroenterol.* **2010**, *105*, 525–539. [CrossRef] [PubMed]
29. Chan, W.; Chen, A.; Tiao, D. Medication adherence in inflammatory bowel disease. *Intestig. Res.* **2017**, *15*, 434–445. [CrossRef] [PubMed]
30. D'Amico, F.; Rahier, J.F.; Leone, S.; Peyrin-Biroulet, L.; Danese, S. Views of patients with inflammatory bowel disease on the COVID-19 pandemic: A global survey. *Lancet Gastroenterol. Hepatol.* **2020**, *5*, 631–632. [CrossRef]
31. Korean Association for the Study for Intestinal Disease (KASID). Available online: https://www.kasid.org/board/list.html?num=1648&start=0&sort=top%20desc,num%20desc&code=ilban&key=&keyword (accessed on 25 January 2022).
32. Lee, Y.J.; Kim, S.E.; Park, Y.E. SARS-CoV-2 vaccination for adult patients with inflammatory bowel disease: Expert consensus statement by KASID. *Korean J. Gastroenterol.* **2021**, *78*, 117–128. [CrossRef]
33. Stone, M.L.; Feng, M.; Forster, E.M. COVID-19 Pandemic Increased Anxiety Among Patients with Inflammatory Bowel Disease: A Patient Survey in a Tertiary Referral Center. *Dig. Dis. Sci.* **2021**, 1–6. [CrossRef]

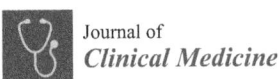

Article

Liver Function Tests in COVID-19: Assessment of the Actual Prognostic Value

Urszula Tokarczyk [1,*], Krzysztof Kaliszewski [1,*], Anna Kopszak [2], Łukasz Nowak [3], Karolina Sutkowska-Stępień [1], Maciej Sroczyński [1], Monika Sępek [1], Agata Dudek [1], Dorota Diakowska [4], Małgorzata Trocha [5], Damian Gajecki [6], Jakub Gawryś [6], Tomasz Matys [6], Justyna Maciejiczek [7], Valeriia Kozub [7], Roman Szalast [7], Marcin Madziarski [8], Anna Zubkiewicz-Zarębska [9], Krzysztof Letachowicz [10], Katarzyna Kiliś-Pstrusińska [11], Agnieszka Matera-Witkiewicz [12], Michał Pomorski [13], Marcin Protasiewicz [14], Janusz Sokołowski [15], Barbara Adamik [16], Krzysztof Kujawa [2], Adrian Doroszko [6], Katarzyna Madziarska [10,†] and Ewa Anita Jankowska [17,†]

1 Clinical Department of General, Minimally Invasive and Endocrine Surgery, Wroclaw Medical University, Borowska Street 213, 50-556 Wroclaw, Poland; karolina.sutkowska@onet.pl (K.S.-S.); maciej.sroczynski@o2.pl (M.S.); moniasep@wp.pl (M.S.); agatadudek7@gmail.com (A.D.)
2 Statistical Analysis Center, Wroclaw Medical University, Marcinkowski Street 2-6, 50-368 Wroclaw, Poland; anna.kopszak@umw.edu.pl (A.K.); krzysztof.kujawa@umw.edu.pl (K.K.)
3 Clinical Department of Urology and Urological Oncology, Wroclaw Medical University, Borowska Street 213, 50-556 Wroclaw, Poland; lllukasz.nowak@gmail.com
4 Department of Basic Science, Faculty of Health Science, Wroclaw Medical University, Bartel Street 5, 51-618 Wroclaw, Poland; dorota.diakowska@umw.edu.pl
5 Department of Pharmacology, Wroclaw Medical University, Mikulicz-Radecki Street 2, 50-345 Wroclaw, Poland; malgorzata.trocha@umw.edu.pl
6 Clinical Department of Internal and Occupational Diseases, Hypertension and Clinical Oncology, Wroclaw Medical University, Borowska 213, 50-556 Wroclaw, Poland; damian.gajecki@umw.edu.pl (D.G.); jakub.gawrys@umw.edu.pl (J.G.); tomasz.matys@umw.edu.pl (T.M.); adrian.doroszko@umw.edu.pl (A.D.)
7 Clinical Department of Internal Medicine, Pneumology and Allergology, Wroclaw Medical University, M. Skłodowskiej-Curie Street 66, 50-369 Wroclaw, Poland; justynamaciejiczej@umw.edu.pl (J.M.); vkozub@usk.wroc.pl (V.K.); romanszalast@gmail.com (R.S.)
8 Clinical Department of Rheumatology and Internal Medicine, Wroclaw Medical University, Borowska Street 213, 50-556 Wroclaw, Poland; madziarski.marcin@gmail.com
9 Clinical Department of Gastroenterology and Hepatology, Wroclaw Medical University, Borowska Street 213, 50-556 Wroclaw, Poland; anna.zubkiewicz-zarebska@umw.edu.pl
10 Clinical Department of Nephrology and Transplantation Medicine, Wroclaw Medical University, Borowska Street 213, 50-556 Wroclaw, Poland; krzysztof.letachowicz@umw.edu.pl (K.L.); katarzyna.madziarska@umw.edu.pl (K.M.)
11 Clinical Department of Pediatric Nephrology, Wroclaw Medical University, Borowska Street 213, 50-556 Wroclaw, Poland; katarzyna.kilis-pstrusinska@umw.edu.pl
12 Screening Laboratory of Biological Activity Assays and Collection of Biological Material, Faculty of Pharmacy, Wroclaw Medical University, Borowska Street 211A, 50-556 Wroclaw, Poland; agnieszka.matera-witkiewicz@umw.edu.pl
13 Clinical Department of Gynecology and Obstetrics, Wroclaw Medical University, Borowska Street 213, 50-556 Wroclaw, Poland; michal.pomorski@umw.edu.pl
14 Clinical Department and Clinic of Cardiology, Wroclaw Medical University, Borowska Street 213, 50-556 Wroclaw, Poland; marcin.protasiewicz@umw.edu.pl
15 Department of Emergency Medicine, Wroclaw Medical University, Borowska Street 213, 50-556 Wroclaw, Poland; janusz.sokolowski@umw.edu.pl
16 Clinical Department of Anaesthesiology and Intensive Therapy, Wroclaw Medical University, Borowska Street 213, 50-556 Wroclaw, Poland; barbara.adamik@umw.edu.pl
17 University Hospital in Wroclaw, Institute of Heart Diseases, Wroclaw Medical University, Borowska Street 213, 50-556 Wroclaw, Poland; ewa.jankowska@umw.edu.pl
* Correspondence: urszula.tokarczyk@student.umw.edu.pl (U.T.); krzysztof.kaliszewski@umw.edu.pl (K.K.); Tel.: +48-723-781-491 (U.T.); +48-71-734-30-00 (K.K.); Fax: +48-71-734-30-00 (K.K.)
† These authors contributed equally to this work.

Citation: Tokarczyk, U.; Kaliszewski, K.; Kopszak, A.; Nowak, Ł.; Sutkowska-Stępień, K.; Sroczyński, M.; Sępek, M.; Dudek, A.; Diakowska, D.; Trocha, M.; et al. Liver Function Tests in COVID-19: Assessment of the Actual Prognostic Value. *J. Clin. Med.* **2022**, *11*, 4490. https://doi.org/10.3390/jcm11154490

Academic Editor: Hemant Goyal

Received: 4 April 2022
Accepted: 29 July 2022
Published: 1 August 2022

Publisher's Note: MDPI stays neutral with regard to jurisdictional claims in published maps and institutional affiliations.

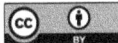

Copyright: © 2022 by the authors. Licensee MDPI, Basel, Switzerland. This article is an open access article distributed under the terms and conditions of the Creative Commons Attribution (CC BY) license (https://creativecommons.org/licenses/by/4.0/).

Abstract: Deviations in laboratory tests assessing liver function in patients with COVID-19 are frequently observed. Their importance and pathogenesis are still debated. In our retrospective study, we analyzed liver-related parameters: aspartate aminotransferase (AST), alanine aminotransferase (ALT), alkaline phosphatase (ALP), gamma-glutamyltransferase (GGT), total bilirubin (TBIL), albumin, co-morbidities and other selected potential risk factors in patients admitted with SARS-CoV-2 infection to assess their prognostic value for intensive care unit admission, mechanical ventilation necessity and mortality. We compared the prognostic effectiveness of these parameters separately and in pairs to the neutrophil-to-lymphocyte ratio (NLR) as an independent risk factor of in-hospital mortality, using the Akaike Information Criterion (AIC). Data were collected from 2109 included patients. We created models using a sample with complete laboratory tests n = 401 and then applied them to the whole studied group excluding patients with missing singular variables. We estimated that albumin may be a better predictor of the COVID-19-severity course compared to NLR, irrespective of comorbidities ($p < 0.001$). Additionally, we determined that hypoalbuminemia in combination with AST (OR 1.003, p = 0.008) or TBIL (OR 1.657, p = 0.001) creates excellent prediction models for in-hospital mortality. In conclusion, the early evaluation of albumin levels and liver-related parameters may be indispensable tools for the early assessment of the clinical course of patients with COVID-19.

Keywords: COVID-19; SARS-CoV-2; severity of COVID-19; hospitalized patients; risk factors; liver

1. Introduction

Coronavirus disease 2019 (COVID-19) caused by Severe Acute Respiratory Syndrome Coronavirus 2 (SARS-CoV-2) was first reported to the World Health Organization on 30 December 2019 in Wuhan. [1–3]. The symptoms of COVID-19 are predominantly related to the pulmonary tract and are manifested by dry cough, fever, fatigue and headache [4]. However, the virus may also lead to a systemic and multi-organ disease causing extra-pulmonary manifestations involving the cardiovascular, hematological, renal, gastrointestinal and hepatobiliary, neurological, ophthalmological and dermatological systems [5]. According to the meta-analysis, the most common gastrointestinal manifestations include anorexia, diarrhea and nausea. Additionally, vomiting, abdominal pain and abdominal distension can be observed [6].

The liver's involvement in patients with COVID-19 is still the subject of dispute, especially due to the fact that 76% of patients present liver biochemistry abnormalities, usually mild to moderate [7,8]. A multicenter retrospective study by Wuhan revealed that acute liver injury (ALI) occurs later in the course of COVID-19 (day 17 IQR, 13–23) and follows the development of ARDS [9]. The latest research shows that ALI is more common than initially thought and may occur in up to 22.8% of patients [10]. The potential mechanism of hepatocyte damage remains unclear. Direct damage can be mediated by angiotensin converting enzyme 2 (ACE2) receptors and cellular serine protease called TMPRSS2, which is needed to prime the Spike protein for cell entrance [11]. These receptors are expressed in only 3% of hepatocytes, whereas their presence in cholangiocytes reaches 60% of cells [12–14]. However, L-SIGN, which is a liver-specific membrane receptor binding to ACE2, may be excessively expressed in infected sinusoid cells [15]. Thus, it may constitute a bridge for SARS-CoV-2 to infect hepatocytes. Other considered receptors include CD147, which can be overexpressed in an inflammatory process. The affinity between CD147 and the SARS-CoV-2 spike protein was shown in in vitro studies [16]. Sun et al. suggest probable patomechanisms as immune-mediated damage, hypoxic damage and drug-induced liver injury [17]. Additionally, studies focused on the impact of preexisting non-alcoholic fatty liver disease (NAFLD) on the severe course of COVID-19 suggest that obesity associated with NAFLD can contribute to the polarization of macrophages into M1 proinflammatory macrophages, which may exacerbate SARS-CoV-2 infection [18]. Thus, it seems that the liver impairment caused by COVID-19 is likely of multifactorial origin.

The substantial majority of studies focused on COVID-19-associated liver abnormalities evaluate peak levels of liver enzymes, such as aspartate aminotransferase (AST), alanine aminotransferase (ALT), alkaline phosphatase (ALP), gamma-glutamyl transferase (GGT), total bilirubin (TBIL) and albumin [9,19,20]. They showed a predominance of parenchymal liver injury based on the prevalence of elevated AST and ALT [21]. Studies considering liver biochemistry at baseline seem to confirm this tendency [22,23]. Significant elevations in ALP are uncommonly recorded despite strong cholangiocyte ACE2 expression, with mildly raised GGT levels seen in up to 50% of patients [7,22–24]. Nevertheless, the clinical significance of these observations remains inconclusive. There are still some lacking answers, especially regarding the impact of previously taken medications.

The clinical course and outcome of patients with COVID-19 and liver abnormalities require further investigation, given the alterations in liver function tests and liver impairment in pathological findings in patients with COVID-19. Furthermore, the association between liver enzymes and worse outcomes, including COVID-19-related in-hospital fatalities, should also be analyzed.

In our retrospective study, we aimed to develop a predictive model for COVID-19 patients based on baseline data, including liver abnormalities especially associated with potential biliary tract damage, hoping to find a new objective path to forecast the progression of COVID-19 to severe and lethal forms while excluding the influence of comorbidities.

2. Materials and Methods

2.1. Study Population and Data Collection

All procedures were performed in accordance with the ethical standards of Wroclaw Medical University (Poland) and with the 1964 Helsinki Declaration and its later amendments. The study protocol was approved by the Commission of Bioethics at Wroclaw Medical University (No: KB-444/2021).

This study enrolled 2184 adult patients admitted to the University Hospital in Wroclaw (USW) with positive SARS-CoV-2 real-time PCR (RT-PCR) from March 2020 to November 2021. Generic data included the following characteristics: gender, age, prior history of hypertension, diabetes, asthma, chronic obstructive pulmonary disease (COPD), dementia, stroke/transient ischemic attack (TIA), chronic kidney disease, myocardial infraction, heart failure, chronic liver disease, solid malignant disease, leukemia, lymphoma and active acquired immunodeficiency syndrome (AIDS). Further information about smoking status and length of hospital stay was collected. Patients with accompanying chronic liver disease, such as chronic hepatitis, cirrhosis with or without portal hypertension, and fatty liver disease ($n = 74$), were excluded from the analysis. Admission values of laboratory tests including liver enzymes such as AST, ALT, ALP, GGT, TBIL and albumin were examined as a main subject of our survey. Further data collection included a complete blood count with differential used to calculate neutrophil-to-lymphocyte ratio (NLR), which is an independent risk factor of in-hospital mortality [25]. Endpoints for COVID-19 severity were defined as: (1) admission to the ICU, (2) intubation and (3) death.

2.2. Statistical Analysis

Categorical variables are presented as numbers and percentages. Means and standard deviations were used to present the central tendency of the continuous variables. The normal distribution of these variables was verified using the Shapiro–Wilk test. The chi-square test was used to determine the association between the two categorical variables. Reviewing the percentage of patients whose parameters related to liver function were abnormal, we considered only the group without liver diseases in a previous history ($n = 2109$). To analyze the association between liver function tests and the severity of disease, logistic regression was used adjusting for comorbidities: hypertension, diabetes, asthma, COPD, dementia, stroke/TIA in patient history, chronic kidney disease, myocardial infarction in patient history, heart failure, leukemia, lymphoma and solid malignant disease in order of additional assessment of their influence on COVID-19 severity in our population and a potential ability to interfere with the objective assessment of liver-related parameters as predictors. Additionally, adjustment was performed for length of hospital stay and smoking history, which is considered an independent risk factor for worse outcomes in COVID-19 disease [26]. In the above-mentioned logistic regression, we assessed only patients who had complete laboratory tests, which is the reason for the sample size variation ($n = 401$). In further analyses, we created models composed of pairs formed by laboratory parameters (AST, ALT, ALP, GGT, TBIL, albumin) in various configurations using the same adjustments as in the previous analysis to find the best predictors that could be objective laboratory indicators of the severe course of COVID-19, regardless of comorbidities and other factors mentioned above. The accuracy of multivariate models evaluating single parameters related to the liver and their double combinations was assessed using the Nagelkerke coefficient. The best models were selected using the Akaike Information Criterion (AIC) and then applied to the whole sample ($n = 2109$), excluding patients with missing data. Receiver operating characteristic (ROC) curves were calculated to present a comparison between the models.

All statistical analyses were performed using the Statistica 13.3 package and R software, version 4.1.1 (2021-08-10, R Foundation for Statistical Computing). Statistical significance was determined at $p < 0.05$.

3. Results

3.1. Clinical Characteristics

The baseline clinical characteristics of the COVID-19 patients from our cohort are summarized in Table 1. The median age was 64 years and 50.4% were female. In our sample, men statistically significantly more frequently met fatal outcomes, were admitted to ICU and required invasive respiratory support. The most prevalent underlying medical conditions were arterial hypertension (46.8%), diabetes mellitus of any kind (23.6%), heart failure (11.7%) and chronic kidney disease (10.6%). Hypertension and diabetes were significantly more frequent in the groups for all endpoints. Furthermore, myocardial infraction in the patient history co-occurred with mechanical ventilation requirements and fatal outcomes. In the group of deceased patients, the prevalence of dementia, stroke/TIA in the past, chronic kidney disease, heart failure and solid malignant disease was also statistically relevant.

Table 1. Baseline demographic data and comorbidities of 2184 patients hospitalized due to COVID-19.

	All Patients	ICU Admission	p-Value	Mechanical Ventilation	p-Value	Fatal Outcome	p-Value
	$n = 2184$	$n = 214$		$n = 215$		$n = 326$	
		% 9.8		% 9.8		% 14.9	
Age, median	64 (46–73)	64 (52–70)		65 (54–71)		72.5 (65–84)	
Gender, n (%)			<0.001		<0.001		<0.001
Female	1102 (50.4%)	71 (6.4%)		70 (6.4%)		129 (11.7%)	
Male	1082 (49.5%)	143 (13.2%)		145 (13.4%)		197 (18.2%)	
Underlying comorbidities, n (%)							
Hypertension	1022 (46.8%)	125 (5.7%)	<0.001	130 (5.95%)	<0.001	219 (10%)	<0.001
Diabetes	516 (23.6%)	75 (3.4%)	<0.001	79 (3.6%)	<0.001	122 (5.6%)	<0.001
Asthma	85 (3.9%)	12 (0.6%)	0.172	11 (0.5%)	0.328	14 (0.6%)	0.684
COPD	75 (3.4%)	5 (0.2%)	0.353	6 (0.3%)	0.585	18 (0.8%)	0.025
Dementia	132 (6%)	3 (0.1%)	0.003	6 (0.3%)	0.035	49 (2.2%)	<0.001
Stroke/TIA in patient history	164 (7.5)	13 (0.6%)	0.402	16 (0.7%)	0.969	35 (1.6%)	0.017
Chronic kidney disease	231 (10.6)	21 (1%)	0.702	22 (1%)	0.863	72 (3.3%)	<0.001
Myocardial infraction in patient history	191 (8.7%)	28 (1.3%)	0.018	32 (1.5%)	<0.001	74 (3.4%)	<0.001
Heart failure	255 (11.7%)	33 (1.5%)	0.072	33 (1.5%)	0.077	89 (4.1%)	<0.001
Chronic liver disease	74 (3.4%)	7 (0.3%)	0.802	5 (0.2%)	0.83	12 (0.6%)	0.508
Solid malignant disease	151 (6.9%)	10 (0.5%)	0.098	10 (0.5%)	0.096	42 (1.9%)	<0.001
Leukemia	19 (0.9%)	6 (0.3%)	0.001	4 (0.2%)	0.1	8 (0.4%)	0.001
Lymphoma	18 (0.8%)	0 (0%)	0.200	0 (0%)	0.2	6 (0.3%)	0.03
AIDS	2 (0.1%)	0 (0%)	0.641	0 (0%)	0.640	0 (0%)	0.553
Smoking status, n (%)	193 (8.8%)	15 (0.7%)	0.606	15 (0.7%)	0.606	41 (1.9%)	0.004
Active smoker	117 (5.4%)	6 (0.3%)		6 (0.3%)		11 (0.5%)	
Former smoker	76 (3.5%)	9 (0.4%)		9 (0.4%)		30 (1.4%)	
Length of hospital stay days, median	9 (2–16)	18 (9–27)		16 (6–26)		13 (5–21)	

Values for continuous variables were showed as or median (Q25–Q75). ICU: intensive care unit; COPD: chronic obstructive pulmonary disease; TIA: transient ischemic attack; AIDS: active acquired immunodeficiency syndrome.

3.2. Clinical Course and Outcome

Out of the 2184 patients with SARS-CoV-2 infection that were included in our cohort, 214 (9.8%) required treatment in the ICU and 215 (9.8%) underwent mechanical ventilation. The total fatality rate among patients with COVID-19 was 14.9%. The median time of hospital stay was 9 days, yet it varied between groups of patients with certain outcomes (Table 1).

3.3. Liver Biochemistry Abnormalities

Liver test abnormalities were defined as the deviation of the following liver enzymes in serum: AST > 31 U/L, ALT > 35 U/L, GGT > 38 U/L, ALP > 150 U/L, ALP < 40 U/L, TBIL > 1.2 mg/dL, albumin < 3.5 g/L and albumin > 5.2 g/L. As COVID-19 is a new, emerging infectious disease, guidance or consensus on liver injury classifications is lacking.

Median values and percentages of abnormal laboratory tests at the time of hospital admission are presented in Table 2.

Table 2. Labolatory parameters of patients on admission $n = 2109$.

	Median (IQR)	Abnormal (%)
AST (0–31 U/L)	37 (24–62)	38.9
ALT (0–35 U/L)	29 (18–50)	29.3
GGT (0–38 U/L)	42 (24–83)	33.2
ALP (40–150 U/L)	65 (51–95)	6.2
TBIL (0.2–1.2 mg/dL)	0.6 (0.5–0.8)	6.7
Albumin (3.5–5.2 g/L)	3.1 (2.7–3.5)	21.1
Neu (2.5×10^3–6×10^3/mm^3) ($\times 10^3$)	5.5 (3.5–8.4)	34.0
Lym (1.5×10^3–3.5×10^3/mm^3) ($\times 10^3$)	1.0 (0.7–1.4)	46.7
NLR	5.9 (3.1–10.8)	

IQR: Interquartial Range; AST: aspartate aminotransferase; ALT: alanine aminotransferase; GGT: gamma-glutamyltransferase; ALP: alkaline phosphatase; TBIL: total bilirubin; Neu: neutrophil; Lym: lymphocyte; NLR: neutrophil-to-lymphocyte ratio.

3.4. Association of Liver Biochemistry Abnormalities at Admission with COVID-19 Severity

In this section, we described the results obtained from testing models adjusted for comorbidities and potential risk factors (hypertension, diabetes, asthma, COPD, dementia, stroke/TIA in patient history, chronic kidney disease, myocardial infarction in patient history, heart failure, leukemia, lymphoma and solid malignant disease, smoking history and length of hospital stay), including single liver-related parameters and their double combinations. The sample in that part consisted of patients who had complete results of all laboratory tests considered in our research ($n = 401$).

Elevation of AST at admission was observed in 38.9% ($n = 2109$, Table 2). The AST model showed statistical significance for all endpoints at the significance level $p < 0.001$, but its role within the model was determined as significant only for COVID-19-related death (Table 3). Similar observations were made for AST models in combination with GGT, ALT, ALP, TBIL and albumin (Supplementary Materials Tables S11, S15 and S17–S19).

Table 3. The role of liver-related laboratory parameters in models containing potential risk factors and their impact on outcome.

	ICU Admission			Mechanical Ventilation			Fatal Outcome		
	OR	95% CI	p-Value	OR	95% CI	p-Value	OR	95% CI	p-Value
Liver biochemistry abnormality									
AST	1.000	0.998–1.000	0.6	1.000	0.999–1.000	0.32	1.004	1.001–1.010	0.008
ALT	1.000	0.998–1.000	0.55	1.000	0.999–1.000	0.46	1.002	0.999–1.00	0.133
GGT	1.000	0.999–1.000	0.74	1.000	0.999–1.000	0.60	1.001	0.999–1.000	0.220
ALP	0.999	0.996–1.000	0.41	0.999	0.996–1.000	0.29	1.002	0.999–1.00	0.087
TBIL	0.965	0.698–1.270	0.81	0.985	0.717–1.300	0.92	1.598	1.188–2.250	0.004
albumin	0.281	0.172–0.450	<0.001	0.247	0.148–0.400	<0.001	0.233	0.143–0.370	<0.001
NLR	1.033	1.015–1.060	0.001	1.032	1.014–1.050	0.001	1.031	1.011–1.060	0.006

Stated are the OR (Odds Ratio), 95% CI (Confidence Interval) and p-values for laboratory parameters, each in single model adjusted for comorbidities. A full model description is available in Supplementary Materials Tables S1–S7.

ICU: intensive care unit; AST: aspartate aminotransferase; ALT: alanine aminotransferase; GGT: gamma-glutamyltransferase; ALP: alkaline phosphatase; TBIL: total bilirubin; NLR: neutrophil-to-lymphocyte ratioAST combined with ALT revealed better predictive value for death than NLR, with $p < 0.001$ for the model and $p = 0.002$, OR 1.009, $p = 0.03$, OR 0.992 for the following parameters (Supplementary Materials Table S17).

Deviation in ALT, GGT and ALP levels were observed in 29.3%, 33.2% and 6.2% respectively (Table 2). Models that contain these parameters achieved a statistically significant predictive value $p < 0.001$ (Supplementary Materials Tables S3, S4 and S6). However, in none of them, ALT, GGT or ALP were significant within the model, both alone (Table 3) or together with other characteristics (Supplementary Materials Tables S6, S8, S10, S12–S16, S18 and S20–S22).

TBIL elevation at admission was observed in a relatively small proportion of patients ($n = 2109$, Table 2), but it was associated significantly with higher mortality. The model for fatal outcome including TBIL reached a p-value at the level of<0.001, and TBIL significance was described as $p = 0.004$, OR 1.598. Interestingly, the model including TBIL and AST turned out to have a greater predictive value for death than the model containing NLR (Table 4), with p-value = 0.023, OR 1.471 for TBIL, and $p = 0.038$, OR 1.003 for AST (Supplementary Materials Table S19).

Table 4. Comparison of the models with single parameters and their double combinations adjusted for comorbidities and potential risk factors according to AIC for individual endpoints.

	ICU-Admission			Mechanical Ventilation			Fatal Outcome	
	Model	AIC		Model	AIC		Model	AIC
1	albumin+ALP	439.0	1	albumin	426.2	1	albumin+TBIL	455.1
2	albumin	439.2	2	albumin+ALP	426.2	2	albumin+AST	456.8
3	albumin+ALT	440.7	3	albumin+ALT	427.3	3	albumin+ALT	462.1
4	albumin+TBIL	441.0	4	albumin+AST	427.5	4	albumin	464.1
5	albumin+AST	441.2	5	albumin+TBIL	428.0	5	albumin+GGT	464.7
6	albumin+GGT	441.2	6	albumin+GGT	428.1	6	albumin+ALP	464.7
7	NLR	456.3	7	NLR	448.4	7	AST+ALT	493.2
8	ALP	469.8	8	AST	461.1	8	AST+TBIL	493.5
9	ALT	470.4	9	AST+ALP	461.5	9	NLR	497.0
10	AST	470.4	10	ALP	461.6	10	AST	497.2
11	GGT	470.5	11	ALT	461.6	11	TBIL+GGT	497.2
12	TBIL	470.6	12	GGT	461.9	12	TBIL	497.5
13	AST+ALP	470.9	13	TBIL	462.1	13	TBIL+ALT	497.7
14	ALP+GGT	470.9	14	ALP+GGT	462.4	14	AST+ALP	498.7
15	ALP+ALT	471.0	15	ALP+ALT	462.6	15	AST+GGT	499.1
16	ALP+TBIL	471.6	16	AST+TBIL	462.8	16	ALP+TBIL	499.5
17	TBIL+GGT	472.1	17	AST+GGT	463.1	17	ALP+ALT	504.6
18	AST+TBIL	472.1	18	AST+ALT	463.1	18	ALP	504.6
19	TBIL+ALT	472.2	19	ALP+TBIL	463.3	19	ALT	504.7
20	ALT+GGT	472.2	20	TBIL+GGT	463.4	20	ALT+GGT	505.8
21	ALT+AST	472.3	21	ALT+GGT	463.4	21	GGT	506.4
22	AST+GGT	472.3	22	TBIL+ALT	463.5	22	TBIL+GGT	506.5

AIC: Akaike Information Criterion; ICU: intensive care unit; AST: aspartate aminotransferase; ALT: alanine aminotransferase; GGT: gamma-glutamyltransferase; ALP: alkaline phosphatase; TBIL: total bilirubin; NLR: neutrophil-to-lymphocyte ratio.

Deviation in albumin levels on admission was presented by 21.1% of patients ($n = 2109$, Table 2). Hypoalbuminemia as a single test, as the only one of all investigated parameters, was statistically significantly associated with all three endpoints (Table 3). Remarkably, each of these models showed by far the highest predictive value for all the variables included (Supplementary Materials Table S7).

Albumin combined with each of the examined characteristics (AST, ALT, GGT, ALP and TBIL) produced a stronger predictive model for all endpoint tests than NLR, according to the AIC (Table 4). Albumin was the most important component examined in each of these tests, with a statistically significant effect on the final test result at the $p < 0.0001$ level (Supplementary Materials Tables S8–11 and S16).

ALP together with albumin performed better than albumin alone for ICU admission (Table 4), but a careful examination reveals that ALP was not statistically significant ($p = 0.199$, Supplementary Materials Table S8).

In the overview of models predicting the necessity of mechanical ventilation, we observed a similar distribution as in the case of ICU admission; however, for this particular outcome, the model using albumin without additional parameters works as well as the model combining albumin with ALP (Table 4).

The albumin-TBIL model ($p < 0.001$, Supplementary Materials Table S9) and albumin together with AST ($p < 0.001$, Supplementary Materials Table S11) were found to be the greatest predictors of fatal outcome (Table 4).

TBIL and albumin were the most important covariates in the model ($p = 0.003$, OR 1.705, $p = 0.001$, OR 0.228, respectively), outweighing the potential of other comorbidities (Supplementary Materials Table S9). In the model combining albumin and AST, the predictive value of both factors within the model was statistically significant ($p < 0.001$, OR 0.233, $p = 0.009$, OR 1.003, respectively, Supplementary Materials Table S11).

Models examining the combination of albumin with other parameters (ALT, GGT, ALP) for fatal outcomes also performed better than the model with NLR (Table 4), while the inclusion of GGT and ALP seems to lower the value of the model compared to the one considering albumin alone (Table 4, Supplementary Materials Tables S8 and S16). ALT in combination with albumin fares better than albumin; however, ALT does not reach statistical significance within the model ($p = 0.09$, OR 1.002, Supplementary Materials Table S10).

The comorbidities and risk factors with a statistically significant ($p < 0.05$) impact on ICU admission and mechanical ventilation were chronic kidney disease (OR < 1) and length of hospital stay (OR > 1) (Supplementary Materials Tables S1–S22).

Within models testing the influence of included factors on the risk of death due to COVID-19, the most important ($p < 0.05$) were hypertension (OR > 1), dementia (OR > 1), myocardial infarction in the past (OR > 1) and leukemia (OR > 1). The laboratory parameters that always achieved greater statistical significance within the models for this endpoint were NLR and albumin (Supplementary Materials Tables S1, S7–S11 and S16).

3.5. Best Predictive Models

In this section, we present models with the highest predictive value for severe COVID-19, selected on the basis of $n = 401$ sample tests and examined on the entire population of patients included in the study ($n = 2109$), while excluding those with missing desired laboratory data. This means that samples tested in each model consisted of slightly different groups of patients, which is the reason for variation in statistical significance analyzed parameters, comorbidities and risk factors (hypertension, diabetes, asthma, COPD, dementia, stroke/TIA in patient history, chronic kidney disease, myocardial infarction in patient history, heart failure, leukemia, lymphoma and solid malignant disease, smoking history and length of hospital stay, Tables 5–7).

Table 5. The best models to predict ICU admission in COVID-19 tested on larger groups of patients.

ICU Admission								
Variables	OR	95% CI		p-Value	Sample Size n	NG	LR p-Value	AIC
		25%	75%					
Model: albumin+ALP	36.810	8.245	177.080	<0.0001	459	0.292	<0.0001	518.2
ALP	0.997	0.994	1.000	0.101				
albumin	0.277	0.176	0.420	<0.0001				
Hypertension	1.103	0.675	1.810	0.694				
Diabetes-1	0.243	0.012	1.570	0.207				
Diabetes-2	1.504	0.824	2.740	0.182				
Diabetes-3	1.881	0.754	4.650	0.170				
Diabetes-4	2.234	0.588	8.410	0.228				
Diabetes-5	<0.001	<0.001	<0.001	0.997				
Asthma	1.837	0.579	5.700	0.290				
COPD	0.236	0.033	1.050	0.088				
Dementia	0.061	0.009	0.230	<0.001				
Stroke/TIA in patient history	0.650	0.257	1.540	0.341				
Chronic kiedney disease	0.279	0.138	0.540	<0.001				
Active smoker	0.706	0.192	2.300	0.576				
Former smoker	0.279	0.069	0.910	0.047				
Myocardial infraction in patient history	1.704	0.802	3.630	0.164				
Heart failure	0.959	0.473	1.910	0.905				
Leukemia	4.327	0.946	21.070	0.058				
Solid malignant disease without metastases	0.863	0.317	2.260	0.767				
Solid malignant disease with metastases	<0.001	<0.001	>1000	0.988				
Lymphoma	<0.001	<0.001	>1000	0.989				
Lenght of hospital stay	1.007	0.993	1.020	0.341				
Variables	OR	95% CI		p-Value	Sample Size n	NG	LR p-Value	AIC
		25%	75%					
Model: albumin	21.583	6.137	79.200	<0.0001	621	0.276	<0.0001	666
albumin	0.295	0.200	0.430	<0.0001				
Hypertension	1.055	0.685	1.630	0.808				
Diabetes-1	0.224	0.012	1.300	0.168				
Diabetes-2	1.751	1.038	2.950	0.035				
Diabetes-3	1.782	0.809	3.870	0.146				
Diabetes-4	2.423	0.730	8.030	0.142				
Diabetes-5	<0.001	<0.001	>1000	0.994				
Asthma	1.749	0.708	4.260	0.218				
COPD	0.514	0.142	1.610	0.274				
Dementia	0.068	0.015	0.210	<0.001				
Stroke/TIA in patient history	0.748	0.329	1.600	0.468				
Chronic kiedney disease	0.263	0.139	0.470	<0.001				
Active smoker	0.773	0.268	2.070	0.618				
Former smoker	0.352	0.105	1.000	0.065				
Myocardial infraction in patient history	1.495	0.780	2.840	0.221				
Heart failure	0.861	0.467	1.560	0.625				
Leukemia	4.333	1.092	17.900	0.036				
Solid malignant disease without metastases	0.532	0.217	1.200	0.144				
Solid malignant disease with metastases	<0.001	<0.001	>1000	0.984				
Lymphoma	<0.001	<0.001	>1000	0.987				
Lenght of hospital stay	1.006	0.994	1.020	0.333				

OR: Odds Ratio; 95% CI: Confidence Interval; NG: Nagelkerke pseudo R2; LR: Likelihood Ratio; AIC: Akaike Information Criterion; ICU: intensive care unit; ALP: alkaline phosphatase; Diabetes-1:diabetes mellitus type 1, including LADA; Diabetes-2: diabetes mellitus type 2 treated with oral medications; Diabetes-3: diabetes mellitus type 2 treated with insulin; Diabtes-4: prediabetes; Diabtes-5: gestational diabetes; COPD: chronic obstructive pulmonary disease; TIA: transient ischemic attack.

Table 6. The best models to predict nesscesity of mechanical ventilation in COVID-19 tested on larger groups of patients.

Mechanical Ventilation								
	OR	95% CI		p-Value	Sample Size n	NG	LR p-Value	AIC
Variables		25%	75%					
Model: albumin+ALP	50.933	11.113	253.280	<0.0001	459	0.298	<0.0001	507.8
ALP	0.998	0.994	1.000	0.121				
albumin	0.244	0.154	0.380	<0.0001				
Hypertension	1.334	0.810	2.210	0.259				
Diabetes-1	0.244	0.012	1.590	0.209				
Diabetes-2	1.331	0.723	2.440	0.356				
Diabetes-3	2.102	0.828	5.330	0.115				
Diabetes-4	2.232	0.582	8.530	0.233				
Diabetes-5	<0.001	<0.001	<0.001	0.997				
Asthma	1.342	0.404	4.180	0.616				
COPD	0.410	0.080	1.610	0.230				
Dementia	0.057	0.008	0.220	<0.001				
Stroke/TIA in patient history	0.735	0.287	1.760	0.502				
Chronic kiedney disease	0.270	0.131	0.530	<0.001				
Active smoker	0.765	0.208	2.500	0.668				
Former smoker	0.211	0.043	0.760	0.030				
Myocardial infraction in patient history	1.622	0.751	3.500	0.216				
Heart failure	0.649	0.309	1.320	0.241				
Leukemia	1.515	0.266	7.180	0.611				
Solid malignant disease without metastases	0.739	0.260	1.970	0.555				
Solid malignant disease with metastases	<0.001	<0.001	>1000	0.987				
Lymphoma	<0.001	<0.001	>1000	0.988				
Lenght of hospital stay	1.005	0.991	1.020	0.497				
	OR	95% CI		p-Value	Sample Size n	NG	LR p-Value	AIC
Variables		25%	75%					
Model: albumin	23.245	6.524	86.500	<0.0001	621	0.266	<0.0001	657.3
albumin	0.284	0.192	0.410	<0.0001				
Hypertension	1.228	0.794	1.900	0.356				
Diabetes-1	0.233	0.012	1.360	0.180				
Diabetes-2	1.677	0.990	2.830	0.053				
Diabetes-3	2.286	1.043	4.980	0.037				
Diabetes-4	2.721	0.826	8.980	0.095				
Diabetes-5	<0.001	<0.001	>1000	0.994				
Asthma	1.572	0.627	3.820	0.322				
COPD	0.512	0.142	1.610	0.273				
Dementia	0.072	0.016	0.220	<0.001				
Stroke/TIA in patient history	0.800	0.351	1.720	0.577				
Chronic kiedney disease	0.294	0.157	0.530	<0.001				
Active smoker	0.731	0.243	2.000	0.556				
Former smoker	0.356	0.104	1.030	0.073				
Myocardial infraction in patient history	1.686	0.880	3.210	0.112				
Heart failure	0.647	0.345	1.190	0.167				
Leukemia	1.770	0.399	7.030	0.426				
Solid malignant disease without metastases	0.488	0.191	1.120	0.108				
Solid malignant disease with metastases	<0.001	<0.001	>1000	0.984				
Lymphoma	<0.001	<0.001	>1000	0.987				
Lenght of hospital stay	1.000	0.989	1.010	0.953				

OR: Odds Ratio; 95% CI: Confidence Interval; NG: Nagelkerke pseudo R2; LR: Likelihood Ratio; AIC: Akaike Information Criterion; ALP: alkaline phosphatase; Diabetes-1:diabetes mellitus type 1, including LADA; Diabetes-2: diabetes mellitus type 2 treated with oral medications; Diabetes-3: diabetes mellitus type 2 treated with insulin; Diabtes-4: prediabetes; Diabtes-5: gestational diabetes; COPD: chronic obstructive pulmonary disease; TIA: transient ischemic attack.

Table 7. The best models to predict fatal outcomes in COVID-19 tested on larger groups of patients.

Fatal Outcome

Variables	OR	95% CI 25%	75%	p-Value	Sample Size n	NG	LR p-Value	AIC
Model: albumin+TBIL	26.886	7.227	105.600	<0.0001	582	0.291	<0.0001	645
TBIL	1.657	1.249	2.290	0.001				
albumin	0.229	0.151	0.340	<0.0001				
Hypertension	1.538	0.982	2.420	0.061				
Diabetes-1	0.800	0.159	3.190	0.764				
Diabetes-2	1.814	1.071	3.070	0.026				
Diabetes-3	1.723	0.819	3.580	0.146				
Diabetes-4	3.292	0.895	11.440	0.063				
Diabetes-5	<0.001	<0.001	>1000	0.984				
Asthma	1.191	0.432	3.040	0.723				
COPD	0.806	0.259	2.360	0.700				
Dementia	1.473	0.709	3.070	0.298				
Stroke/TIA in patient history	0.916	0.449	1.820	0.804				
Chronic kiedney disease	0.614	0.354	1.050	0.077				
Active smoker	1.110	0.405	2.880	0.835				
Former smoker	0.818	0.283	2.200	0.699				
Myocardial infraction in patient history	2.904	1.609	5.310	<0.001				
Heart failure	1.313	0.750	2.290	0.337				
Leukemia	6.608	1.617	30.450	0.010				
Solid malignant disease without metastases	1.017	0.443	2.240	0.967				
Solid malignant disease with metastases	0.286	0.065	1.010	0.068				
Lymphoma	1.895	0.338	8.780	0.431				
Lenght of hospital stay	0.974	0.960	0.990	<0.001				
Variables	OR	CI 95% 25%	75%	p-Value	Sample Size n	NG	LR p-Value	AIC
Model: albumin+AST	38.776	10.422	152.550	<0.0001	603	0.305	<0.0001	661.5
albumin	0.213	0.140	0.310	<0.0001				
AST	1.003	1.001	1.010	0.008				
Hypertension	1.573	1.009	2.460	0.046				
Diabetes-1	1.021	0.276	3.450	0.973				
Diabetes-2	1.685	1.007	2.810	0.046				
Diabetes-3	1.533	0.724	3.200	0.258				
Diabetes-4	3.133	0.838	11.120	0.079				
Diabetes-5	<0.001	<0.001	>1000	0.980				
Asthma	1.011	0.363	2.600	0.983				
COPD	0.823	0.267	2.390	0.725				
Dementia	1.550	0.749	3.220	0.237				
Stroke/TIA in patient history	0.925	0.454	1.840	0.827				
Chronic kiedney disease	0.717	0.414	1.220	0.228				
Active smoker	1.267	0.484	3.190	0.621				
Former smoker	0.693	0.250	1.780	0.461				
Myocardial infraction in patient history	2.751	1.542	4.970	0.001				
Heart failure	1.520	0.882	2.610	0.129				
Leukemia	6.975	1.720	32.450	0.008				
Solid malignant disease without metastases	1.250	0.566	2.690	0.572				
Solid malignant disease with metastases	0.537	0.159	1.640	0.289				
Lymphoma	1.829	0.331	8.470	0.454				
Lenght of hospital stay	0.975	0.962	0.990	<0.001				

OR: Odds Ratio; 95% CI: Confidence Interval; NG: Nagelkerke pseudo R2; LR: Likelihood Ratio; AIC: Akaike Information Criterion; ICU: intensive care unit; TBIL: total bilirubin; AST: aspartate aminotransferase; Diabetes-1:diabetes mellitus type 1, including LADA; Diabates-2: diabetes mellitus type 2 treated with oral medications; Diabetes-3: diabetes mellitus type 2 treated with insulin; Diabtes-4: prediabetes; Diabtes-5: gestational diabetes; COPD: chronic obstructive pulmonary disease; TIA: transient ischemic attack.

Within the models predicting the risk of ICU admission, which revealed the greatest impact on final outcome, the most important was hypoalbuminemia (OR < 0.3, $p < 0.0001$ for both models, Table 5). This time, despite the larger group of patients analyzed in the study, the model including ALP achieved better results than the model containing albumin as the only laboratory parameter, according to AIC. Moreover, the lack of statistical significance of ALP was confirmed. The better accuracy of the model containing ALP may result from the consideration of an additional parameter and a certain cooperation of ALP and albumin. Their reduced values may indicate cachexia and malnutrition.

Regarding mechanical ventilation as an endpoint, the reduced albumin level was assessed as the most powerful predictor in the models (Table 6).

The best model to predict COVID-19-related death became the one including albumin and TBIL, with albumin significance at the level of OR 0.229, $p < 0.0001$, and TBIL OR 1.657, $p = 0.001$ (Table 7). The model analyzing albumin and AST accompanied by other potential risk factors presented slightly worse according to AIC, but again both laboratory tests had influence (albumin OR 0.213, $p < 0.0001$, AST OR 1.003, $p = 0.008$, Table 7). Figure 1 shows the relationships between the best models for all endpoints.

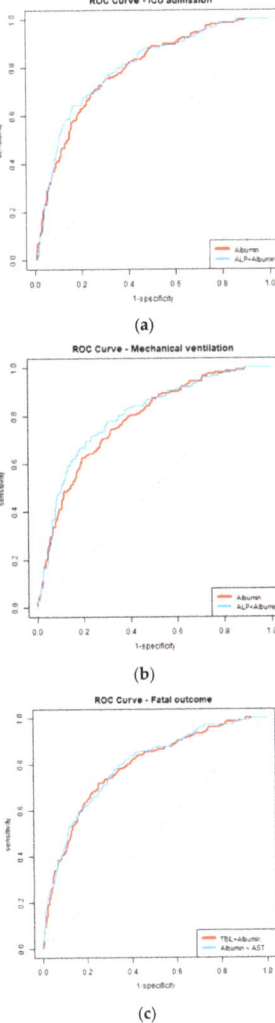

Figure 1. ROC curves presenting relationships between best models for endpoints (**a**) ICU admission, (**b**) mechanical ventilation, and (**c**) fatal outcome. The models, apart from the laboratory parameters, were adjusted for hypertension, diabetes, asthma, COPD, dementia, stroke/TIA in patient history, chronic kidney disease, myocardial infarction in patient history, heart failure, leukemia, lymphoma and solid malignant disease, smoking history and length of hospital stay.

4. Discussion

COVID-19, since it arose in Wuhan, China, has become a major public health concern all over the world. Early recognition of the severe course is an exclusive problem that is of vital importance for the management and use of medical facilities. In this situation, the search for a reliable combination of laboratory parameters that can be prognostic factors is definitely justified.

Lately, it has become evident that liver abnormalities are present in a relevant proportion of COVID-19 patients and correlate with worse outcomes [27]. The pattern of liver injury is predominantly hepatocellular or mixed-type and presents as aminotransferases and GGT elevation [21–24]. Nevertheless, we still do not have a sufficient explanation for this phenomenon. Direct viral effects on the liver have been discussed [12–14,17,28–30] since ACE2 is expressed in a subset of cholangiocytes, while expression in hepatocytes is low [12–14]. However, findings regarding the increased expression of ACE2 in liver cells due to hypoxia and inflammatory conditions should be mentioned [31,32]. Further potential mechanisms include liver damage through ACE2 receptors expressed in endothelial cells [33], but it has been confirmed that ACE2 is absent in sinusoidal endothelial cells [17]. The contribution of the CD47 receptor and the interactions between the L-SIGN receptor and ACE2 are other theories that should be mentioned [15,16]. Considering aminotranses, we need to note that the source of the elevated AST may be not the liver but the muscle or cardiac injury, which was suggested previously [34]. A study performed by Bloom et al. showed that there is moderate correlation between muscle injury markers such as creatine kinase, lactate dehydrogenase and AST elevation [35]. On the other hand, drug-induced liver injury is a possible contributing factor, based on recent studies. In the present research, we used only baseline parameters for prognostication, which allowed us to exclude the hepatotoxic potential of a wide array of drugs (e.g., redemsivir) used to treat COVID-19, mostly in off-label fashion. However, since many patients have chronic diseases, it is likely that chronic medications are taken. Therefore, in our multivariate models, we considered comorbidities, assessed their impact on the final value of the model and compared them with the influence of considered laboratory tests.

At the time of hospital admission, patients presented with liver biochemistry abnormalities 38.9% of AST, 29.3% of ALT, 33.2% of GGT, 21.1% of albumin, 6.7% of TBIL and 6.2% of ALP (Table 2).

The increased values of AST and ALT have already been widely commented on in the literature.

Lei et al. [9] reported a connection between liver injury based on markers of hepatic injury and inpatient mortality, specifically an association between AST abnormality and risk of death during hospitalization. Ramachandran et al. [36] claimed that elevated AST or ALT levels among hospitalized COVID-19 patients were associated with higher rates of mechanical ventilation but were not significant independent predictors of more severe disease. Pazgan-Simon et al. presented a rife elevation of ALT and AST at baseline, with no correlation with higher mortality [22]. In our cohort, AST was the most frequently elevated liver-related parameter, consistent with previously reported results. It has a significant predictive value for death in the course of COVID-19, but in the studied model, the presence of myocardial infarction in the patient's history was more statistically significant ($p = 0.008$, OR 1.006 vs. $p = 0.003$, OR 2.805, respectively). That could bring us to the conclusion that AST may be elevated due to extrahepatic causes, such as exacerbation of previously existing coronary artery disease (CAD) already described in COVID-19 patients [37] or be the result of liver damage caused by chronic statin use due to CAD. AST in combination with TBIL outperformed the model with NLR, according to the AIC, but in this case, again, the most important factor in the model was myocardial infarction in the past ($p = 0.003$, OR 1.446 vs. $p = 0.038$, OR 1.0004 for AST, $p = 0.023$, OR 1.068 for TBIL). Nevertheless, it should be noted that elevated TBIL and AST levels on admission are independently associated with in-hospital death in patients with COVID-19.

ALT elevation is predominantly observed in hepatocellular injuries. Viral hepatitis classically leads to an ALT variation, which has also been reported in many studies focused on COVID-19 as more common than ALP or TBIL elevation but less common than AST, which does not match the viral pattern [21,24,35,38–40]. Bloom et al. [35] proved a strong correlation between AST and ALT, which may suggest that real hepatocellular injury is a predominant source of aminotransferase elevation. That conclusion is in line with the theory of cytokine-mediated injury or hypoxia proposed not only for COVID-19 [17,35,41] but also for influenza [42]. In our study, elevated ALT was observed in 29.3% of patients at baseline, which is comparable to the previously mentioned papers. In each model, ALT was not independently associated with the final outcome, besides combination with AST predicting death, in which it achieved significance at the level of $p = 0.026$, OR 0.986. This finding may support the theory that AST has a source other than the liver and that deviations in AST and ALT in COVID-19 patients are unrelated.

Hypoalbuminemia is a typical trait of all severely ill patients and is often related to inflammatory diseases, mainly due to increased vascular permeability (with increased albumin distribution volume) and a shortened albumin half-life. A low albumin level is a negative prognostic indication in hyperinflammatory conditions such as trauma, shock or infection and has been linked to poor outcomes and a shorter life expectancy [43]. The processes causing hypoalbuminemia in COVID-19 have not yet been fully investigated and described. Albumin is produced in the liver, but it has been subject to dispute as to whether its insufficiency in COVID-19 could be caused by liver dysfunction. According to the study performed by Huang et al. [44], this occurrence cannot be explained solely by liver damage as a result of hepatocellular dysfunction; nonetheless, they did not find any correlation between AST and ALT elevation and worse outcomes, which might be explained by population differences.

The literature often addresses hypoalbuminemia in severe COVID-19 [24,45,46], but the prognostic value of albumin is still underestimated. According to our research, lower albumin levels on admission can predict COVID-19 outcomes irrespective of most co-morbidities and better than NLR. Our results emphasize the remarkable effectiveness of albumin as a predictor of intubation necessity. Models tested on a smaller group of patients $n = 401$, which included albumin, turned out to be a better indicator of COVID-19 severity than the NLR for all endpoints and, along with TBIL, the best model to predict the risk of death, which aligns with Weber and colleagues' findings [24]. Similarly, hypoalbuminemia, in combination with variation in ALP, became the best combination to assess the risk of a patient's admission to the ICU.

The albumin level confirmed its prognostic efficiency during testing the models on larger groups of patients (Tables 5–7).

Moreover, according to the results of our study, attention should be paid to the assessment of TBIL and AST levels, whose significance was confirmed during testing on larger samples (Table 7). Although some of the variables considered exceeded their importance, each of them turned out to be significant, so they can be independent predictors of death in the course of COVID-19, working better when assessed in combination with albumin.

The majority of the available data show that the cholestatic pattern of injury is less common in COVID-19 patients than AST and ALT, but mildly raised GGT levels can be seen in up to 50% of patients [7,21–24,35,38–40]. In our study, GGT, ALP and TBIL were varied in 33.2%, 6.2% and 6.7% of patients, respectively.

GGT elevation and its predictive value in terms of COVID-19 severity have been widely commented upon recently. Shao et al. reported that elevated GGT and CRP levels were associated with a longer hospital stay [47]. Kasapoglu and colleagues determined that elevated serum GGT levels, but not aminotransferases, at admission were associated with the increased risk of ICU admission and mortality [48], while Weber et al. claimed that AST, ALT, GGT and albumin correlated strongly with COVID-19-related death [24]. Our results show that, despite the fact that elevated GGT is frequently observed at baseline, it is not the best predictor for COVID-19 severity. Elevated ALP levels are rather rare among patients admitted to hospital for COVID-19, and worldwide prevalence reaches 4% [21,24,35]. In our study, abnormal ALP was observed in a similar percentage. Although uncommon, it should not be neglected. Da et al., in their study, assessed the effect of cholestasis, defined as the serum ALP level > 3x upper normal limits (UNL), on the mortality of COVID-19 patients [49]. Our research did not reveal any statistically significant effect of ALP on COVID-19 severity, neither in models with ALP alone nor in different combinations, tested both, on sample $n = 401$ or $n = 459$ (Tables 3, 5 and 6). Consideration of an extra parameter, as well as a certain corporation of ALP and albumin, whose lower levels may suggest cachexia and malnutrition, could result in improved accuracy of the model comprising ALP (Tables 4–6).

Bilirubin, a natural end product of haeme catabolism, has long been recognized as a protective molecule with powerful antioxidant, anti-inflammatory, and other bioactivities [50]. Liu et al. [51] observed that a low percentage of COVID-19 patients had elevated bilirubin levels, and this group tended to have a worse outcome and a more severe illness. Furthermore, those with greater TBIL levels at admission had a higher mortality risk. Ding et al. [52] found that abnormal AST and direct bilirubin baseline and peak are associated with in-hospital fatal outcomes. Weber et al. [24] claimed that TBIL elevation was the most predictive single factor of COVID-19-related death. In our study, the most influential singular factor remained hypoalbuminemia, but hypoalbuminemia and TBIL elevation on admission became the best predictive model for in-hospital mortality due to COVID-19. Moreover, it is necessary to consider the predictive ability of the TBIL and AST combination, which value exceeded the model for NLR and the fact that the role of each parameter in the model also proves to have a significant impact on final fatal outcome.

Referring to the observed impact of comorbidities and potential risk factors, the opposite effect of chronic kidney disease on the risk of admission to the ICU and intubation was noted. In the analysis with the endpoint of death due to COVID-19, chronic kidney disease did not show statistical significance; however, the OR also took a value < 1 (Table 7, Supplementary Materials Tables S1–S22). This observation is in contrast to the currently available data [53,54]. The reason for this unexpected remark may be the sample size and the precise group of patients who had performed admission tests. Similar observations were made for smoking history (Tables 5 and 6), contrary to popular claims [37,55]. Dementia was shown to be adversely linked with the risk of ICU admission and invasive respiratory support in our cohort, but not with the risk of mortality due to SARS-CoV-2 infection (OR > 1, Table 7). Although the lack of significance may be due to the small size of the research group, the tendency of dementia to indicate COVID-19-related death is visible and consistent with previous observations [56]. CVD and type 2 diabetes mellitus are well-known risk factors for the severe course of COVID-19, and our survey for these comorbidities is compatible [57,58]. Leukemia was also significantly associated with mortality, in line with earlier considerations [59], and our group had a strong influence on the risk of admission to the ICU.

In this research, patients with chronic liver diseases known as chronic hepatitis, cirrhosis and fatty liver were excluded from the analysis. This allowed us for an objective assessment of the liver function of COVID-19 patients on admission, but at the same time made it impossible to investigate in depth the impact of these comorbidities on the severe course of the disease. However, this influence was reported previously by Galiero et al. in a large multicenter study [60].

Our study had several limitations. First, due to the retrospective nature of the study, the results of the laboratory tests on admission were incomplete. This caused a constraint of the sample to $n = 401$ during the creation of adequate and reliable models that were later implemented on the entire group of patients included in the study ($n = 2109$). Second, we investigated test results obtained at admission to the hospital, which caused an inability to analyze further fluctuations in the parameters in the course of the disease. Moreover, in our study, we did not include the international normalized ratio (INR), which could be a useful tool to assess liver function and to complete our conclusions. In our study, we excluded patients with chronic liver diseases, which did not allow us to evaluate how SARS-CoV-2 infection affects disease progression or how the deterioration of liver functioning in these cases might affect the course of COVID-19. Finally, because the study was single-center, a certain selectivity of the analyzed group may have resulted in bias. Therefore, prospective, long-term studies are necessary to verify the validity of our observations and conclusions.

5. Conclusions

In our study, we attempted to find predictive factors for the severe course of SARS-CoV-2 infection, which is important for risk classification, optimizing hospital resource redistribution, and guiding healthcare strategies.

Our observations emphasize that hypoalbuminemia is a strong predictor of severe COVID-19 course and, in combination with AST or TBIL, has a remarkable association with mortality. This is the most important finding for clinicians because the assessment of the albumin, AST and TBIL levels at admission is an inexpensive, quick test that can be performed in most patients and allows for a more accurate prognosis in the course of SARS-CoV-2 infection.

Moreover, based on our results, we suspect that the liver may not be the source of the elevated AST level, which is often observed in COVID-19 patients. Deviated AST on admission should draw our attention to the feasible risk of exacerbation of CVD and cannot be underestimated; however, further research is required to fully explore this assumption.

Despite the presence of abundant ACE-2 receptors in cholangiocytes, the parameters associated with cholestasis did not appear to be useful in the early risk assessment of severe COVID-19. GGT and ALP were not found to be predictors of worse outcomes; nonetheless, elevated TBIL levels, although rare, are a significant predictor of death in the course of SARS-CoV-2 infection.

Overall, the early determination of biochemical parameters in COVID-19 patients can provide important prognostic information. Decreased albumin, high AST and TBIL levels should be alarming as potentially associated with a severe course of the disease.

Supplementary Materials: The following supporting information can be downloaded at: https://www.mdpi.com/article/10.3390/jcm11154490/s1; Table S1: Model for NLR adjusted for comorbidities and potential risk factors, Table S2: Model for TBIL adjusted for comorbidities and potential risk factors, Table S3: Model for ALP adjusted for comorbidities and potential risk factors, Table S4: Model for ALT adjusted for comorbidities and potential risk factors, Table S5: Model for AST adjusted for comorbidities and potential risk factors, Table S6: Model for GGT adjusted for comorbidities and potential risk factors, Table S7: Model for albumin adjusted for comorbidities and potential risk factors, Table S8: Model for ALP and albumin adjusted for comorbidities and potential risk factors, Table S9: Model for TBIL and albumin adjusted for comorbidities and potential risk factors, Table S10. Model for ALT and albumin adjusted for comorbidities and potential risk factors, Table S11. Model for AST and albumin adjusted for comorbidities and potential risk factors, Table S12: Model for GGT and TBIL adjusted for comorbidities and potential risk factors, Table S13: Model for GGT and ALP adjusted for comorbidities and potential risk factors, Table S14. Model for GGT and ALT adjusted for comorbidities and potential risk factors, Table S15: Model for GGT and AST adjusted for comorbidities and potential risk factors, Table S16: Model for GGT and albumin adjusted for comorbidities and potential risk factors, Table S17: Model for ALT and AST adjusted for comorbidities and potential risk factors, Table S18: Model for ALP and AST adjusted for comorbidities and potential risk factors, Table S19: Model for TBIL and AST adjusted for comorbidities and potential risk factors, Table S20: Model for ALT and ALP adjusted for comorbidities and potential risk factors, Table S21: Model for TBIL and ALT adjusted for comorbidities and potential risk factors, Table S22: Model for TBIL and ALT adjusted for comorbidities and potential risk factors.

Author Contributions: Conceptualization: U.T.; Data acquisition: U.T., K.K. (Krzysztof Kaliszewski), A.K. and K.K. (Krzysztof Kujawa); Formal analysis: U.T., K.K. (Krzysztof Kaliszewski), A.K. and K.K. (Krzysztof Kujawa); Investigation: U.T., K.K. (Krzysztof Kaliszewski), A.K. and K.K. (Krzysztof Kujawa); Methodology: U.T., K.K. (Krzysztof Kaliszewski), A.K. and K.K. (Krzysztof Kujawa); Project administration: U.T. and K.K. (Krzysztof Kaliszewski); Resources: U.T., K.K. (Krzysztof Kaliszewski),

Ł.N., K.S.-S., M.S. (Maciej Sroczyński), M.S. (Monika Sępek), A.D. (Agata Dudek), D.D., M.T., D.G., J.G., T.M., J.M., V.K., R.S., M.M., A.Z.-Z., K.L., K.K.-P., A.M.-W., M.P. (Michał Pomorski), M.P. (Marcin Protasiewicz), J.S. and B.A.; Supervision: U.T., K.K. (Krzysztof Kaliszewski), A.D. (Adrian Doroszko), K.M. and E.A.J.; Validation: U.T., K.K. (Krzysztof Kaliszewski) and A.K.; Writing the original draft: U.T., A.K. and K.K. (Krzysztof Kaliszewski); Writing, reviewing and editing: U.T., K.K. (Krzysztof Kaliszewski), A.K. and K.K. (Krzysztof Kujawa). All authors have read and agreed to the published version of the manuscript.

Funding: This research received no external funding.

Institutional Review Board Statement: The study was conducted according to the guidelines of the Declaration of Helsinki and approved by the Bioethics Committee of Wroclaw Medical University, Wroclaw, Poland (Signature number: KB-444/2021).

Informed Consent Statement: All patients provided informed consent, which stipulated that results may be used for research purposes.

Data Availability Statement: The datasets used and/or analyzed during the current study are available from the corresponding author upon reasonable request.

Acknowledgments: The authors are grateful to all the staff and the patients at the study center who contributed to this work.

Conflicts of Interest: The authors declare no conflict of interest.

References

1. World Health Organization. *Coronavirus Disease 2019 (COVID 19). Situation Report-72*; World Health Organization: Geneva, Switzerland, 2020.
2. World Health Organization. *Coronavirus Disease (COVID-19) Pandemic*; World Health Organization: Geneva, Switzerland, 2020; Volume 2020.
3. European Centre for Disease Prevention and Control. *Novel Coronavirus in China*; World Health Organization: Geneva, Switzerland, 2020.
4. Wang, D.; Hu, B.; Hu, C.; Zhu, F.; Liu, X.; Zhang, J.; Wang, B.; Xiang, H.; Cheng, Z.; Xiong, Y.; et al. Clinical Characteristics of 138 Hospitalized Patients with 2019 Novel Coronavirus–Infected Pneumonia in Wuhan, China. *JAMA* **2020**, *323*, 1061–1069. [CrossRef]
5. Gupta, A.; Madhavan, M.; Sehgal, K.; Nair, N.; Mahajan, S.; Sehrawat, T.; Bikdeli, B.; Ahluwalia, N.; Ausiello, J.; Wan, E.; et al. Extrapulmonary manifestations of COVID-19. *Nat. Med.* **2020**, *26*, 1017–1032. [CrossRef]
6. Zarifian, A.; Zamiri Bidary, M.; Arekhi, S.; Rafiee, M.; Gholamalizadeh, H.; Amiriani, A.; Ghaderi, M.S.; Khadem-Rezaiyan, M.; Amini, M.; Ganji, A. Gastrointestinal and hepatic abnormalities in patients with confirmed COVID-19: A systematic review and meta-analysis. *J. Med. Virol.* **2020**, *93*, 336–350. [CrossRef]
7. Cai, Q.; Huang, D.; Yu, H.; Zhu, Z.; Xia, Z.; Su, Y.; Li, Z.; Zhou, G.; Gou, J.; Qu, J.; et al. COVID-19: Abnormal Liver Function Tests. *J. Hepatol.* **2020**, *73*, 566–574. [CrossRef]
8. Zhang, C.; Shi, L.; Wang, F.-S. Liver Injury in COVID-19: Management and Challenges. *Lancet Gastroenterol. Hepatol.* **2020**, *5*, 428–430. [CrossRef]
9. Lei, F.; Liu, Y.; Zhou, F.; Qin, J.; Zhang, P.; Zhu, L.; Zhang, X.; Cai, J.; Lin, L.; Ouyang, S.; et al. Longitudinal Association between Markers of Liver Injury and Mortality in COVID-19 in China. *Hepatology* **2020**, *72*, 389–398. [CrossRef]
10. Harapan, H.; Fajar, J.; Supriono, S.; Soegiarto, G.; Wulandari, L.; Seratin, F.; Prayudi, N.; Dewi, D.; Monica Elsina, M.; Atamou, L.; et al. The prevalence, predictors and outcomes of acute liver injury among patients with COVID-19: A systematic review and meta-analysis. *Rev. Med. Virol.* **2021**, *32*, 2304. [CrossRef]
11. Hoffmann, M.; Kleine-Weber, H.; Schroeder, S.; Krüger, N.; Herrler, T.; Erichsen, S.; Schiergens, T.; Herrler, G.; Wu, N.; Nitsche, A.; et al. SARS-CoV-2 Cell Entry Depends on ACE2 and TMPRSS2 and Is Blocked by a Clinically Proven Protease Inhibitor. *Cell* **2020**, *181*, 271–280. [CrossRef]
12. Qi, F.; Qian, S.; Zhang, S.; Zhang, Z. Single Cell RNA Sequencing of 13 Human Tissues Identify Cell Types and Receptors of Human Coronaviruses. *Biochem. Biophys. Res. Commun.* **2020**, *526*, 135–140. [CrossRef]
13. Hamming, I.; Timens, W.; Bulthuis, M.; Lely, A.; Navis, G.; van Goor, H. Tissue Distribution of ACE2 Protein, the Functional Receptor for SARS Coronavirus. A First Step in Understanding SARS Pathogenesis. *J. Pathol.* **2004**, *203*, 631–637. [CrossRef]
14. Uhlen, M.; Fagerberg, L.; Hallstrom, B.M.; Lindskog, C.; Oksvold, P.; Mardinoglu, A.; Sivertsson, A.; Kampf, C.; Sjostedt, E.; Asplund, A.; et al. Tissue-Based Map of the Human Proteome. *Science* **2015**, *347*, 1260419. [CrossRef]
15. Kondo, Y.; Larabee, J.; Gao, L.; Shi, H.; Shao, B.; Hoover, C.; McDaniel, J.; Ho, Y.; Silasi-Mansat, R.; Archer-Hartmann, S.; et al. L-SIGN is a receptor on liver sinusoidal endothelial cells for SARS-CoV-2 virus. *JCI Insight* **2021**, *6*, e148995. [CrossRef]
16. Wang, K.; Chen, W.; Zhang, Z.; Deng, Y.; Lian, J.; Du, P.; Wei, D.; Zhang, Y.; Sun, X.; Gong, L.; et al. CD147-spike protein is a novel route for SARS-CoV-2 infection to host cells. *Signal Transduct. Target. Ther.* **2020**, *5*, 283. [CrossRef] [PubMed]

17. Sun, J.; Aghemo, A.; Forner, A.; Valenti, L. COVID-19 and Liver Disease. *Liver Int.* **2020**, *40*, 1278–1281. [CrossRef] [PubMed]
18. Vranić, L.; Radovan, A.; Poropat, G.; Mikolašević, I.; Milić, S. Non-Alcoholic Fatty Liver Disease and COVID-19–Two Pandemics Hitting at the Same Time. *Medicina* **2020**, *57*, 1057. [CrossRef] [PubMed]
19. Phipps, M.M.; Barraza, L.H.; LaSota, E.D.; Sobieszczyk, M.E.; Pereira, M.R.; Zheng, E.X.; Fox, A.N.; Zucker, J.; Verna, E.C. Acute Liver Injury in COVID-19: Prevalence and Association with Clinical Outcomes in a Large U.S. Cohort. *Hepatol.* **2020**, *72*, 807–817. [CrossRef] [PubMed]
20. Da, B.L.; Kushner, T.; El Halabi, M.; Paka, P.; Khalid, M.; Uberoi, A.; Lee, B.T.; Perumalswami, P.V.; Rutledge, S.M.; Schiano, T.D.; et al. Liver Injury in Patients Hospitalized with Coronavirus Disease 2019 Correlates with Hyperinflammatory Response and Elevated Interleukin-6. *Hepatol. Commun.* **2020**, *5*, 177–188. [CrossRef]
21. Wijarnpreecha, K.; Ungprasert, P.; Panjawatanan, P.; Harnois, D.M.; Zaver, H.B.; Ahmed, A.; Kim, D. COVID-19 and Liver Injury: A Meta-Analysis. *Eur. J. Gastroenterol. Hepatol.* **2020**, *33*, 990–995. [CrossRef]
22. Pazgan-Simon, M.; Serafińska, S.; Kukla, M.; Kucharska, M.; Zuwała-Jagiełło, J.; Buczyńska, I.; Zielińska, K.; Simon, K. Liver Injury in Patients with COVID-19 without Underlying Liver Disease. *J. Clin. Med.* **2022**, *11*, 308. [CrossRef]
23. Guan, W.; Ni, Z.; Hu, Y.; Liang, W.; Ou, C.; He, J.; Liu, L.; Shan, H.; Lei, C.; Hui, D.S.C.; et al. Clinical Characteristics of Coronavirus Disease 2019 in China. *N. Engl. J. Med.* **2020**, *382*, 1708–1720. [CrossRef] [PubMed]
24. Weber, S.; Hellmuth, J.C.; Scherer, C.; Muenchhoff, M.; Mayerle, J.; Gerbes, A.L. Liver Function Test Abnormalities at Hospital Admission Are Associated with Severe Course of SARS-CoV-2 Infection: A Prospective Cohort Study. *Gut* **2021**, *70*, 1925–1932. [CrossRef] [PubMed]
25. Liu, Y.; Du, X.; Chen, J.; Jin, Y.; Peng, L.; Wang, H.H.X.; Luo, M.; Chen, L.; Zhao, Y. Neutrophil-To-Lymphocyte Ratio as an Independent Risk Factor for Mortality in Hospitalized Patients with COVID-19. *J. Infect.* **2020**, *81*, 6–12. [CrossRef] [PubMed]
26. Shastri, M.D.; Shukla, S.D.; Chong, W.C.; KC, R.; Dua, K.; Patel, R.P.; Peterson, G.M.; O'Toole, R.F. Smoking and COVID-19: What We Know so Far. *Respir. Med.* **2021**, *176*, 106237. [CrossRef] [PubMed]
27. Jothimani, D.; Venugopal, R.; Abedin, M.F.; Kaliamoorthy, I.; Rela, M. COVID-19 and the Liver. *J. Hepatol.* **2020**, *73*, 1231–1240. [CrossRef] [PubMed]
28. Bertolini, A.; Peppel, I.P.; Bodewes, F.A.J.A.; Moshage, H.; Fantin, A.; Farinati, F.; Fiorotto, R.; Jonker, J.W.; Strazzabosco, M.; Verkade, H.J.; et al. Abnormal Liver Function Tests in Patients with COVID-19: Relevance and Potential Pathogenesis. *Hepatology* **2020**, *72*, 1864–1872. [CrossRef] [PubMed]
29. Wang, Y.; Liu, S.; Liu, H.; Li, W.; Lin, F.; Jiang, L.; Li, X.; Xu, P.; Zhang, L.; Zhao, L.; et al. SARS-CoV-2 Infection of the Liver Directly Contributes to Hepatic Impairment in Patients with COVID-19. *J. Hepatol.* **2020**, *73*, 807–816. [CrossRef]
30. Zhao, B.; Ni, C.; Gao, R.; Wang, Y.; Yang, L.; Wei, J.; Lv, T.; Liang, J.; Zhang, Q.; Xu, W.; et al. Recapitulation of SARS-CoV-2 Infection and Cholangiocyte Damage with Human Liver Ductal Organoids. *Protein Cell* **2020**, *11*, 771–775. [CrossRef]
31. Paizis, G. Chronic Liver Injury in Rats and Humans Upregulates the Novel Enzyme Angiotensin Converting Enzyme 2. *Gut* **2005**, *54*, 1790–1796. [CrossRef] [PubMed]
32. Gkogkou, E.; Barnasas, G.; Vougas, K.; Trougakos, I.P. Expression Profiling Meta-Analysis of ACE2 and TMPRSS2, the Putative Anti-Inflammatory Receptor and Priming Protease of SARS-CoV-2 in Human Cells, and Identification of Putative Modulators. *Redox Biol.* **2020**, *36*, 101615. [CrossRef]
33. Portincasa, P.; Krawczyk, M.; Machill, A.; Lammert, F.; Di Ciaula, A. Hepatic Consequences of COVID-19 Infection. Lapping or Biting? *European J. Intern. Med.* **2020**, *77*, 18–24. [CrossRef]
34. Fix, O.K.; Hameed, B.; Fontana, R.J.; Kwok, R.M.; McGuire, B.M.; Mulligan, D.C.; Pratt, D.S.; Russo, M.W.; Schilsky, M.L.; Verna, E.C.; et al. Clinical Best Practice Advice for Hepatology and Liver Transplant Providers during the COVID-19 Pandemic: AASLD Expert Panel Consensus Statement. *Hepatology* **2020**, *72*, 287–304. [CrossRef]
35. Bloom, P.P.; Meyerowitz, E.A.; Reinus, Z.; Daidone, M.; Gustafson, J.; Kim, A.Y.; Schaefer, E.; Chung, R.T. Liver Biochemistries in Hospitalized Patients with COVID-19. *Hepatology* **2020**, *73*, 890–900. [CrossRef]
36. Ramachandran, P.; Perisetti, A.; Gajendran, M.; Chakraborti, A.; Narh, J.T.; Goyal, H. Increased Serum Aminotransferase Activity and Clinical Outcomes in Coronavirus Disease 2019. *J. Clin. Exp. Hepatol.* **2020**, *10*, 533–539. [CrossRef] [PubMed]
37. Szarpak, L.; Mierzejewska, M.; Jurek, J.; Kochanowska, A.; Gasecka, A.; Truszewski, Z.; Pruc, M.; Blek, N.; Rafique, Z.; Filipiak, K.J.; et al. Effect of Coronary Artery Disease on COVID-19—Prognosis and Risk Assessment: A Systematic Review and Meta-Analysis. *Biology* **2022**, *11*, 221. [CrossRef] [PubMed]
38. Hundt, M.A.; Deng, Y.; Ciarleglio, M.M.; Nathanson, M.H.; Lim, J.K. Abnormal Liver Tests in COVID-19: A Retrospective Observational Cohort Study of 1,827 Patients in a Major U.S. Hospital Network. *Hepatology* **2020**, *72*, 1169–1176. [CrossRef] [PubMed]
39. Wang, Y.; Shi, L.; Wang, Y.; Yang, H. An Updated Meta-Analysis of AST and ALT Levels and the Mortality of COVID-19 Patients. *Am. J. Emerg. Med.* **2021**, *40*, 208–209. [CrossRef]
40. Hwaiz, R.; Merza, M.; Hamad, B.; HamaSalih, S.; Mohammed, M.; Hama, H. Evaluation of Hepatic Enzymes Activities in COVID-19 Patients. *Int. Immunopharmacol.* **2021**, *97*, 107701. [CrossRef]
41. Nardo, A.D.; Schneeweiss-Gleixner, M.; Bakail, M.; Dixon, E.D.; Lax, S.F.; Trauner, M. Pathophysiological Mechanisms of Liver Injury in COVID-19. *Liver Int.* **2021**, *41*, 20–32. [CrossRef]
42. Papic, N.; Pangercic, A.; Vargovic, M.; Barsic, B.; Vince, A.; Kuzman, I. Liver Involvement during Influenza Infection: Perspective on the 2009 Influenza Pandemic. *Influenza Other Respir. Viruses* **2011**, *6*, 2–5. [CrossRef]

43. Fulks, M.; Stout, R.L.; Dolan, V.F. Albumin and all-cause mortality risk in insurance applicants. *J. Insur. Med.* **2010**, *42*, 11–17.
44. Huang, J.; Cheng, A.; Kumar, R.; Fang, Y.; Chen, G.; Zhu, Y.; Lin, S. Hypoalbuminemia Predicts the Outcome of COVID-19 Independent of Age and Co-Morbidity. *J. Med. Virol.* **2020**, *92*, 2152–2158. [CrossRef]
45. Soetedjo, N.N.M.; Iryaningrum, M.R.; Damara, F.A.; Permadhi, I.; Sutanto, L.B.; Hartono, H.; Rasyid, H. Prognostic Properties of Hypoalbuminemia in COVID-19 Patients: A Systematic Review and Diagnostic Meta-Analysis. *Clin. Nutr. ESPEN* **2021**, *45*, 120–126. [CrossRef]
46. Zhang, Y.; Zheng, L.; Liu, L.; Zhao, M.; Xiao, J.; Zhao, Q. Liver Impairment in COVID-19 Patients: A Retrospective Analysis of 115 Cases from a Single Center in Wuhan City, China. *Liver Int.* **2020**, *40*, 2095–2103. [CrossRef]
47. Shao, T.; Tong, Y.; Lu, S.; Jeyarajan, A.J.; Su, F.; Dai, J.; Shi, J.; Huang, J.; Hu, C.; Wu, L.; et al. Gamma-Glutamyltransferase Elevation Is Frequent in Patients with COVID-19: A Clinical Epidemiologic Study. *Hepatol. Commun.* **2020**, *4*, 1744–1750. [CrossRef]
48. Kasapoglu, B.; Yozgat, A.; Tanoglu, A.; Can, G.; Sakin, Y.S.; Kekilli, M. Gamma-Glutamyl-Transferase May Predict COVID-19 Outcomes in Hospitalised Patients. *Int. J. Clin. Pract.* **2021**, *75*, e14933. [CrossRef]
49. Da, B.L.; Suchman, K.; Roth, N.; Rizvi, A.; Vincent, M.; Trindade, A.J.; Bernstein, D.; Satapathy, S.K. Cholestatic Liver Injury in COVID-19 Is a Rare and Distinct Entity and Is Associated with Increased Mortality. *J. Intern. Med.* **2021**, *290*, 470–472. [CrossRef] [PubMed]
50. Boon, A.-C.; Bulmer, A.C.; Coombes, J.S.; Fassett, R.G. Circulating Bilirubin and Defense against Kidney Disease and Cardiovascular Mortality: Mechanisms Contributing to Protection in Clinical Investigations. *Am. J. Physiol.-Ren. Physiol.* **2014**, *307*, 123–136. [CrossRef]
51. Liu, Z.; Li, J.; Long, W.; Zeng, W.; Gao, R.; Zeng, G.; Chen, D.; Wang, S.; Li, Q.; Hu, D.; et al. Bilirubin Levels as Potential Indicators of Disease Severity in Coronavirus Disease Patients: A Retrospective Cohort Study. *Front. Med.* **2020**, *7*, 598870. [CrossRef] [PubMed]
52. Ding, Z.; Li, G.; Chen, L.; Shu, C.; Song, J.; Wang, W.; Wang, Y.; Chen, Q.; Jin, G.; Liu, T.; et al. Association of Liver Abnormalities with In-Hospital Mortality in Patients with COVID-19. *J. Hepatol.* **2021**, *74*, 1295–1302. [CrossRef]
53. D'Marco, L.; Puchades, M.J.; Romero-Parra, M.; Gimenez-Civera, E.; Soler, M.J.; Ortiz, A.; Gorriz, J.L. Coronavirus Disease 2019 in Chronic Kidney Disease. *Clin. Kidney J.* **2020**, *13*, 297–306. [CrossRef]
54. Council, E.-E.; Ortiz, A.; Cozzolino, M.; Fliser, D.; Fouque, D.; Goumenos, D.; Massy, Z.A.; Rosenkranz, A.R.; Rychlık, I.; Soler, M.J.; et al. Chronic Kidney Disease Is a Key Risk Factor for Severe COVID-19: A Call to Action by the ERA-EDTA. *Nephrol. Dial. Transplant.* **2021**, *36*, 87–94. [CrossRef] [PubMed]
55. Reddy, R.K.; Charles, W.N.; Sklavounos, A.; Dutt, A.; Seed, P.T.; Khajuria, A. The Effect of Smoking on COVID-19 Severity: A Systematic Review and Meta-Analysis. *J. Med. Virol.* **2020**, *93*, 1045–1056. [CrossRef] [PubMed]
56. Tahira, A.C.; Verjovski-Almeida, S.; Ferreira, S.T. Dementia Is an Age-Independent Risk Factor for Severity and Death in COVID-19 Inpatients. *Alzheimer's Dement. J. Alzheimer's Assoc.* **2021**, *17*, 1818–1831. [CrossRef] [PubMed]
57. Barron, E.; Bakhai, C.; Kar, P.; Weaver, A.; Bradley, D.; Ismail, H.; Knighton, P.; Holman, N.; Khunti, K.; Sattar, N.; et al. Associations of Type 1 and Type 2 Diabetes with COVID-19-Related Mortality in England: A Whole-Population Study. *Lancet Diabetes Endocrinol.* **2020**, *8*, 813–822. [CrossRef]
58. Fang, L.; Karakiulakis, G.; Roth, M. Are Patients with Hypertension and Diabetes Mellitus at Increased Risk for COVID-19 Infection? *Lancet Respir. Med.* **2020**, *8*, 21. [CrossRef]
59. Mato, A.R.; Roeker, L.E.; Lamanna, N.; Allan, J.N.; Leslie, L.; Pagel, J.M.; Patel, K.; Osterborg, A.; Wojenski, D.; Kamdar, M.; et al. Outcomes of COVID-19 in Patients with CLL: A Multicenter International Experience. *Blood* **2020**, *136*, 1134–1143. [CrossRef]
60. Galiero, R.; Pafundi, P.; Simeon, V.; Rinaldi, L.; Perrella, A.; Vetrano, E.; Caturano, A.; Alfano, M.; Beccia, D.; Nevola, R.; et al. Impact of chronic liver disease upon admission on COVID-19 in-hospital mortality: Findings from COVOCA study. *PLoS ONE* **2020**, *15*, 0243700. [CrossRef]

Review

Mechanisms Leading to Gut Dysbiosis in COVID-19: Current Evidence and Uncertainties Based on Adverse Outcome Pathways

Laure-Alix Clerbaux [1,*], Julija Fillipovska [2], Amalia Muñoz [3], Mauro Petrillo [4], Sandra Coecke [1], Maria-Joao Amorim [5,6] and Lucia Grenga [7]

[1] European Commission, Joint Research Centre (JRC), 21027 Ispra, Italy
[2] Independent Researcher, 6000 Ohrid, North Macedonia
[3] European Commission, Joint Research Centre (JRC), 2440 Geel, Belgium
[4] Seidor Italy SRL, 20219 Milano, Italy
[5] Instituto Gulbenkian de Ciência, 2780-156 Oeiras, Portugal
[6] Católica Medical School, Católica Biomedical Research Centre, Universidade Católica Portuguesa, 1649-023 Lisbon, Portugal
[7] Département Médicaments et Technologies pour la Santé, Commissariat à l'Énergie Atomique et Aux Énergies Alternatives (CEA), Institut National de Recherche pour l'Agriculture, l'Alimentation et l'Environnement (INRAE), Université Paris-Saclay, 30200 Bagnols-sur-Cèze, France
* Correspondence: laure-alix.clerbaux@ec.europa.eu

Abstract: Alteration in gut microbiota has been associated with COVID-19. However, the underlying mechanisms remain poorly understood. Here, we outlined three potential interconnected mechanistic pathways leading to gut dysbiosis as an adverse outcome following SARS-CoV-2 presence in the gastrointestinal tract. Evidence from the literature and current uncertainties are reported for each step of the different pathways. One pathway investigates evidence that intestinal infection by SARS-CoV-2 inducing intestinal inflammation alters the gut microbiota. Another pathway links the binding of viral S protein to angiotensin-converting enzyme 2 (ACE2) to the dysregulation of this receptor, essential in intestinal homeostasis—notably for amino acid metabolism—leading to gut dysbiosis. Additionally, SARS-CoV-2 could induce gut dysbiosis by infecting intestinal bacteria. Assessing current evidence within the Adverse Outcome Pathway framework justifies confidence in the proposed mechanisms to support disease management and permits the identification of inconsistencies and knowledge gaps to orient further research.

Keywords: SARS-CoV-2 infection; COVID-19; gut dysbiosis; microbiota; gastrointestinal disorders; intestinal inflammation; ACE2 dysregulation

1. Introduction

Coronavirus disease 2019 (COVID-19) caused by severe acute respiratory syndrome coronavirus 2 (SARS-CoV-2) is still a global public health emergency. A better understanding of the mechanisms underlying the progression and severity of the disease is needed. Particularly, COVID-19 is markedly heterogeneous in terms of clinical outcomes, with a high variation at the individual level. Poor clinical outcomes in COVID-19 patients were notably associated with elderliness and certain pre-existing medical conditions, including but not limited to diabetes, cardiovascular diseases, obesity, and high LDH levels [1–5]. Older age and the comorbidities mentioned above are associated with alterations in the gut microbiota [6–8]. Besides, COVID-19 patients exhibit fecal microbiome alterations compared to controls [9–12]. These changes correlated to COVID-19 severity [12]. Gut dysbiosis, defined as a reduction in gut microbiota diversity or the depletion of beneficial bacteria with an enrichment of the pathogenic ones, may alter susceptibility to SARS-CoV-2 infection [13–15]. This is aligned with the evidence that many pathophysiological dimensions of diseases are underpinned by the gut microbiota, especially in chronic inflammatory diseases [16] such as inflammatory bowel diseases (IBD). Although the exact etiologies of IBD remain uncertain, many studies have provided important insights into the central role of gut dysbiosis and barrier dysfunction in inflammatory status [17,18]. The gut microbiota plays an essential role in the education and functions of both the local and systemic immune systems. Besides, emerging evidence has demonstrated important cross-talks between the gut microbiota and many other organs via communication axes such as the gut–lung [19], gut–liver [20,21], and gut–brain [22] axes. Notably, gut dysbiosis during respiratory viral infection has been shown to worsen pulmonary symptoms [23]. Similarly, gut dysbiosis and disrupted intestinal barrier can cause neurological inflammation [22] or hepatic inflammation through the translocation of endotoxins and bacteria via the portal vein [24]. Consistently, taking into account gut microbiome-mediated mechanisms may help depict a comprehensive overview of COVID-19 pathogenesis. Exploring how gut dysbiosis as a pre-existing condition in some COVID-19 patients mechanistically influences the disease progression and impacts the clinical outcomes might help identify high-risk patients, and has been discussed elsewhere [5]. Here, we aim to investigate how SARS-CoV-2 might directly alter the gut microbiota, thus considering gut dysbiosis as a direct consequence of the virus in the gastrointestinal (GI) tract. Recently, animal studies have provided evidence for a direct impact of SARS-CoV-2 infection on the gut microbiota. A study conducted in transgenic mice expressing human ACE2 showed that the gut microbiome is affected by SARS-CoV-2 in a dose-dependent manner after intranasal inoculation [25]. In Syrian hamsters, SARS-CoV-2 infection was associated with mild intestinal inflammation, relative alteration of the intestinal barrier property, and alteration of the gut microbiota [26]. SARS-CoV-2 infection in nonhuman primates was associated with changes in the gut microbiota composition and functional activity [27]. However, despite the dynamic research, the underlying pathways leading to gut dysbiosis in COVID-19 are still poorly understood.

To contribute to deciphering these mechanisms, the Joint Research Centre of the European Commission initiated an interdisciplinary project, the CIAO project, to model the pathogenesis of COVID-19 using the Adverse Outcome Pathway (AOP) framework [28–31]. The AOP approach is well established in regulatory toxicology [32] but is innovatively applied here to a viral disease of high societal relevance. The project relies on the assumption that an AOP-driven organization of the relevant knowledge will improve the integration of the tsunami of data on COVID-19 [28]. The AOP approach does not capture all the details in a biological pathway, but aims for a pragmatic identification of successively linked key events (KE) that represent essential steps in a pathway leading to an adverse outcome [33–36]. A key event describes a measurable and essential change in a biological system that can be quantified in experimental or clinical settings [32]. The AOP framework also provides a structured approach for the evaluation of the level of evidence currently available to ascertain the causal relationships between pairs of successive key events [37]. AOPs do not build on the correlation between two events but gather and weigh the evidence for their causal relationship. Because of this mechanistic and causal description of the pathways, AOPs help elucidate the pathophysiological mechanisms also by learning from other diseases, such as IBD or respiratory virus-related diseases presenting gut dysbiosis. Finally, an AOP integrates knowledge across the different biological levels (from molecular, cellular, tissue, organ, and up to organism level). While research tends to compartmentalize in silos, this pandemic calls for an interdisciplinary integration of data from the different experimental systems. Hence, the AOP approach allows the structured review and organization of rapidly growing relevant *in vitro*, *in vivo*, and clinical data. Assessing the evidence currently available using the AOP framework permits the identification of critical inconsistencies and knowledge gaps guiding future research needs. The AOPs are steered by the Organization for Economic Co-operation and Development (OECD), which maintains a centralized online platform called AOP wiki (https://aopwiki.org/ accessed on 29 June 2022), where information captured in AOPs is openly accessible. Numbers in the text refer to these AOP-wiki pages (Table 1).

Table 1. AOP-wiki pages.

KER1739	https://aopwiki.org/events/1739	accessed on 29 June 2022
KER1738	https://aopwiki.org/events/1738	accessed on 29 June 2022
KER1847	https://aopwiki.org/events/1847	accessed on 29 June 2022
KER1901	https://aopwiki.org/events/1901	accessed on 29 June 2022
KER1493	https://aopwiki.org/events/1493	accessed on 29 June 2022
KER1497	https://aopwiki.org/events/1497	accessed on 29 June 2022
KER1954	https://aopwiki.org/events/1954	accessed on 29 June 2022
KER2311	https://aopwiki.org/events/2311	accessed on 29 June 2022

This study was conducted as part of the CIAO project (https://www.ciao-covid.net/ accessed on 29 June 2022) aiming to provide a holistic overview of the COVID-19 pathogenesis through the Adverse Outcome Pathway framework, offering scientists from different fields an international platform to collaborate across disciplines [1]. Here, we outlined three putative pathways initiated by SARS-CoV-2 presence in the gut leading to gut dysbiosis. We applied the AOP approach to analyze the weight of available evidence supporting the causality of the key event relationships (KER) involved in the proposed pathways. For each causal step, we first described the biological plausibility, then we explored the existing literature and data qualitatively and quantitatively supporting this link, and finally, we highlighted the current inconsistencies, uncertainties, and knowledge gaps. Ultimately, we discussed the potential implication of each pathway for disease management.

2. Enteric SARS-CoV-2 Presence Leads to Intestinal Inflammation Altering Gut Microbiota

2.1. SARS-CoV-2 Entry into Enterocytes Leads to Intestinal Inflammation

The biological plausibility, evidence, and uncertainties for a productive SARS-CoV-2 enteric infection (an active replication in the GI tract) inducing intestinal inflammation are described in detail elsewhere [38]. Briefly, following binding to the ACE2 receptor (KE1739), SARS-CoV-2 enters into enterocytes (KE1738) and might replicate (KE1847) after antagonizing the antiviral response (KE1901). Viral infection induces the secretion of pro-inflammatory mediators (KE1493), which recruit inflammatory cells (KE1497). SARS-CoV-2 enters into enterocytes via binding to the ACE2 receptor and cleavage, preferentially by transmembrane serine protease 2 (TMPRSS2) at the plasma membrane. Enterocytes in the small intestine express the highest levels of ACE2 in the human body [39,40], and co-express TMPRSS2, indicating potential enteric infection [39,41,42]. ACE2-KO intestinal organoids were fully resistant to SARS-CoV-2 infection [43], suggesting that ACE2 is the entry receptor for SARS-CoV-2 in intestinal cells *in vitro*. Following cellular entry, SARS-CoV-2 induces an antiviral response [44]. The timely production of type I interferons by host cells is critical for limiting viral replication and promoting antiviral immunity [45]. While a body of evidence points towards a productive enteric infection, it is not firmly established that SARS-CoV-2 can actively replicate in the human intestine [38]. Specific conditions, such as viral load, comorbidities, age, medication, inflammatory status, fasted–fed status, or pre-existing dysbiosis, might render the GI epithelium permissive to SARS-CoV2 infection [38]. In addition to interferon, viral infection induces the release of pro-inflammatory cytokines, such as interleukins (IL) and tumor necrosis factor (TNF) alpha by epithelial cells [27,46]. Pro-inflammatory signaling recruits immune cells to the gut. This local inflammatory response due to viral entry into cells and potential active replication might alter the gut microbiota (Figure 1).

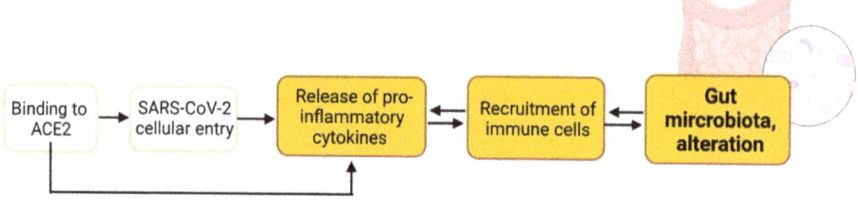

Figure 1. Spike proteins of SARS-CoV-2 virus binding to ACE2 receptor expressed in enterocytes mediates viral entry inducing intestinal inflammation (release of pro-inflammatory mediators and recruitment of inflammatory cells) leading to alteration of gut microbiota. Created with Biorender.com.

2.2. Binding to Enteric ACE2 Leads to Intestinal Inflammation

Functional studies based on colitis animal models have indicated that the modulation of ACE2 expression itself affects the severity of intestinal inflammation. ACE2 deficiency causes enhanced susceptibility to dextran sodium sulfate-induced colitis [47], suggesting that ACE2 plays a protective role in colitis. Moreover, Ang (1–7) treatment alleviates colitis progression, whereas the blockade of Mas aggravates the disease [48], indicating the protective role of the ACE2/Ang (1–7)/Mas axis. In contrast, treatment with the ACE2 inhibitor GL1001 reduces the severity of colitis [49], suggesting that ACE2 plays a pathogenic role in intestinal inflammation. During SARS-CoV-2 infection, the downregulation of ACE2 would potentially result in unopposed functions of Ang II and decreased levels of Ang (1–7), thereby shifting the balance toward the pro-inflammatory side [50,51]. In IBD, reduced small bowel but elevated colonic ACE2 levels are associated with inflammation, suggesting compartmentalization of ACE2-related biology in the small intestine and colon inflammation [52]. Further studies are needed to assess if intestinal ACE2 dysregulation due to the interaction with SARS-CoV-2/S proteins leads to intestinal inflammation.

2.3. Intestinal Inflammation Leads to Alteration of Gut Microbiota

Biological plausibility. Intestinal inflammation is associated with aerobic conditions, biological sources from dying epithelial cells, and mucus thickness, which provide an optimal environment for the growth of microorganisms. Dysbiosis is defined as a reduction in microbial diversity and a combination of the loss of beneficial bacteria and a rise in pathogenic ones (KE1954).

Evidence. Plasma concentrations of inflammatory cytokines correlated with gut microbiota composition in studies on COVID-19 patients [10]. Several studies in other diseases provided evidence that an inflamed gut microenvironment induces gut microbiota alterations [53–57]. The alteration is often characterized by blooms of normally low-abundance and harmful bacterial species (e.g., *Enterobacteriaceae*) that are capable of utilizing nutrients found more abundantly in the inflamed gut, while other families of symbiotic bacteria succumb to the inflammatory environmental changes [53–57].

Feedback loop. A causal role for gut microbes in generating an inflammatory phenotype was demonstrated. Germ-free mice receiving microbial transfers from insulin-resistant mice exhibited more inflammation than mice receiving microbial transfers from controls [58]. In humans, abundant reports highlight the role of gut microbiota in the pathogenesis of inflammatory diseases such as asthma, type 1 and type 2 diabetes mellitus, and obesity [59–61]. Antibiotic-resistant *Klebsiella* species can lead to inflammation in genetically susceptible hosts [62]. Adherent-invasive *E. coli*, commonly reported as enriched in IBD, increases chemokine secretion (IL-8/CCL20 levels). Other *Enterobacteriaceae* species, namely *Citrobacter rodentium* and *Salmonella*, utilize virulence factors to induce intestinal inflammation, which subsequently confers a growth advantage for these pathogens in the intestinal lumen to compete with beneficial bacteria [63–65]. Some bacteria produce short-chain fatty acids with anti-inflammatory properties [66–68]. *Faecalibacterium pausnitizii*, reduced in

IBD [69], convert acetate to butyrate, which facilitates the regeneration of colonocytes, thus maintaining intestinal integrity [49] and the balance between Th7 and Treg cells to prevent intestinal inflammation [70]. The reduction of butyrate-producing bacteria contributes to intestinal inflammation; notably, T_{reg} cells were shown to be activated by butyrate, blocking an excessive proinflammatory response [71]. Butyrate can exert an anti-inflammatory effect in part by suppressing the activation of NF-κB [72], a transcription factor that regulates the inflammatory and innate immune responses [73]. In addition, butyrate strongly inhibits the interferon-gamma (IFN-γ) signaling to ameliorate inflammation [74]. Butyrate also targets peroxisome proliferator-activated receptor-γ (PPARγ) to prevent colon inflammation [75]. IL-10-deficient mice developing enterocolitis when maintained in conventional conditions showed no evidence of colitis when kept in a germ-free environment, suggesting that resident enteric bacteria are necessary for immune system activation in these mice [47]. Anaerobic and mutually exclusive *Bacteroides* species could dominate the microbiota and exert commensal, mutualistic, or pathogenic behaviors depending on host–microbe interactions, bio-geographical location, and nutritional availability. As a known pathobiont in IBD, *Bacteroides vulgatus* activates NF-kB pathways, and some strains are important for colonization and persistence in CD. Similarly, entero-toxigenic *B. fragilis* has been shown to promote intestinal inflammation and possibly colon carcinogenesis through the activation of NF-kB [76], resulting in increased pro-inflammatory cytokine levels, such as IL-8/CXCL8. The composition of the gut microbiome has been associated with the severity of COVID-19, possibly via its immune-modulatory properties. Gut commensals with known immunomodulatory potential, such as *F. prausnitzii*, *Eubacterium rectale*, and *Bifidobacterium adolescentis*, were found to be significantly under-represented in COVID-19 patients compared with healthy controls, and were associated with disease severity after taking account of antibiotic use and patient age [10]. Furthermore, the microbial imbalance found in COVID-19 patients was also associated with raised levels of inflammatory cytokines such as C-reactive protein The inflammatory phenotype could represent a risk factor in SARS-CoV-2 infection.

Uncertainties, inconsistencies, and gaps. Disturbances of the microbiota are evident in inflammatory diseases. However, despite encouraging evidence from animal models in which inflammatory conditions were successfully treated via gut microbiota manipulation, data from human trials are less conclusive. It is still unclear from human studies whether the alteration in the microbial community is a cause or consequence of inflammation. A higher degree of resolution of microbiome analysis matched with lifestyle factors, heterogeneity of the host genotype, and epigenome, is likely to be required to advance the understanding of host–microbe interactions.

The gut microbiota also play an important role in the production of interleukin-22 (IL-22) in the gut, which is central to the induction of antimicrobial peptides, and promotes the protective functions of the epithelial barrier [50]. Klooster et al. [77] showed that intestinal viral infections induce IL-22 expression by T cells stimulated by IFNβ1-mediated IL-7 production by epithelial cells and IL-6 production by fibroblasts. Their findings suggest that IL-22 modulates genes involved in viral entry and replication. Specifically, IL-22 inhibits the expression of the viral entry receptors, ACE2 and TMPRSS2, while increasing the expression of antiviral proteins [77]. Although IL-22 is well-known for its role in bacterial defense, there are limited and conflicting data on the importance and regulation of IL-22 in intestinal viral defense.

2.4. Potential Implication for Disease Management

The persistence of gut microbiota dysbiosis after disease resolution in COVID-19 could contribute to persistent symptoms, highlighting a need to understand how gut microorganisms are involved in inflammation and COVID-19. Notably, it remains unknown whether inflammation-associated gut microorganisms enriched in COVID-19 play an active part in the disease or flourish opportunistically due to a depletion of other gut microorganisms. Follow-ups of patients with COVID-19 (e.g., 3 months to 1 year after clearing the virus) are needed to address questions related to (i) the duration of gut microbiota dysbiosis post-recovery, (ii) the link between microbiota dysbiosis and long-term persistent symptoms, and (iii) whether the enrichment/depletion of specific gut microorganisms predisposes recovered individuals to future health problems.

3. Intestinal ACE2 Dysregulation Inducing Gut Dysbiosis

Research in the last few years has highlighted the key role of ACE2 in intestinal homeostasis by influencing multiple processes [78–81], including the modulation of gut microbiota [82–84]. Therefore, it is plausible that the binding of the viral S protein to ACE2 in the gut may lead to the dysregulation of physiological functions such as alteration of the GI amino acid (AA) metabolism, altering the gut microbiota (Figure 2).

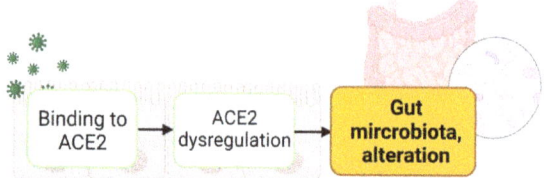

Figure 2. Virus binding to ACE2 expressed in enterocytes induces ACE2 dysregulation leading to alteration in gut microbiota. Created with Biorender.com.

3.1. Binding of S Proteins to Enteric ACE2 Induces Intestinal ACE2 Dysregulation

Biological plausibility. The binding of S proteins to ACE2 is likely to impede the physiological functions of ACE2. In the gut, ACE2 modulates the local renin–angiotensin signaling (RAS) system in a paracrine and autocrine manner, mediating cell-specific growth, proliferation, and metabolic activity [83]. Little is known about the potential role of intestinal ACE2 in modulating the local KKS system in the gut. The role of ACE2 as a chaperone for neutral AA transporters in the intestines is its most studied RAS-independent and non-enzymatic function [85,86]. ACE2 and ACE, components of the RAS system, are present in the intestine. Intestinal ACE2 stabilizes the transporter B^0AT1 (Slc6a19), which mediates the uptake of neutral dietary AA, such as tryptophan (Trp), into intestinal cells in a sodium-dependent manner [86]. ACE2 has also been proposed to interact functionally with sodium-dependent imino transporter 1 (SIT1), a luminal L-proline transporter expressed in small intestine enterocytes [78]. Therefore, it is plausible that SARS-CoV-2 binding might interfere with ACE2 association with AA transporters and their function.

Evidence. Extensive evidence exists for ACE2 dysregulation as a result of interaction with the viral S proteins in different cells and tissues, with changes in ACE2 mRNA expression, protein levels, and enzymatic activity (KER2311). Evidence for ACE2 protein down-regulation mediated by viral S proteins comes from lung and liver-derived cell systems [79,80] which monitored ACE2 protein levels in whole cell lysates. Membrane and cellular ACE2 protein down-regulation following treatment with SARS-CoV-1 S protein have also been demonstrated in studies with kidney cell lines that concomitantly monitored and showed increased ACE2 enzymatic activity in the extracellular compartment [81,87,88]. In these non-GI test systems, the decrease of the full-length ACE2 cellular protein is due to S-protein-mediated cleavage of ACE2 by cellular proteases (TACE/ADAM17). The precise role of ACE2 cleavage and shedding in SARS-CoV and SARS-CoV-2 viral entry and/or maturation of infective particles remains to be elucidated. ACE2 down-regulation at the transcriptional level has been reported in kidney biopsies from deceased patients [89] and in GI tract-derived organoids [90]. Using a single-cell transcriptomics approach and multiplex single-molecule RNA fluorescence in situ hybridization (FISH), ACE2 mRNA down-regulation was observed in both ileal- and colon-derived 2D organoids infected with SARS-CoV-2 (relative to mock infected organoids) [90]. Tissue-specific differences were noted. In ileum-derived organoids, ACE2 mRNA was down-regulated in the bystander cells (cells not showing active SARS-CoV-2 replication as judged by detection of viral RNA) whereas in the colon-derived bystander cells, ACE2 was comparable to mock/uninfected cells. This difference may also be due to the method applied to determine the threshold for distinguishing actively infected and bystander cells (which also contained detectable viral RNA). Nataf and Pays (2021) [91] reported profound but transient down-regulation of ACE2 mRNA in SARS-CoV-2-infected differentiated human intestinal organoids compared to controls. Interestingly, they also reported decreased B^0AT1 mRNA, which requires ACE2 for its membrane expression and function [86]. The mRNA levels for both ACE2 and B^0AT1 returned to baseline by 60 hpi. Nataf and Pays [91] re-analyzed the mRNA expression levels generated in a study by Lamers et al. [46] but reported results from earlier time points.

Evidence for up-regulation of ACE2 (mRNA and protein) following interaction with SARS-CoV-2 S proteins is available in a significant number of studies with non-GI-infected tissues or *in vitro* cell systems (KER2311). In differentiated human small intestinal 3D organoids (DIF) infected with SARS-CoV-2, a modest ACE2 mRNA up-regulation was reported [46]. The DIF showed significantly higher levels of ACE2 expression compared to expanding organoids (EO). Data in this study shows ACE2 mRNA down-regulation in the DIF organoids [91]. SARS-CoV infection up-regulated ACE2 mRNA at 24 and 60 hpi in EO while the data for SARS-CoV-2 in EO showed up-regulation of ACE2 mRNA at 60 hpi only. Up-regulation of both ACE2 mRNA (~3×) and protein (1.3×) in 2D differentiated Caco-2-derived infected with SARS-CoV-2 were observed compared to uninfected cells [78]. Up-regulation was noted when the viral titer was at saturation. ACE2 mRNA up-regulation was also reported with SARS-CoV-2 in human colon 3D organoids [92].

Uncertainties, inconsistencies, and gaps. Evidence supports the high plausibility of ACE2 dysregulation in the GI tract due to the interaction with SARS-CoV-2. However, direct evidence for ACE2 dysregulation resulting from S protein binding rather than viral replication in the gut or in gut-derived systems is currently lacking. In addition, there are inconsistencies in the evidence that need further consideration.

The apparent inconsistencies regarding the direction and magnitude of ACE2 dysregulation in the different studies (using various test systems) may reflect the dynamic and temporal components of the dysregulation. The latter could be driven not only by the interaction of ACE2 with the surface viral components, but also by the interaction of the replicating viral components with the innate immunity response elements, particularly in the test systems using replicating viruses. ACE2 mRNA down-regulation in SARS-CoV2-treated GI-derived organoids was reported in enterocytes actively replicating the virus [90]. A second study also reported profound but transient ACE mRNA downregulation [91]. Contrary evidence for SARS-CoV2 mediating up-regulation of ACE2 mRNA in GI organoids [46,92,93] is consistent with similar studies in many other tissue/organ systems (KER2311) and with the finding that *ace2* is an Interferon Stimulated Gene (ISG) in airway epithelial cells [94] and in colon enterocytes [92]. These studies also demonstrated a time concordance of ACE2 mRNA up-regulation with stimulation of ISG response in the infected organoids [46,92,93]. Interestingly, a scRNAseq study by Triana et al. [90] found that SARS-CoV2 exposure induced distinct proinflammatory and ISG expression profiles in infected and bystander cells in the organoid. Expression of ISGs was pronounced in bystander cells, while the infected cells showed strong NFkB/TNF-mediated pro-inflammatory response but limited production of ISGs. This suggests that while SARS-CoV-2 may activate ISG by paracrine signaling, it may suppress the autocrine action of interferon i.e. induction of ISG, including ACE2, in infected cells. This would be consistent with ACE2 down-regulation in the infected cells observed in this study. In addition, this may explain why in some studies ACE2 mRNA down-regulation can be observed under certain conditions and at some (earlier) time points of replication. Furthermore, the causal relationship between an observed increase in ACE2 mRNA and dysregulation at protein and enzymatic levels remains to be elucidated. Indeed, most recently Harnik et al. [95] examined the spatial discordances between mRNAs and proteins in the intestinal epithelium and their significance for the interpretation of transcriptomic data. In addition, in the intestines of SARS-CoV-2-

infected Hamsters, mRNA expression of ACE2 was up-regulated and ACE2 function was decreased [26]. Such apparent discordances have also been reported in the heart and lung tissue of mice and humans (KE1854).

The identification of alternative forms of ACE2 mRNA and protein, an N-terminus truncated dACE2, which appears to have a distinct transcriptional regulation profile compared to flACE2 [95–97], may also account for some of the observed inconsistencies. A detailed analysis of experimental conditions in the past, and careful design of probes and primers in future studies would be informative. Interestingly, concomitant down- and up-regulation of 97kD and 80kD anti-ACE2 polyclonal Ab-reacting proteins have been detected in human colon adenocarcinoma cell line HT29 [98]. Considering only one form of ACE2 relevant, the authors concluded that ACE2 was down-regulated in mature differentiated enterocytes compared to undifferentiated ones. This is in contrast to all the studies described above which demonstrated that the highest level of ACE2 (both mRNA and protein) were detected in the mature enterocytes and at the brush borders of the intestine and 3D organoids [46,90,92,93]. The inconsistencies disused above clearly illustrate the need for careful characterization of the test systems to facilitate robust interpretation of the results.

The majority of studies have focused on ACE2 mRNA levels, while protein and functional analyses are often lacking, particularly in the GI system. The novel gut-derived organoid systems could help address this gap by monitoring the level and cell distribution of ACE2 protein as well as its function as B^0AT1 chaperon, by monitoring the membrane expression and the transporter function of B^0AT1. In addition, treatment with S protein and with non-replicating SARS-CoV-2 pseudoviruses [98] may better address any potential direct effect of S-binding on ACE2 dysregulation. Indeed, it remains to be elucidated if S protein alone can elicit ACE2 dysregulation, as this would mean that a nonviable virus reaching the gut lumen would be sufficient to induce such a mechanism. Finally, a development of more complex organoid systems that would also include microbiota and/or elements of the immune system is needed to better examine ACE2 dysregulation by SARS-CoV2, but also the effects of such dysregulation at higher organizational levels and in conjunction with the other elements of the RAS system. Finally, evidence of up- or down-regulation of ACE2 in the GI tract of SARS-CoV-2-infected patients was not available. Examining potentially existing or generating GI-specific transcriptomic, proteomic and biomarker databases of COVID-19 patents may help address some of these uncertainties. This again highlights the importance of interdisciplinary collaboration between basic, translational, and clinical researchers.

3.2. Enteric ACE2 Dysregulation Leads to Gut Microbiota Alteration

Biological plausibility. ACE2 co-expresses with several AA transporters in enterocytes, such as B^0AT1 for Trp [99] and SIT-1 for proline [78,100,101]. Thus, in the gut, ACE2 modulates dietary AA transport. Trp regulates the secretion of antimicrobial peptides by Paneth cells through the mTOR pathway [102]. Those antimicrobial peptides impact the composition and diversity of the microbiota [12,103]. In addition, the gut microbiota is influenced by the host intestinal AA metabolism as bacteria of the gut use dietary AA for protein synthesis [104–106]. Alteration of dietary AA transport due to viral S proteins binding to ACE2 could modify the ratio of AA-fermenting bacterial species and their metabolic pathways. Metabolism of AA by gut bacteria results in the formation of diverse metabolites, several of which are considered deleterious (nitrosamines, heterocyclic amines, and hydrogen sulfides), while others are beneficial, such as short-chain fatty acids (SCFA), namely butyrate, propionic acid, and acetic acid. Finally, as a regulator of local RAS, ACE2 receptor hijacked by the viral S proteins could lead to reduced ACE2 cleavage of AngII, an increase in local Ang II levels, and Ang 1-7 decrease resulting in luminal activation of ATR1 [107], enhancing permeability [99], and impacting gut microbiota. In addition, the GI RAS appears to be involved in numerous processes in the gut including AA, fluid, and electrolyte absorption and secretion [108].

Evidence. Some evidence linking ACE2-mediated altered dietary AA (such as Trp) and gut dysbiosis exist. Ace2 KO mice lack B⁰AT1 [86] and exhibited reduced Trp serum levels, along with downregulated expression of the mTOR pathway, inducing impaired expression of small intestinal antimicrobial peptides, and resulting in altered gut microbiota, which was re-established by Trp supplementation [109]. Exacerbated diabetes-induced dysbiosis was also observed in ACE2 KO/y-Akita mice [110]. ACE2 is also a co-receptor of SIT-1 transporting proline. ACE2 KO mice showed decreased intestinal proline absorption [111,112], not reflecting an increase of intestinal permeability but an alteration of the selective aspect of the intestinal barrier. In fecal microbiota of COVID-19 patients, the abundance of opportunistic pathogens was higher, and SCFA-producing bacterial populations were lower compared to healthy controls [9,113], suggesting that intestinal AA metabolism is altered. There is preclinical evidence of the presence of all RAS components in the GI tract [108,114]. Evidence also indicates a complex association between gut microbiota, ACE2 expression, and Vitamin D in COVID-19 severity. Vitamin D contributes to the regulation of the gut microbiome by maintaining microbial diversity and by promoting the growth of beneficial commensal strains of *Bifida* and *Fermicutus*. In addition, Vitamin D is a negative regulator for renin expression and interacts with the RAS/ACE/ACE-2 signaling axis [115].

Feedback loop. Interestingly, the gut microbiota seems to influence Ace2 expression and activity. A study found that several *Streptococcus* spp. increased the level of ACE2 protein in mammalian cells [116]. In patients, *Coprobacillus* enrichment—associated with clinical severity of COVID-19 [12] has been shown to upregulate colonic ACE2 in mice [48,117]. The abundance of specific gut bacteria such as certain Bacteroides species (*Bacteroides dorei*, *Bacteroides thetaiotaomicron*, *Bacteroides massiliensis*, and *Bacteroides ovatus*) was associated with a reduction in ACE2 expression in the mouse gut [48,117] and negatively correlated with fecal SARS-CoV-2 load [12], suggesting that they may limit the ability of SARS-CoV-2 to enter enterocytes [48]. In addition, gnotobiotic rats colonized with 9 bacterial phyla showed a decrease in colonic Ace2 expression compared to germ-free rats [118].

Uncertainties, inconsistencies, and gaps. Evidence linking altered levels/functions of ACE2 with altered uptake of dietary AA (Trp and/or proline) and alteration in gut microbiota needs to be further evaluated. One could examine Trp levels in ACE2-infected mice and assess dysbiosis with or without Trp supplementation. The use of S proteins, non-replicating SARS-CoV-2 pseudoviruses, or SARS-CoV-2 viruses might be informative as well as further exploration of the pro- and prebiotic effects on ACE2 regulation. In addition, not enough evidence is available so far regarding the intestinal RAS following ACE2 dysregulation in COVID-19.

3.3. Potential Implications for Disease Management

Many forms of diarrheal disease depend on the dysregulation of intestinal ion transporters, and an imbalance between secretory and absorptive functions of the intestinal epithelium [119]. It is tempting to consider that infectious dysbiosis and diarrhea might be effectively targeted by small molecules that act specifically on transporters implicated in the disease. Indeed, efforts are already ongoing to identify such molecules and some promising candidates have been identified [120,121], but they seem to be focused on exploring the ACE2–Spike protein interaction rather than ACE2 function/activity alone, or RAS-related function which is critical for cardiovascular homeostasis [122]. Similar approaches screening for the intestinal-specific functions of ACE2 may help in the management of gut dysbiosis during COVID-19 and potentially other ACE2-mediated gut dysfunctions. Based on the AOP outlined above, screening for modulating factors of ACE2 function that alter gut microbiota would be an informative target focus. Recognizing that testing or modeling systems that include microbiota are not yet fully available, the evidence analysis in the AOP justifies efforts needed for their development.

4. SARS-CoV-2 Infection of Microbial Bacteria Driving Gut Dysbiosis

In the gut, human cells might not be the sole SARS-CoV-2 targets. SARS-CoV-2 infection of human gut bacteria might be another mechanism driving dysbiosis in COVID-19 patients (Figure 3).

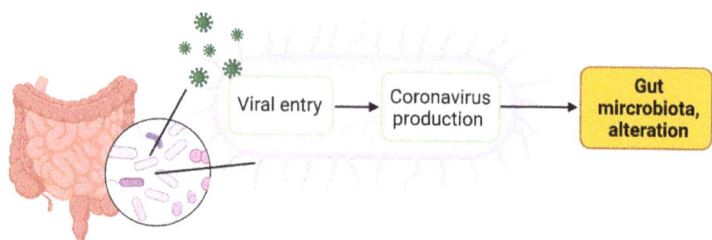

Figure 3. SARS-CoV2 infection of gut microbial bacteria might drive alteration in the gut microbiota. Created with Biorender.com.

4.1. Viral Entry in Gut Bacteria Leads to Coronavirus Production in Bacteria

Biological plausibility. Bacteriophages are viruses that infect prokaryotic hosts, such as bacteria of the gut microbiome. Typically, a phage virion binds to the host cell surface using a phage receptor-binding protein triggering the insertion of its genome into the host [123].

Evidence. A series of serine protease TMPRSS2 and peptidyl peptidase with high similarity to ACE2 peptidase domain were identified in silico in bacteria of the *Proteobacteria* phylum [124]. Transmission electron microscopy analysis showed the presence of SARS-CoV-2 particles on the surface and inside gut bacteria obtained from COVID-19 patients [125], consistent with a viral tropism for gut bacteria [13]. SARS-CoV-2 replication has been observed outside the human body in bacterial growth medium, following bacterial growth, and reduced by antibiotics administration [13].

Uncertainties, inconsistencies, and gaps. A virus able to infect at the same time eukaryotic and prokaryotic cells has never been described before. In addition, enveloped bacteriophages are not very common. The best-known family (*Cystoviridae*) is lipid-containing with three double-stranded RNA (ds-RNA) genome segments: resembling the family *Reoviridae*, cystoviruses served as a simple model for reovirus assembly, but *Cystoviridae* genome packaging mechanism have not yet fully elucidated [126]. Looking for taxa potentially acting as a receptor for the virus would be really informative. Evidence of two bacterial species susceptible to being infected by SARS-CoV-2 has been recently reported [125]. However, the full picture of SARS-CoV-2-susceptible human gut bacterial species is lacking [13].

4.2. Coronavirus Production in Gut Bacteria Leads to Alteration of Gut Microbiota

Biological plausibility. Bacteriophages can shape bacterial communities by predation or by horizontal gene transfer through transduction. Besides, viruses can modulate microbiota function by modulating their metabolism.

Evidence. Altered microbiota compositions were found to be independent of the presence of SARS-CoV-2 in the respiratory tract, disease severity, and GI symptoms, but correlated with GI levels of SARS-CoV-2 RNA [127].

Uncertainties, inconsistencies and gaps. There is a wealth of literature on the role of bacteriophages within the human gut. However, there are still large areas that require further investigation, and if fully elucidated, could trigger beneficial treatments for human diseases, similar to what we are currently seeing with the bacterial component of the human microbiome [128]. A key issue is that current analysis tends to focus on the known annotated component of viral datasets [129,130] and the need for reproducible methods limiting bias at the different steps. Furthermore, besides taxonomy, investigating the metabolomic alteration following SARS-CoV-2 infection *in vitro* would help to provide evidence of the causal link between bacterial coronavirus production and dysbiosis.

4.3. Potential Implications for Disease Management

This proposed mechanism might have a direct effect on human health. If the virus is hosted by bacteria in the gut microbiome, eliminating the bacterial host with appropriate antibiotics might kill the virus [131]. The efficacy of some antibiotics (like rifaximin and azithromycin) in reducing viral RNA load to negligible levels in *in vitro* fecal microbiota cultures obtained from stool samples of SARS-CoV-2-positive individuals has been reported [13,132]. However, a better understanding via the AOP concept of these complex interactions makes prevention or adequate therapeutic interventions mechanism-based, taking into account different modulating factors [123]. In this regard, multidisciplinary approaches that couple tests on the efficacy of antimicrobials with proteomic and electron microscopy image analyses would be beneficial to shed light on the potential viral tropism of SARS-CoV-2 for gut bacteria.

5. Central Role of Gut Microbiota in COVID-19 and Potential Modulation

The three above proposed pathways leading to an alteration of gut microbiota following SARS-CoV-2 presence in the gut lumen are non-mutually exclusive but rather interconnected (Figure 4).

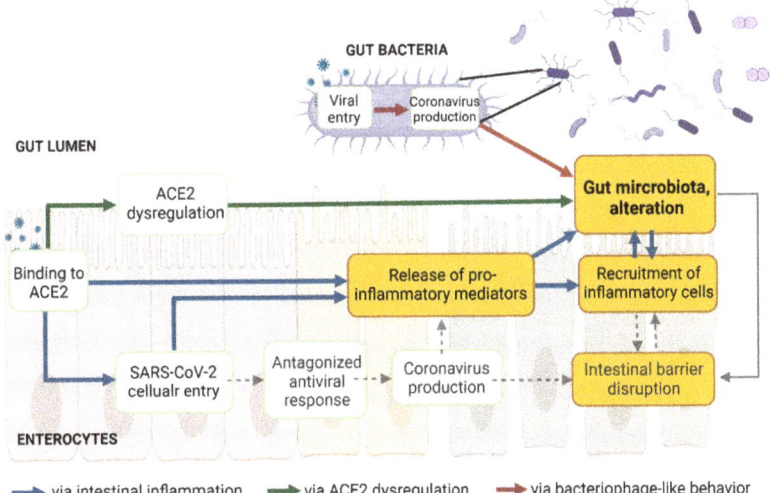

Figure 4. The three proposed pathways leading to gut dysbiosis following SARS-CoV-2 presence in the gut lumen are not mutually exclusive but might be interconnected. Created with Biorender.com.

5.1. Gut Microbiota and Intestinal Barrier Integrity in COVID-19

Together with the mucosal barrier and the cellular immune system, the intestinal epithelial cell monolayer and the tight junction proteins act simultaneously as a physical barrier against harmful external substances, as well as a selective barrier. Increased intestinal permeability, a sign of an impaired barrier function, enhances the translocation of gut bacteria and bacterial toxins from the intestinal lumen into the systemic circulation. The gut microbiota ensures intestinal barrier integrity through diverse mechanisms [48] (Figure 4, dashed grey lines). Beneficial butyrate-producing bacteria are proposed to maintain intestinal integrity, as butyrate, a short-chain fatty acid (SCFA), facilitates the regeneration of healthy colonocytes [49]. A reduced relative proportion of bacteria producing SCFA was observed in Syrian hamsters infected with SARS-CoV-2, compared to non-infected controls, with a transient decrease in systemic SCFA amounts [26]. Decreases in the abundance of butyrate-producing bacteria and a decline in SCFA were observed in severe COVID-19 [10,12,133]. Besides the reduction of beneficial bacteria, the overgrowth of pathobionts, such as *Escherichia coli* or *Salmonella enterica*, disrupts intestinal barrier function [134–136]. Outgrowth of pathogenic *Prevotella* has been associated with reduced mucus secretion, one crucial protective layer of the intestinal barrier [137]. Blooms of pathogenic bacteria have been observed in hospitalized COVID-19 patients, along with the translocation of gut bacteria into the blood [25]. Lowered levels of butyrate-producers and higher levels of opportunistic pathogens (including *E. coli* and *S. enterica*) were observed in COVID-19 patients compared with H1N1 patients and healthy controls [9]. In addition, gut microbiota composition correlated with plasma levels of tissue damage markers, altered tight junctions, and microbial translocation in COVID-19 patients [10]. Finally, the colonic mucus barrier is shaped by the composition of the gut microbiota [138]. Alteration of the gut microbiota might contribute to disrupting the mucus barrier.

Human intestinal organoid co-cultures with microbes could represent useful systems to investigate the protective function of bacteria on gut permeability upon SARS-CoV-2 infection [139]. In addition, similar to the treatment of other diseases, treating SARS-CoV-2 infected mice or Syrian hamsters with SCFA supplementation [26,51], prebiotics, or probiotics (such as *Lactobacillus reuteri* in rodents), [140] and evaluating the intestinal permeability (dextran and bacterial translocation) in parallel with microbiota omics could strengthen our understanding of the relationship between gut microbiota and the intestinal barrier in COVID-19 pathophysiology.

5.2. Central Role of the Gut (Microbiota) in COVID-19 and Long COVID

Dysbiosis, intestinal inflammation, and leaky gut are intimately interconnected (Figure 4) and intestinal homeostasis is increasingly recognized as an underpinning clinical driver in several noncommunicable diseases as well as in COVID-19. Accumulating evidence supports that altered gut microbiota and associated leaky gut may contribute to the GI symptoms and the cytokine storm and multiorgan complications in COVID-19 [141,142]. In critically ill patients with sepsis and respiratory distress, bacterial translocation is widely documented [143,144]. Higher plasma levels of gut permeability markers were found in COVID-19 patients, along with abnormal presence of gut bacteria in the blood [145,146]. These markers correlated with higher levels of C-reactive peptide (a marker of hyperinflammation) and with a higher mortality rate [146]. Serum levels of lipopolysaccharide-binding protein were higher in patients with severe COVID-19 and were associated with circulating inflammation biomarkers [147]. Altered intestinal homeostasis induces diarrhea [148], which is the digestive symptom most commonly reported in COVID-19 patients [149–153].

Despite the well-documented prevalence of GI symptoms and the high rate of SARS-CoV-2 fecal RNA shedding, the isolation of replication-competent virus from fecal samples has not been reproducibly and systematically demonstrated [38]. The biological, clinical, and epidemiological relevance of SARS-CoV-2 shedding remains unclear [154]. SARS-CoV-2 shedding in stools has been reported from one week to seven months after diagnosis [154,155]. The prolonged presence of viral RNA in feces [154], but not in respiratory samples, and its association with GI symptoms suggests that SARS-CoV-2 infects the GI tract, and that this infection can be prolonged in a subset of individuals with COVID-19. SARS-CoV-2 infection leading to perturbation of the gut microbiome may contribute to the underlying etiology of GI symptoms observed in COVID-19 and long COVID [45,156]. Alteration in the gut microbiome persists long after a patient recovers, suggesting that the gut microbiome may play an important role in long COVID [157]. Long COVID or post-acute COVID-19 syndrome (PACS) is rapidly emerging across the globe and many studies following patients who have recovered from the respiratory effects of COVID-19 identified persistent GI sequelae, including dysbiosis [154,155,158]. While the pathogenesis of long COVID is still under intense investigation, on the four current leading hypotheses [45], it is interesting to note that gut dysbiosis is considered as one of them [157,159]. A comprehensive understanding of the dynamics of fecal clearance of SARS-CoV-2 RNA and its link with gut dysbiosis is currently lacking. Further studies are needed as the gut microbiota could serve as a potential prognosis indicator and could be therapeutically valuable.

5.3. Potential Modulation of Gut Microbiota to Mitigate COVID-19

In light of the current insight into the central role of the gut in COVID-19 and long COVID, modulating the gut microbiota to improve disease prevention and management may be relevant. First, fecal microbiota transplantation (FMT) enables stool infusion from a healthy individual to a severely ill patient to restore intestinal microbial balance [160]. So far, FMT has been remarkably successful in the treatment of *Clostridium difficile* infection, but much less in treating other conditions, such as IBD or metabolic disorders. COVID-19 being an infectious disease and not an inflammatory disorder, FMT could be more successful [141]. However, COVID-19 could potentially be transmitted via FMT, particularly from asymptomatic donors who tested negative for the presence of the virus in their respiratory tract but positive in their stools [161]. No cases of COVID-19 transmission through FMT have been reported so far, but only FMT products generated from stools donated before December/November 2019 were used according to the FDA and Hong Kong recommendations, respectively. Secondly, gut microbiota modulation with probiotics, prebiotics, or diet and therapies preventing gut barrier defects may represent easy-to-implement strategies to mitigate COVID-19 [162]. Clinical trials of probiotics with expected anti-inflammatory effects for preventing or treating SARS-CoV-2 infection are currently ongoing [163]. Next-generation probiotics focusing on butyrate-producing bacteria, or simply increasing the daily intake of dietary fiber are proposed as potential beneficial approaches for COVID-19 patients [141]. A few reports cite indirect evidence for the association between probiotics and COVID-19, primarily based on previous coronaviruses and other viral infections [164,165]. The health benefits of prebiotics to the GI tract, including the inhibition of pathogens and stimulation of the immune system, are due to their ability to modulate the composition and activity of human microbiota [166–168]. However, to date, there is no information directly linking prebiotics to COVID-19 infections, although an indirect effect may be hypothesized [169]. Thus, using conventional probiotics is not currently warranted, but is considered promising, and a better understanding of SARS-CoV-2 pathogenesis and its mutual effect on gut microbiota is needed. More generally, diet is obviously a factor impacting gut microbiota [170–173]. Dietary adaptation may be the easiest method to be implemented in the preventive arsenal against COVID-19 and for general health improvement [141].

6. Conclusions and Future Perspectives

Here we explored the evidence currently available in the literature supporting that SARS-CoV-2 induces intestinal inflammation, dysregulates intestinal ACE2 physiological functions, and/or infects gut bacteria, as three potential interconnected mechanisms leading to gut dysbiosis in COVID-19. Based on the current insights into the underlying mechanisms, we discussed the potential implications for disease management in infected patients. In addition, the alterations in the gut microbial community are observed long after the respiratory syndrome is resolved, and thus a better understanding of the underlying mechanisms is needed to capture the potentially important role of microbiota in long COVID. The approach applied also permits identifying knowledge gaps and proposes methods to perform further research. Notably, examining potentially existing or generating GI-specific transcriptomic, proteomic, and biomarker databases of COVID-19 patents may help address some of these uncertainties. Large-scale population-based studies are warranted to validate with more confidence these pathways, and intervention studies could help to explore the roles of gut microbiota alteration in COVID-19 pathogenesis. In addition, it remains unclear to what extent the gut microbiota composition as an outcome of COVID-19 is influenced by clinical management due to the variability across COVID-19 treatments. Due to all these current uncertainties, there is a need to continue the interdisciplinary collaboration between basic, translational, and clinical researchers.

Author Contributions: L.-A.C. conceptualized the manuscript and edited the figures. All authors contributed to an in-depth review of the literature and the writing of the different parts of the manuscript. All authors have read and agreed to the published version of the manuscript.

Funding: This research was funded by Fundação para a Ciência e Tecnologia through CEECIND/02373/2020 for M.-J.A. For the others, this research received no external funding.

Acknowledgments: The work was performed under the JRC Exploratory Research project CIAO—*Modelling COVID-19 pathogenesis using the Adverse Outcome Pathways*.

Conflicts of Interest: The authors declare no conflict of interest.

Disclaimer: This study is solely associated with participating individual scientists, and their expressions of interest and opinions; it does not represent the official position of any institution.

References

1. Williamson, E.J.; Walker, A.J.; Bhaskaran, K.; Bacon, S.; Bates, C.; Morton, C.E.; Curtis, H.J.; Mehrkar, A.; Evans, D.; Inglesby, P.; et al. Factors associated with COVID-19-related death using OpenSAFELY. *Nature* **2020**, *584*, 430–436. [CrossRef] [PubMed]
2. Chidambaram, V.; Tun, N.L.; Haque, W.Z.; Majella, M.G.; Sivakumar, R.K.; Kumar, A.; Hsu, A.T.-W.; Ishak, I.A.; Nur, A.A.; Ayeh, S.K.; et al. Factors associated with disease severity and mortality among patients with COVID-19: A systematic review and meta-analysis. *PLoS ONE* **2020**, *15*, e0241541. [CrossRef]
3. Mudatsir, M.; Fajar, J.K.; Wulandari, L.; Soegiarto, G.; Ilmawan, M.; Purnamasari, Y.; Mahdi, B.A.; Jayanto, G.D.; Suhendra, S.; Setianingsih, Y.A.; et al. Predictors of COVID-19 severity: A systematic review and meta-analysis. *F1000Research* **2020**, *9*, 1107. [CrossRef] [PubMed]
4. Nishiga, M.; Wang, D.W.; Han, Y.; Lewis, D.B.; Wu, J.C. COVID-19 and cardiovascular disease: From basic mechanisms to clinical perspectives. *Nat. Rev. Cardiol.* **2020**, *17*, 543–558. [CrossRef] [PubMed]
5. Clerbaux, L.-A.; Albertini, M.C.; Amigó, N.; Beronius, A.; Bezemer, G.F.G.; Coecke, S.; Daskalopoulos, E.P.; del Giudice, G.; Greco, D.; Grenga, L.; et al. Factors Modulating COVID-19: A Mechanistic Understanding Based on the Adverse Outcome Pathway Framework. *J. Clin. Med.* **2022**, *11*, 4464. [CrossRef] [PubMed]
6. Ragonnaud, E.; Biragyn, A. Gut microbiota as the key controllers of "healthy" aging of elderly people. *Immun. Ageing* **2021**, *18*, 2. [CrossRef] [PubMed]
7. Bosco, N.; Noti, M. The aging gut microbiome and its impact on host immunity. *Genes Immun.* **2021**, *22*, 289–303. [CrossRef]
8. Vodnar, D.-C.; Mitrea, L.; Teleky, B.-E.; Szabo, K.; Călinoiu, L.-F.; Nemeş, S.-A.; Martău, G.-A. Coronavirus Disease (COVID-19) Caused by (SARS-CoV-2) Infections: A Real Challenge for Human Gut Microbiota. *Front. Cell. Infect. Microbiol.* **2020**, *10*, 575559. [CrossRef]
9. Gu, S.; Chen, Y.; Wu, Z.; Chen, Y.; Gao, H.; Lv, L.; Guo, F.; Zhang, X.; Luo, R.; Huang, C.; et al. Alterations of the Gut Microbiota in Patients with Coronavirus Disease 2019 or H1N1 Influenza. *Clin. Infect. Dis.* **2020**, *71*, 2669–2678. [CrossRef]
10. Yeoh, Y.K.; Zuo, T.; Lui, G.C.-Y.; Zhang, F.; Liu, Q.; Li, A.Y.; Chung, A.C.; Cheung, C.P.; Tso, E.Y.; Fung, K.S.; et al. Gut microbiota composition reflects disease severity and dysfunctional immune responses in patients with COVID-19. *Gut* **2021**, *70*, 698–706. [CrossRef]
11. Cheung, C.C.L.; Goh, D.; Lim, X.; Tien, T.Z.; Lim, J.C.T.; Lee, J.N.; Tan, B.; Tay, Z.E.A.; Wan, W.Y.; Chen, E.X.; et al. Residual SARS-CoV-2 viral antigens detected in GI and hepatic tissues from five recovered patients with COVID-19. *Gut* **2022**, *71*, 226–229. [CrossRef] [PubMed]
12. Zuo, T.; Zhang, F.; Lui, G.C.Y.; Yeoh, Y.K.; Li, A.Y.L.; Zhan, H.; Wan, Y.; Chung, A.C.K.; Cheung, C.P.; Chen, N.; et al. Alterations in Gut Microbiota of Patients with COVID-19 During Time of Hospitalization. *Gastroenterology* **2020**, *159*, 944–955.e948. [CrossRef]
13. Petrillo, M.; Brogna, C.; Cristoni, S.; Querci, M.; Piazza, O.; Eede, G.V.D. Increase of SARS-CoV-2 RNA load in faecal samples prompts for rethinking of SARS-CoV-2 biology and COVID-19 epidemiology. *F1000Research* **2021**, *10*, 370. [CrossRef] [PubMed]
14. Sarkar, A.; Harty, S.; Moeller, A.H.; Klein, S.L.; Erdman, S.E.; Friston, K.J.; Carmody, R.N. The gut microbiome as a biomarker of differential susceptibility to SARS-CoV-2. *Trends Mol. Med.* **2021**, *27*, 1115–1134. [CrossRef]
15. Schult, D.; Reitmeier, S.; Koyumdzhieva, P.; Lahmer, T.; Middelhoff, M.; Erber, J.; Schneider, J.; Kager, J.; Frolova, M.; Horstmann, J.; et al. Gut bacterial dysbiosis and instability is associated with the onset of complications and mortality in COVID-19. *Gut Microbes* **2022**, *14*, 2031840. [CrossRef]
16. Spor, A.; Koren, O.; Ley, R. Unravelling the effects of the environment and host genotype on the gut microbiome. *Nat. Rev. Microbiol.* **2011**, *9*, 279–290. [CrossRef] [PubMed]
17. Zhang, Y.-J.; Li, S.; Gan, R.-Y.; Zhou, T.; Xu, D.-P.; Li, H.-B. Impacts of Gut Bacteria on Human Health and Diseases. *Int. J. Mol. Sci.* **2015**, *16*, 7493–7519. [CrossRef]
18. Sartor, R.B. Mechanisms of Disease: Pathogenesis of Crohn's disease and ulcerative colitis. *Nat. Clin. Pr. Gastroenterol. Hepatol.* **2006**, *3*, 390–407. [CrossRef]
19. Dang, A.T.; Marsland, B.J. Microbes, metabolites, and the gut–lung axis. *Mucosal Immunol.* **2019**, *12*, 843–850. [CrossRef]
20. Tripathi, A.; Debelius, J.; Brenner, D.A.; Karin, M.; Loomba, R.; Schnabl, B.; Knight, R. The gut–liver axis and the intersection with the microbiome. *Nat. Rev. Gastroenterol. Hepatol.* **2018**, *15*, 397–411. [CrossRef]

21. Manzoor, R.; Ahmed, W.; Afify, N.; Memon, M.; Yasin, M.; Memon, H.; Rustom, M.; Al Akeel, M.; Alhajri, N. Trust Your Gut: The Association of Gut Microbiota and Liver Disease. *Microorganisms* **2022**, *10*, 1045. [CrossRef] [PubMed]
22. Mitrea, L.; Nemes, S.A.; Szabo, K.; Teleky, B.E.; Vodnar, D.C. Guts Imbalance Imbalances the Brain: A Review of Gut Microbiota Association with Neurological and Psychiatric Disorders. *Front. Med.* **2022**, *9*, 813204. [CrossRef] [PubMed]
23. Manna, S.; Baindara, P.; Mandal, S.M. Molecular pathogenesis of secondary bacterial infection associated to viral infections including SARS-CoV-2. *J. Infect. Public Health* **2020**, *13*, 1397–1404. [CrossRef] [PubMed]
24. Chen, J.; Hall, S.; Vitetta, L. Altered gut microbial metabolites could mediate the effects of risk factors in COVID-19. *Rev. Med. Virol.* **2021**, *31*, 1–13. [CrossRef]
25. Venzon, M.; Bernard-Raichon, L.; Klein, J.; Axelrad, J.; Hussey, G.; Sullivan, A.; Casanovas-Massana, A.; Noval, M.; Valero-Jimenez, A.; Gago, J.; et al. Gut microbiome dysbiosis during COVID-19 is associated with increased risk for bacteremia and microbial translocation. *Res. Sq.* **2021**. [CrossRef]
26. Sencio, V.; Machelart, A.; Robil, C.; Benech, N.; Hoffmann, E.; Galbert, C.; Deryuter, L.; Heumel, S.; Hantute-Ghesquier, A.; Flourens, A.; et al. Alteration of the gut microbiota following SARS-CoV-2 infection correlates with disease severity in hamsters. *Gut Microbes* **2022**, *14*, 2018900. [CrossRef]
27. Sokol, H.; Contreras, V.; Maisonnasse, P.; Desmons, A.; Delache, B.; Sencio, V.; Machelart, A.; Brisebarre, A.; Humbert, L.; Deryuter, L.; et al. SARS-CoV-2 infection in nonhuman primates alters the composition and functional activity of the gut microbiota. *Gut Microbes* **2021**, *13*, 1893113. [CrossRef]
28. Nymark, P.; Sachana, M.; Leite, S.B.; Sund, J.; Krebs, C.E.; Sullivan, K.; Edwards, S.; Viviani, L.; Willett, C.; Landesmann, B.; et al. Systematic Organization of COVID-19 Data Supported by the Adverse Outcome Pathway Framework. *Front. Public Health* **2021**, *9*, 638605. [CrossRef]
29. Wittwehr, C.; Amorim, M.J.; Clerbaux, L.A.; Krebs, C.; Landesmann, B.; Macmillan, D.S.; Nymark, P.; Ram, R.; Garcia-Reyero, N.; Sachana, M.; et al. Understanding COVID-19 through adverse outcome pathways–2nd CIAO AOP Design Workshop. *ALTEX* **2021**, *38*, 351–357. [CrossRef]
30. Clerbaux, L.-A.; Amigó, N.; Amorim, M.J.; Bal-Price, A.; Leite, S.B.; Beronius, A.; Bezemer, G.F.G.; Bostroem, A.-C.; Carusi, A.; Coecke, S.; et al. COVID-19 through Adverse Outcome Pathways: Building networks to better understand the disease—3rd CIAO AOP Design Workshop. *ALTEX* **2022**, *39*, 322–335. [CrossRef]
31. CIAO. Modelling the Pathogenesis of COVID-19 Using the Adverse Outcome Pathway Framework. Available online: www.ciao-covid.net (accessed on 29 June 2022).
32. OECD. Users' Handbook supplement to the Guidance Document for developing and assessing Adverse Outcome Pathways. In *OECD Series on Adverse Outcome Pathways*; OECD Publishing: Paris, France, 2018. [CrossRef]
33. Draskau, M.K.; Spiller, C.M.; Boberg, J.; Bowles, J.; Svingen, T.; Kam, M. Developmental biology meets toxicology: Contributing reproductive mechanisms to build adverse outcome pathways. *Mol. Hum. Reprod.* **2020**, *26*, 111–116. [CrossRef] [PubMed]
34. Siwicki, A.K.; Terech-Majewska, E.; Grudniewska, J.; Malaczewska, J.; Kazun, K.; Lepa, A. Influence of deltamethrin on nonspecific cellular and humoral defense mechanisms in rainbow trout (*Oncorhynchus mykiss*). *Environ. Toxicol. Chem.* **2010**, *29*, 489–491. [CrossRef] [PubMed]
35. Villeneuve, D.L.; Crump, D.; Garcia-Reyero, N.; Hecker, M.; Hutchinson, T.H.; Lalone, C.A.; Landesmann, B.; Lettieri, T.; Munn, S.; Nepelska, M.; et al. Adverse Outcome Pathway (AOP) Development I: Strategies and Principles. *Toxicol. Sci.* **2014**, *142*, 312–320. [CrossRef] [PubMed]
36. Villeneuve, D.L.; Crump, D.; Garcia-Reyero, N.; Hecker, M.; Hutchinson, T.H.; Lalone, C.A.; Landesmann, B.; Lettieri, T.; Munn, S.; Nepelska, M.; et al. Adverse Outcome Pathway Development II: Best Practices. *Toxicol. Sci.* **2014**, *142*, 321–330. [CrossRef]
37. Svingen, T.; Villeneuve, D.L.; Knapen, D.; Panagiotou, E.M.; Draskau, M.K.; Damdimopoulou, P.; O'Brien, J.M. A Pragmatic Approach to Adverse Outcome Pathway Development and Evaluation. *Toxicol. Sci.* **2021**, *184*, 183–190. [CrossRef]
38. Clerbaux, L.A.; Muñoz, A.; Soares, H.; Petrillo, M.; Albertini, M.C.; Lanthier, N.; Grenga, L.; Amorim, M.J. Gut as an alternative entry route for SARS-CoV-2: Current evidence and uncertainties of productive enteric infection in COVID-19. *J. Clin. Med.* **2022**. submitted.
39. Hamming, I.; Timens, W.; Bulthuis, M.L.C.; Lely, A.T.; Navis, G.J.; van Goor, H. Tissue distribution of ACE2 protein, the functional receptor for SARS coronavirus. A first step in understanding SARS pathogenesis. *J. Pathol.* **2004**, *203*, 631–637. [CrossRef]
40. Suárez-Fariñas, M.; Tokuyama, M.; Wei, G.; Huang, R.; Livanos, A.; Jha, D.; Levescot, A.; Irizar, H.; Kosoy, R.; Cording, S.; et al. Intestinal Inflammation Modulates the Expression of ACE2 and TMPRSS2 and Potentially Overlaps with the Pathogenesis of SARS-CoV-2–related Disease. *Gastroenterology* **2021**, *160*, 287–301.e20. [CrossRef]
41. Guo, M.; Tao, W.; Flavell, R.A.; Zhu, S. Potential intestinal infection and faecal–oral transmission of SARS-CoV-2. *Nat. Rev. Gastroenterol. Hepatol.* **2021**, *18*, 269–283. [CrossRef]
42. Lee, J.J.; Kopetz, S.; Vilar, E.; Shen, J.P.; Chen, K.; Maitra, A. Relative Abundance of SARS-CoV-2 Entry Genes in the Enterocytes of the Lower Gastrointestinal Tract. *Genes* **2020**, *11*, 645. [CrossRef]
43. Beumer, J.; Geurts, M.H.; Lamers, M.M.; Puschhof, J.; Zhang, J.; van der Vaart, J.; Mykytyn, A.Z.; Breugem, T.I.; Riesebosch, S.; Schipper, D.; et al. A CRISPR/Cas9 genetically engineered organoid biobank reveals essential host factors for coronaviruses. *Nat. Commun.* **2021**, *12*, 5498. [CrossRef] [PubMed]

44. Stanifer, M.L.; Kee, C.; Cortese, M.; Zumaran, C.M.; Triana, S.; Mukenhirn, M.; Kraeusslich, H.-G.; Alexandrov, T.; Bartenschlager, R.; Boulant, S. Critical Role of Type III Interferon in Controlling SARS-CoV-2 Infection in Human Intestinal Epithelial Cells. *Cell Rep.* **2020**, *32*, 107863. [CrossRef] [PubMed]
45. Merad, M.; Blish, C.A.; Sallusto, F.; Iwasaki, A. The immunology and immunopathology of COVID-19. *Science* **2022**, *375*, 1122–1127. [CrossRef] [PubMed]
46. Lamers, M.M.; Beumer, J.; van der Vaart, J.; Knoops, K.; Puschhof, J.; Breugem, T.I.; Ravelli, R.B.G.; van Schayck, J.P.; Mykytyn, A.Z.; Duimel, H.Q.; et al. SARS-CoV-2 productively infects human gut enterocytes. *Science* **2020**, *369*, 50–54. [CrossRef]
47. Sellon, R.K.; Tonkonogy, S.; Schultz, M.; Dieleman, L.A.; Grenther, W.; Balish, E.; Rennick, D.M.; Sartor, R.B. Resident Enteric Bacteria Are Necessary for Development of Spontaneous Colitis and Immune System Activation in Interleukin-10-Deficient Mice. *Infect. Immun.* **1998**, *66*, 5224–5231. [CrossRef]
48. Hu, J.; Zhang, L.; Lin, W.; Tang, W.; Chan, F.K.; Ng, S.C. Review article: Probiotics, prebiotics and dietary approaches during COVID-19 pandemic. *Trends Food Sci. Technol.* **2021**, *108*, 187–196. [CrossRef]
49. Salvi, P.S.; Cowles, R.A. Butyrate and the Intestinal Epithelium: Modulation of Proliferation and Inflammation in Homeostasis and Disease. *Cells* **2021**, *10*, 1775. [CrossRef]
50. Yang, W.; Yu, T.; Huang, X.; Bilotta, A.J.; Xu, L.; Lu, Y.; Sun, J.; Pan, F.; Zhou, J.; Zhang, W.; et al. Intestinal microbiota-derived short-chain fatty acids regulation of immune cell IL-22 production and gut immunity. *Nat. Commun.* **2020**, *11*, 4457. [CrossRef]
51. Sencio, V.; Gallerand, A.; Machado, M.G.; Deruyter, L.; Heumel, S.; Soulard, D.; Barthelemy, J.; Cuinat, C.; Vieira, A.T.; Barthelemy, A.; et al. Influenza Virus Infection Impairs the Gut's Barrier Properties and Favors Secondary Enteric Bacterial Infection through Reduced Production of Short-Chain Fatty Acids. *Infect. Immun.* **2021**, *89*, e0073420. [CrossRef]
52. Potdar, A.A.; Dube, S.; Naito, T.; Li, K.; Botwin, G.; Haritunians, T.; Li, D.; Casero, D.; Yang, S.; Bilsborough, J.; et al. Altered Intestinal ACE2 Levels Are Associated with Inflammation, Severe Disease, and Response to Anti-Cytokine Therapy in Inflammatory Bowel Disease. *Gastroenterology* **2021**, *160*, 809–822.e7. [CrossRef]
53. Zeng, M.Y.; Inohara, N.; Nuñez, G. Mechanisms of inflammation-driven bacterial dysbiosis in the gut. *Mucosal Immunol.* **2017**, *10*, 18–26. [CrossRef] [PubMed]
54. Ichinohe, T.; Pang, I.K.; Kumamoto, Y.; Peaper, D.R.; Ho, J.H.; Murray, T.S.; Iwasaki, A. Microbiota regulates immune defense against respiratory tract influenza A virus infection. *Proc. Natl. Acad. Sci. USA* **2011**, *108*, 5354–5359. [CrossRef] [PubMed]
55. Ryan, F.J.; Ahern, A.M.; Fitzgerald, R.S.; Laserna-Mendieta, E.J.; Power, E.M.; Clooney, A.G.; O'Donoghue, K.W.; McMurdie, P.J.; Iwai, S.; Crits-Christoph, A.; et al. Colonic microbiota is associated with inflammation and host epigenomic alterations in inflammatory bowel disease. *Nat. Commun.* **2020**, *11*, 1512. [CrossRef] [PubMed]
56. Pickard, J.M.; Zeng, M.Y.; Caruso, R.; Núñez, G. Gut microbiota: Role in pathogen colonization, immune responses, and inflammatory disease. *Immunol. Rev.* **2017**, *279*, 70–89. [CrossRef]
57. Wang, J.; Chen, W.-D.; Wang, Y.-D. The Relationship Between Gut Microbiota and Inflammatory Diseases: The Role of Macrophages. *Front. Microbiol.* **2020**, *11*, 1065. [CrossRef]
58. Vijay-Kumar, M.; Aitken, J.D.; Carvalho, F.A.; Cullender, T.C.; Mwangi, S.; Srinivasan, S.; Sitaraman, S.V.; Knight, R.; Ley, R.E.; Gewirtz, A.T. Metabolic Syndrome and Altered Gut Microbiota in Mice Lacking Toll-Like Receptor 5. *Science* **2010**, *328*, 228–231. [CrossRef]
59. Arrieta, M.-C.; Stiemsma, L.T.; Dimitriu, P.A.; Thorson, L.; Russell, S.; Yurist-Doutsch, S.; Kuzeljevic, B.; Gold, M.J.; Britton, H.M.; Lefebvre, D.L.; et al. Early infancy microbial and metabolic alterations affect risk of childhood asthma. *Sci. Transl. Med.* **2015**, *7*, 307ra152. [CrossRef]
60. Knip, M.; Siljander, H. The role of the intestinal microbiota in type 1 diabetes mellitus. *Nat. Rev. Endocrinol.* **2016**, *12*, 154–167. [CrossRef]
61. Meijnikman, A.S.; Gerdes, V.E.; Nieuwdorp, M.; Herrema, H. Evaluating Causality of Gut Microbiota in Obesity and Diabetes in Humans. *Endocr. Rev.* **2018**, *39*, 133–153. [CrossRef]
62. Atarashi, K.; Suda, W.; Luo, C.; Kawaguchi, T.; Motoo, I.; Narushima, S.; Kiguchi, Y.; Yasuma, K.; Watanabe, E.; Tanoue, T.; et al. Ectopic colonization of oral bacteria in the intestine drives T_H1 cell induction and inflammation. *Science* **2017**, *358*, 359–365. [CrossRef]
63. Lupp, C.; Robertson, M.L.; Wickham, M.E.; Sekirov, I.; Champion, O.L.; Gaynor, E.C.; Finlay, B.B. Host-Mediated Inflammation Disrupts the Intestinal Microbiota and Promotes the Overgrowth of Enterobacteriaceae. *Cell Host Microbe* **2007**, *2*, 119–129. [CrossRef] [PubMed]
64. Barman, M.; Unold, D.; Shifley, K.; Amir, E.; Hung, K.; Bos, N.; Salzman, N. Enteric Salmonellosis Disrupts the Microbial Ecology of the Murine Gastrointestinal Tract. *Infect. Immun.* **2008**, *76*, 907–915. [CrossRef]
65. Kamada, N.; Kim, Y.-G.; Sham, H.P.; Vallance, B.A.; Puente, J.L.; Martens, E.C.; Núñez, G. Regulated Virulence Controls the Ability of a Pathogen to Compete with the Gut Microbiota. *Science* **2012**, *336*, 1325–1329. [CrossRef] [PubMed]
66. Vijay, A.; Kouraki, A.; Gohir, S.; Turnbull, J.; Kelly, A.; Chapman, V.; Barrett, D.A.; Bulsiewicz, W.J.; Valdes, A.M. The anti-inflammatory effect of bacterial short chain fatty acids is partially mediated by endocannabinoids. *Gut Microbes* **2021**, *13*, 1997559. [CrossRef] [PubMed]
67. Schirmer, M.; Smeekens, S.P.; Vlamakis, H.; Jaeger, M.; Oosting, M.; Franzosa, E.A.; Ter Horst, R.; Jansen, T.; Jacobs, L.; Bonder, M.J.; et al. Linking the Human Gut Microbiome to Inflammatory Cytokine Production Capacity. *Cell* **2016**, *167*, 1125–1136.e8. [CrossRef]

68. Tedelind, S.; Westberg, F.; Kjerrulf, M.; Vidal, A. Anti-inflammatory properties of the short-chain fatty acids acetate and propionate: A study with relevance to inflammatory bowel disease. *World J. Gastroenterol.* **2007**, *13*, 2826–2832. [CrossRef]
69. Machiels, K.; Joossens, M.; Sabino, J.; De Preter, V.; Arijs, I.; Eeckhaut, V.; Ballet, V.; Claes, K.; Van Immerseel, F.; Verbeke, K.; et al. A decrease of the butyrate-producing species *Roseburia hominis* and *Faecalibacterium prausnitzii* defines dysbiosis in patients with ulcerative colitis. *Gut* **2014**, *63*, 1275–1283. [CrossRef]
70. Zhou, L.; Zhang, M.; Wang, Y.; Dorfman, R.G.; Liu, H.; Yu, T.; Chen, X.; Tang, D.; Xu, L.; Yin, Y.; et al. Faecalibacterium prausnitzii Produces Butyrate to Maintain Th17/Treg Balance and to Ameliorate Colorectal Colitis by Inhibiting Histone Deacetylase 1. *Inflamm. Bowel Dis.* **2018**, *24*, 1926–1940. [CrossRef]
71. Atarashi, K.; Tanoue, T.; Oshima, K.; Suda, W.; Nagano, Y.; Nishikawa, H.; Fukuda, S.; Saito, T.; Narushima, S.; Hase, K.; et al. Treg induction by a rationally selected mixture of Clostridia strains from the human microbiota. *Nature* **2013**, *500*, 232–236. [CrossRef]
72. Lührs, H.; Gerke, T.; Müller, J.G.; Melcher, R.; Schauber, J.; Boxberger, F.; Scheppach, W.; Menzel, T. Butyrate Inhibits NF-κB Activation in Lamina Propria Macrophages of Patients with Ulcerative Colitis. *Scand. J. Gastroenterol.* **2002**, *37*, 458–466. [CrossRef]
73. Karin, M.; Cao, Y.; Greten, F.; Li, Z.-W. NF-κB in cancer: From innocent bystander to major culprit. *Nat. Rev. Cancer* **2002**, *2*, 301–310. [CrossRef] [PubMed]
74. Klampfer, L.; Huang, J.; Sasazuki, T.; Shirasawa, S.; Augenlicht, L. Inhibition of interferon gamma signaling by the short chain fatty acid butyrate. *Mol. Cancer Res.* **2003**, *11*, 855–862.
75. Kinoshita, M.; Suzuki, Y.; Saito, Y. Butyrate reduces colonic paracellular permeability by enhancing PPARγ activation. *Biochem. Biophys. Res. Commun.* **2002**, *293*, 827–831. [CrossRef]
76. Sears, C.L.; Geis, A.L.; Housseau, F. Bacteroides fragilis subverts mucosal biology: From symbiont to colon carcinogenesis. *J. Clin. Investig.* **2014**, *124*, 4166–4172. [CrossRef]
77. Klooster, J.P.T.; Bol-Schoenmakers, M.; van Summeren, K.; van Vliet, A.L.W.; de Haan, C.A.M.; van Kuppeveld, F.J.M.; Verkoeijen, S.; Pieters, R. Enterocytes, fibroblasts and myeloid cells synergize in anti-bacterial and anti-viral pathways with IL22 as the central cytokine. *Commun. Biol.* **2021**, *4*, 631. [CrossRef]
78. Vuille-Dit-Bille, R.; Camargo, S.; Emmenegger, L.; Sasse, T.; Kummer, E.; Jando, J.; Hamie, Q.M.; Meier, C.F.; Hunziker, S.; Forras-Kaufmann, Z.; et al. Human intestine luminal ACE2 and amino acid transporter expression increased by ACE-inhibitors. *Amino Acids* **2015**, *47*, 693–705. [CrossRef]
79. Patra, T.; Meyer, K.; Geerling, L.; Isbell, T.S.; Hoft, D.F.; Brien, J.; Pinto, A.K.; Ray, R.B.; Ray, R. SARS-CoV-2 spike protein promotes IL-6 trans-signaling by activation of angiotensin II receptor signaling in epithelial cells. *PLoS Pathog.* **2020**, *16*, e1009128. [CrossRef]
80. Lei, Y.; Zhang, J.; Schiavon, C.R.; He, M.; Chen, L.; Shen, H.; Zhang, Y.; Yin, Q.; Cho, Y.; Andrade, L.; et al. SARS-CoV-2 Spike Protein Impairs Endothelial Function via Downregulation of ACE 2. *Circ. Res.* **2021**, *128*, 1323–1326. [CrossRef]
81. Glowacka, I.; Bertram, S.; Herzog, P.; Pfefferle, S.; Steffen, I.; Muench, M.O.; Simmons, G.; Hofmann, H.; Kuri, T.; Weber, F.; et al. Differential Downregulation of ACE2 by the Spike Proteins of Severe Acute Respiratory Syndrome Coronavirus and Human Coronavirus NL63. *J. Virol.* **2010**, *84*, 1198–1205. [CrossRef]
82. Penninger, J.M.; Grant, M.B.; Sung, J.J.Y. The Role of Angiotensin Converting Enzyme 2 in Modulating Gut Microbiota, Intestinal Inflammation, and Coronavirus Infection. *Gastroenterology* **2021**, *160*, 39–46. [CrossRef]
83. Jaworska, K.; Koper, M.; Ufnal, M. Gut microbiota and renin-angiotensin system: A complex interplay at local and systemic levels. *Am. J. Physiol. Gastrointest. Liver Physiol.* **2021**, *321*, G355–G366. [CrossRef] [PubMed]
84. Hashimoto, T.; Perlot, T.; Rehman, A.; Trichereau, J.; Ishiguro, H.; Paolino, M.; Sigl, V.; Hanada, T.; Hanada, R.; Lipinski, S.; et al. ACE2 links amino acid malnutrition to microbial ecology and intestinal inflammation. *Nature* **2012**, *487*, 477–481. [CrossRef] [PubMed]
85. Camargo, S.M.; Vuille-Dit-Bille, R.N.; Meier, C.F.; Verrey, F. ACE2 and gut amino acid transport. *Clin. Sci.* **2020**, *134*, 2823–2833. [CrossRef] [PubMed]
86. Camargo, S.M.; Singer, D.; Makrides, V.; Huggel, K.; Pos, K.M.; Wagner, C.A.; Kuba, K.; Danilczyk, U.; Skovby, F.; Kleta, R.; et al. Tissue-Specific Amino Acid Transporter Partners ACE2 and Collectrin Differentially Interact with Hartnup Mutations. *Gastroenterology* **2009**, *136*, 872–882.e3. [CrossRef]
87. Haga, S.; Nagata, N.; Okamura, T.; Yamamoto, N.; Sata, T.; Yamamoto, N.; Sasazuki, T.; Ishizaka, Y. TACE antagonists blocking ACE2 shedding caused by the spike protein of SARS-CoV are candidate antiviral compounds. *Antivir. Res.* **2010**, *85*, 551–555. [CrossRef]
88. Kuba, K.; Imai, Y.; Rao, S.; Gao, H.; Guo, F.; Guan, B.; Huan, Y.; Yang, P.; Zhang, Y.; Deng, W.; et al. A crucial role of angiotensin converting enzyme 2 (ACE2) in SARS coronavirus–induced lung injury. *Nat. Med.* **2005**, *11*, 875–879. [CrossRef]
89. Volbeda, M.; Jou-Valencia, D.; Heuvel, M.C.V.D.; Knoester, M.; Zwiers, P.J.; Pillay, J.; Berger, S.P.; van der Voort, P.H.J.; Zijlstra, J.G.; van Meurs, M.; et al. Comparison of renal histopathology and gene expression profiles between severe COVID-19 and bacterial sepsis in critically ill patients. *Crit. Care* **2021**, *25*, 202. [CrossRef]
90. Triana, S.; Metz-Zumaran, C.; Ramirez, C.; Kee, C.; Doldan, P.; Shahraz, M.; Schraivogel, D.; Gschwind, A.R.; Sharma, A.K.; Steinmetz, L.M.; et al. Single-cell analyses reveal SARS-CoV-2 interference with intrinsic immune response in the human gut. *Mol. Syst. Biol.* **2021**, *17*, e10232. [CrossRef]
91. Nataf, S.; Pays, L. Molecular Insights into SARS-CoV2-Induced Alterations of the Gut/Brain Axis. *Int. J. Mol. Sci.* **2021**, *22*, 10440. [CrossRef]

92. Heuberger, J.; Trimpert, J.; Vladimirova, D.; Goosmann, C.; Lin, M.; Schmuck, R.; Mollenkopf, H.; Brinkmann, V.; Tacke, F.; Osterrieder, N.; et al. Epithelial response to IFN-γ promotes SARS-CoV-2 infection. *EMBO Mol. Med.* **2021**, *13*, e13191. [CrossRef]
93. Lee, S.; Yoon, G.Y.; Myoung, J.; Kim, S.-J.; Ahn, D.-G. Robust and persistent SARS-CoV-2 infection in the human intestinal brush border expressing cells. *Emerg. Microbes Infect.* **2020**, *9*, 2169–2179. [CrossRef] [PubMed]
94. Ziegler, C.G.K.; Allon, S.J.; Nyquist, S.K.; Mbano, I.M.; Miao, V.N.; Tzouanas, C.N.; Cao, Y.; Yousif, A.S.; Bals, J.; Hauser, B.M.; et al. SARS-CoV-2 Receptor ACE2 Is an Interferon-Stimulated Gene in Human Airway Epithelial Cells and Is Detected in Specific Cell Subsets across Tissues. *Cell* **2020**, *181*, 1016–1035.e19. [CrossRef] [PubMed]
95. Harnik, Y.; Buchauer, L.; Ben-Moshe, S.; Averbukh, I.; Levin, Y.; Savidor, A.; Eilam, R.; Moor, A.E.; Itzkovitz, S. Spatial discordances between mRNAs and proteins in the intestinal epithelium. *Nat. Metab.* **2021**, *3*, 1680–1693. [CrossRef]
96. Onabajo, O.O.; Banday, A.R.; Stanifer, M.L.; Yan, W.; Obajemu, A.; Santer, D.M.; Florez-Vargas, O.; Piontkivska, H.; Vargas, J.M.; Ring, T.J.; et al. Interferons and viruses induce a novel truncated ACE2 isoform and not the full-length SARS-CoV-2 receptor. *Nat. Genet.* **2020**, *52*, 1283–1293. [CrossRef] [PubMed]
97. Jankowski, J.; Lee, H.K.; Wilflingseder, J.; Hennighausen, L. Interferon-regulated genetic programs and JAK/STAT pathway activate the intronic promoter of the short ACE2 isoform in renal proximal tubules. *bioRxiv* **2021**. [CrossRef]
98. Bártová, E.; Legartová, S.; Krejčí, J.; Arcidiacono, O.A. Cell differentiation and aging accompanied by depletion of the ACE2 protein. *Aging* **2020**, *12*, 22495–22508. [CrossRef]
99. Perlot, T.; Penninger, J.M. ACE2—From the renin–angiotensin system to gut microbiota and malnutrition. *Microbes Infect.* **2013**, *15*, 866–873. [CrossRef]
100. Bröer, S. Amino Acid Transport Across Mammalian Intestinal and Renal Epithelia. *Physiol. Rev.* **2008**, *88*, 249–286. [CrossRef]
101. Guo, Y.; Wang, B.; Gao, H.; Gao, L.; Hua, R.; Xu, J.-D. ACE2 in the Gut: The Center of the 2019-nCoV Infected Pathology. *Front. Mol. Biosci.* **2021**, *8*, 708336. [CrossRef]
102. Moal, V.L.-L.; Servin, A.L. The Front Line of Enteric Host Defense against Unwelcome Intrusion of Harmful Microorganisms: Mucins, Antimicrobial Peptides, and Microbiota. *Clin. Microbiol. Rev.* **2006**, *19*, 315–337. [CrossRef]
103. Rajput, S.; Paliwal, D.; Naithani, M.; Kothari, A.; Meena, K.; Rana, S. COVID-19 and Gut Microbiota: A Potential Connection. *Indian J. Clin. Biochem.* **2021**, *36*, 266–277. [CrossRef] [PubMed]
104. Rist, V.T.S.; Weiss, E.; Eklund, M.; Mosenthin, R. Impact of dietary protein on microbiota composition and activity in the gastrointestinal tract of piglets in relation to gut health: A review. *Animal* **2013**, *7*, 1067–1078. [CrossRef] [PubMed]
105. Duncan, S.H.; Iyer, A.; Russell, W.R. Impact of protein on the composition and metabolism of the human gut microbiota and health. *Proc. Nutr. Soc.* **2021**, *80*, 173–185. [CrossRef]
106. Masuoka, H.; Suda, W.; Tomitsuka, E.; Shindo, C.; Takayasu, L.; Horwood, P.; Greenhill, A.R.; Hattori, M.; Umezaki, M.; Hirayama, K. The influences of low protein diet on the intestinal microbiota of mice. *Sci. Rep.* **2020**, *10*, 17077. [CrossRef]
107. Trottein, F.; Sokol, H. Potential Causes and Consequences of Gastrointestinal Disorders during a SARS-CoV-2 Infection. *Cell Rep.* **2020**, *32*, 107915. [CrossRef] [PubMed]
108. Garg, M.; Angus, P.W.; Burrell, L.M.; Herath, C.; Gibson, P.R.; Lubel, J.S. Review article: The pathophysiological roles of the renin-angiotensin system in the gastrointestinal tract. *Aliment. Pharmacol. Ther.* **2012**, *35*, 414–428. [CrossRef]
109. Battagello, D.S.; Dragunas, G.; Klein, M.O.; Ayub, A.L.; Velloso, F.J.; Correa, R.G. Unpuzzling COVID-19: Tissue-related signaling pathways associated with SARS-CoV-2 infection and transmission. *Clin. Sci.* **2020**, *134*, 2137–2160. [CrossRef]
110. Duan, Y.; Prasad, R.; Feng, D.; Beli, E.; Li Calzi, S.; Longhini, A.L.F.; Lamendella, R.; Floyd, J.L.; DuPont, M.; Noothi, S.K.; et al. Bone Marrow-Derived Cells Restore Functional Integrity of the Gut Epithelial and Vascular Barriers in a Model of Diabetes and ACE2 Deficiency. *Circ. Res.* **2019**, *125*, 969–988. [CrossRef]
111. Danilczyk, U.; Sarao, R.; Remy, C.; Benabbas, C.; Stange, G.; Richter, A.; Arya, S.; Pospisilik, J.A.; Singer, D.; Camargo, S.; et al. Essential role for collectrin in renal amino acid transport. *Nature* **2006**, *444*, 1088–1091. [CrossRef]
112. Singer, D.; Camargo, S.; Ramadan, T.; Schäfer, M.; Mariotta, L.; Herzog, B.; Huggel, K.; Wolfer, D.; Werner, S.; Penninger, J.; et al. Defective intestinal amino acid absorption in Ace2 null mice. *Am. J. Physiol. Gastrointest. Liver Physiol.* **2012**, *303*, G686–G695. [CrossRef]
113. Aktas, B. Gut Microbiota Dysbiosis and COVID-19: Possible Links. *Ref. Modul. Food Sci.* **2022**, 535–544. [CrossRef]
114. Spak, E.; Hallersund, P.; Edebo, A.; Casselbrant, A.; Fändriks, L. The human duodenal mucosa harbors all components for a local renin angiotensin system. *Clin. Sci.* **2019**, *133*, 971–982. [CrossRef] [PubMed]
115. Shenoy, S. Gut microbiome, Vitamin D, ACE2 interactions are critical factors in immune-senescence and inflammaging: Key for vaccine response and severity of COVID-19 infection. *Inflamm. Res.* **2022**, *71*, 13–26. [CrossRef] [PubMed]
116. Xiong, D.; Muema, C.; Zhang, X.; Pan, X.; Xiong, J.; Yang, H.; Yu, J.; Wei, H. Enriched Opportunistic Pathogens Revealed by Metagenomic Sequencing Hint Potential Linkages between Pharyngeal Microbiota and COVID-19. *Virol. Sin.* **2021**, *36*, 924–933. [CrossRef]
117. Sokol, H.; Pigneur, B.; Watterlot, L.; Lakhdari, O.; Bermúdez-Humarán, L.G.; Gratadoux, J.-J.; Blugeon, S.; Bridonneau, C.; Furet, J.-P.; Corthier, G.; et al. *Faecalibacterium prausnitzii* is an anti-inflammatory commensal bacterium identified by gut microbiota analysis of Crohn disease patients. *Proc. Natl. Acad. Sci. USA* **2008**, *105*, 16731–16736. [CrossRef]
118. Yang, T.; Chakraborty, S.; Saha, P.; Mell, B.; Cheng, X.; Yeo, J.-Y.; Mei, X.; Zhou, G.; Mandal, J.; Golonka, R.; et al. Gnotobiotic Rats Reveal That Gut Microbiota Regulates Colonic mRNA of Ace2, the Receptor for SARS-CoV-2 Infectivity. *Hypertension* **2020**, *76*, e1–e3. [CrossRef]

119. Das, S.; Jayaratne, R.; Barrett, K.E. The Role of Ion Transporters in the Pathophysiology of Infectious Diarrhea. *Cell. Mol. Gastroenterol. Hepatol.* **2018**, *6*, 33–45. [CrossRef]
120. Day, C.J.; Bailly, B.; Guillon, P.; Dirr, L.; Jen, F.E.-C.; Spillings, B.L.; Mak, J.; von Itzstein, M.; Haselhorst, T.; Jennings, M.P. Multidisciplinary Approaches Identify Compounds that Bind to Human ACE2 or SARS-CoV-2 Spike Protein as Candidates to Block SARS-CoV-2–ACE2 Receptor Interactions. *mBio* **2021**, *12*. [CrossRef]
121. Xiong, J.; Xiang, Y.; Huang, Z.; Liu, X.; Wang, M.; Ge, G.; Chen, H.; Xu, J.; Zheng, M.; Chen, L. Structure-Based Virtual Screening and Identification of Potential Inhibitors of SARS-CoV-2 S-RBD and ACE2 Interaction. *Front. Chem.* **2021**, *9*, 740702. [CrossRef]
122. Prada, J.A.H.; Ferreira, A.J.; Katovich, M.J.; Shenoy, V.; Qi, Y.; Santos, R.A.; Castellano, R.K.; Lampkins, A.J.; Gubala, V.; Ostrov, D.A.; et al. Structure-Based Identification of Small-Molecule Angiotensin-Converting Enzyme 2 Activators as Novel Antihypertensive Agents. *Hypertension* **2008**, *51*, 1312–1317. [CrossRef]
123. Sutton, T.D.S.; Hill, C. Gut Bacteriophage: Current Understanding and Challenges. *Front. Endocrinol.* **2019**, *10*, 784. [CrossRef] [PubMed]
124. Ebrahimi, K.H. SARS-CoV-2 spike glycoprotein-binding proteins expressed by upper respiratory tract bacteria may prevent severe viral infection. *FEBS Lett.* **2020**, *594*, 1651–1660. [CrossRef] [PubMed]
125. Petrillo, M.; Querci, M.; Brogna, C.; Ponti, J.; Cristoni, S.; Markov, P.V.; Valsesia, A.; Leoni, G.; Benedetti, A.; Wiss, T.; et al. Evidence of SARS-CoV-2 bacteriophage potential in human gut microbiota. *F1000Research* **2022**, *11*, 292. [CrossRef]
126. Gottlieb, P.; Alimova, A. RNA Packaging in the *Cystovirus* Bacteriophages: Dynamic Interactions during Capsid Maturation. *Int. J. Mol. Sci.* **2022**, *23*, 2677. [CrossRef]
127. Grenga, L.; Gallais, F.; Pible, O.; Gaillard, J.-C.; Gouveia, D.; Batina, H.; Bazaline, N.; Ruat, S.; Culotta, K.; Miotello, G.; et al. Shotgun proteomics analysis of SARS-CoV-2-infected cells and how it can optimize whole viral particle antigen production for vaccines. *Emerg. Microbes Infect.* **2020**, *9*, 1712–1721. [CrossRef]
128. Townsend, E.M.; Kelly, L.; Muscatt, G.; Box, J.D.; Hargraves, N.; Lilley, D.; Jameson, E. The Human Gut Phageome: Origins and Roles in the Human Gut Microbiome. *Front. Cell. Infect. Microbiol.* **2021**, *11*, 643214. [CrossRef]
129. Guerin, E.; Hill, C. Shining Light on Human Gut Bacteriophages. *Front. Cell. Infect. Microbiol.* **2020**, *10*, 481. [CrossRef]
130. Aggarwala, V.; Liang, G.; Bushman, F.D. Viral communities of the human gut: Metagenomic analysis of composition and dynamics. *Mob. DNA* **2017**, *8*, 12. [CrossRef]
131. Zajac, V. Elimination of the new coronavirus and prevention of the second wave of infection. *World J. Adv. Res. Rev.* **2020**, *8*, 148–150. [CrossRef]
132. Brogna, C.; Cristoni, S.; Petrillo, M.; Querci, M.; Piazza, O.; Eede, G.V.D. Toxin-like peptides in plasma, urine and faecal samples from COVID-19 patients. *F1000Research* **2021**, *10*, 550. [CrossRef]
133. Grenga, L.; Pible, O.; Miotello, G.; Culotta, K.; Ruat, S.; Roncato, M.; Gas, F.; Bellanger, L.; Claret, P.; Dunyach-Remy, C.; et al. Taxonomical and functional changes in COVID -19 faecal microbiome could be related to SARS-CoV-2 faecal load. *Environ. Microbiol.* **2022**. [CrossRef] [PubMed]
134. Dean, P.; Kenny, B. Intestinal barrier dysfunction by enteropathogenic Escherichia coli is mediated by two effector molecules and a bacterial surface protein. *Mol. Microbiol.* **2004**, *54*, 665–675. [CrossRef] [PubMed]
135. Viswanathan, V.K.; Koutsouris, A.; Lukic, S.; Pilkinton, M.; Simonovic, I.; Simonovic, M.; Hecht, G. Comparative Analysis of EspF from Enteropathogenic and Enterohemorrhagic *Escherichia coli* in Alteration of Epithelial Barrier Function. *Infect. Immun.* **2004**, *72*, 3218–3227. [CrossRef]
136. Tafazoli, F.; Magnusson, K.-E.; Zheng, L. Disruption of Epithelial Barrier Integrity by *Salmonella enterica* Serovar Typhimurium Requires Geranylgeranylated Proteins. *Infect. Immun.* **2003**, *71*, 872–881. [CrossRef] [PubMed]
137. Larsen, J.M. The immune response to *Prevotella*bacteria in chronic inflammatory disease. *Immunology* **2017**, *151*, 363–374. [CrossRef]
138. Jakobsson, H.E.; Rodríguez-Piñeiro, A.M.; Schütte, A.; Ermund, A.; Boysen, P.; Bemark, M.; Sommer, F.; Bäckhed, F.; Hansson, G.C.; Johansson, M.E.V. The composition of the gut microbiota shapes the colon mucus barrier. *EMBO Rep.* **2015**, *16*, 164–177. [CrossRef]
139. Puschhof, J.; Pleguezuelos-Manzano, C.; Martinez-Silgado, A.; Akkerman, N.; Saftien, A.; Boot, C.; de Waal, A.; Beumer, J.; Dutta, D.; Heo, I.; et al. Intestinal organoid cocultures with microbes. *Nat. Protoc.* **2021**, *16*, 4633–4649. [CrossRef]
140. Dicksved, J.; Schreiber, O.; Willing, B.; Petersson, J.; Rang, S.; Phillipson, M.; Holm, L.; Roos, S. *Lactobacillus reuteri* Maintains a Functional Mucosal Barrier during DSS Treatment Despite Mucus Layer Dysfunction. *PLoS ONE* **2012**, *7*, e46399. [CrossRef]
141. Kim, H.S. Do an Altered Gut Microbiota and an Associated Leaky Gut Affect COVID-19 Severity? *mBio* **2021**, *12*. [CrossRef]
142. Vignesh, R.; Swathirajan, C.R.; Tun, Z.H.; Rameshkumar, M.R.; Solomon, S.S.; Balakrishnan, P. Could Perturbation of Gut Microbiota Possibly Exacerbate the Severity of COVID-19 via Cytokine Storm? *Front. Immunol.* **2020**, *11*, 607734. [CrossRef]
143. Openshaw, P.J. Crossing barriers: Infections of the lung and the gut. *Mucosal Immunol.* **2009**, *2*, 100–102. [CrossRef] [PubMed]
144. Cardinale, V.; Capurso, G.; Ianiro, G.; Gasbarrini, A.; Arcidiacono, P.G.; Alvaro, D. Intestinal permeability changes with bacterial translocation as key events modulating systemic host immune response to SARS-CoV-2: A working hypothesis. *Dig. Liver Dis.* **2020**, *52*, 1383–1389. [CrossRef] [PubMed]
145. Giron, L.B.; Dweep, H.; Yin, X.; Wang, H.; Damra, M.; Goldman, A.R.; Gorman, N.; Palmer, C.S.; Tang, H.-Y.; Shaikh, M.W.; et al. Plasma Markers of Disrupted Gut Permeability in Severe COVID-19 Patients. *Front. Immunol.* **2021**, *12*, 686240. [CrossRef] [PubMed]

146. Prasad, R.; Patton, M.J.; Floyd, J.L.; Fortmann, S.; DuPont, M.; Harbour, A.; Wright, J.; Lamendella, R.; Stevens, B.R.; Oudit, G.Y.; et al. Plasma Microbiome in COVID-19 Subjects: An Indicator of Gut Barrier Defects and Dysbiosis. *Int. J. Mol. Sci.* **2022**, *23*, 9141. [CrossRef] [PubMed]
147. Sun, Z.; Song, Z.-G.; Liu, C.; Tan, S.; Lin, S.; Zhu, J.; Dai, F.-H.; Gao, J.; She, J.-L.; Mei, Z.; et al. Gut microbiome alterations and gut barrier dysfunction are associated with host immune homeostasis in COVID-19 patients. *BMC Med.* **2022**, *20*, 24. [CrossRef] [PubMed]
148. Maguire, M.; Maguire, G. Gut dysbiosis, leaky gut, and intestinal epithelial proliferation in neurological disorders: Towards the development of a new therapeutic using amino acids, prebiotics, probiotics, and postbiotics. *Rev. Neurosci.* **2019**, *30*, 179–201. [CrossRef] [PubMed]
149. Effenberger, M.; Grabherr, F.; Mayr, L.; Schwaerzler, J.; Nairz, M.; Seifert, M.; Hilbe, R.; Seiwald, S.; Scholl-Buergi, S.; Fritsche, G.; et al. Faecal calprotectin indicates intestinal inflammation in COVID-19. *Gut* **2020**, *69*, 1543–1544. [CrossRef]
150. Hayashi, Y.; Wagatsuma, K.; Nojima, M.; Yamakawa, T.; Ichimiya, T.; Yokoyama, Y.; Kazama, T.; Hirayama, D.; Nakase, H. The characteristics of gastrointestinal symptoms in patients with severe COVID-19: A systematic review and meta-analysis. *J. Gastroenterol.* **2021**, *56*, 409–420. [CrossRef]
151. Jin, X.; Lian, J.S.; Hu, J.H.; Gao, J.; Zheng, L.; Zhang, Y.M.; Hao, S.R.; Jia, H.Y.; Cai, H.; Zhang, X.L.; et al. Epidemiological, clinical and virological characteristics of 74 cases of coronavirus-infected disease 2019 (COVID-19) with gastrointestinal symptoms. *Gut* **2020**, *69*, 1002–1009. [CrossRef]
152. Nobel, Y.R.; Phipps, M.; Zucker, J.; Lebwohl, B.; Wang, T.C.; Sobieszczyk, M.E.; Freedberg, D.E. Gastrointestinal Symptoms and Coronavirus Disease 2019: A Case-Control Study from the United States. *Gastroenterology* **2020**, *159*, 373–375.e2. [CrossRef]
153. Redd, W.D.; Zhou, J.C.; Hathorn, K.E.; Mccarty, T.R.; Bazarbashi, A.N.; Thompson, C.C.; Shen, L.; Chan, W.W. Prevalence and Characteristics of Gastrointestinal Symptoms in Patients with Severe Acute Respiratory Syndrome Coronavirus 2 Infection in the United States: A Multicenter Cohort Study. *Gastroenterology* **2020**, *159*, 765–767.e2. [CrossRef] [PubMed]
154. Natarajan, A.; Zlitni, S.; Brooks, E.F.; Vance, S.E.; Dahlen, A.; Hedlin, H.; Park, R.M.; Han, A.; Schmidtke, D.T.; Verma, R.; et al. Gastrointestinal symptoms and fecal shedding of SARS-CoV-2 RNA suggest prolonged gastrointestinal infection. *Med* **2022**, *3*, 371–387.e9. [CrossRef] [PubMed]
155. Wu, Y.; Guo, C.; Tang, L.; Hong, Z.; Zhou, J.; Dong, X.; Yin, H.; Xiao, Q.; Tang, Y.; Qu, X.; et al. Prolonged presence of SARS-CoV-2 viral RNA in faecal samples. *Lancet Gastroenterol. Hepatol.* **2020**, *5*, 434–435. [CrossRef]
156. Brooks, E.F.; Bhatt, A.S. The gut microbiome: A missing link in understanding the gastrointestinal manifestations of COVID-19? *Cold Spring Harb. Mol. Case Stud.* **2021**, *7*, a006031. [CrossRef]
157. Liu, Q.; Mak, J.W.Y.; Su, Q.; Yeoh, Y.K.; Lui, G.C.-Y.; Ng, S.S.S.; Zhang, F.; Li, A.Y.L.; Lu, W.; Hui, D.S.-C.; et al. Gut microbiota dynamics in a prospective cohort of patients with post-acute COVID-19 syndrome. *Gut* **2022**, *71*, 544–552. [CrossRef]
158. Davis, H.E.; Assaf, G.S.; McCorkell, L.; Wei, H.; Low, R.J.; Re'Em, Y.; Redfield, S.; Austin, J.P.; Akrami, A. Characterizing long COVID in an international cohort: 7 months of symptoms and their impact. *eClinicalMedicine* **2021**, *38*, 101019. [CrossRef]
159. Arostegui, D.; Castro, K.; Schwarz, S.; Vaidy, K.; Rabinowitz, S.; Wallach, T. Persistent SARS-CoV-2 Nucleocapsid Protein Presence in the Intestinal Epithelium of a Pediatric Patient 3 Months after Acute Infection. *JPGN Rep.* **2021**, *3*, e152. [CrossRef]
160. Kim, K.O.; Gluck, M. Fecal Microbiota Transplantation: An Update on Clinical Practice. *Clin. Endosc.* **2019**, *52*, 137–143. [CrossRef]
161. Kazemian, N.; Kao, D.; Pakpour, S. Fecal Microbiota Transplantation during and Post-COVID-19 Pandemic. *Int. J. Mol. Sci.* **2021**, *22*, 3004. [CrossRef]
162. Wang, X.; Zhang, P.; Zhang, X. Probiotics Regulate Gut Microbiota: An Effective Method to Improve Immunity. *Molecules* **2021**, *26*, 6076. [CrossRef]
163. Baindara, P.; Chakraborty, R.; Holliday, Z.M.; Mandal, S.M.; Schrum, A.G. Oral probiotics in coronavirus disease 2019: Connecting the gut–lung axis to viral pathogenesis, inflammation, secondary infection and clinical trials. *New Microbes New Infect.* **2021**, *40*, 100837. [CrossRef] [PubMed]
164. Kurian, S.J.; Unnikrishnan, M.K.; Miraj, S.S.; Bagchi, D.; Banerjee, M.; Reddy, B.S.; Rodrigues, G.S.; Manu, M.K.; Saravu, K.; Mukhopadhyay, C.; et al. Probiotics in Prevention and Treatment of COVID-19: Current Perspective and Future Prospects. *Arch. Med. Res.* **2021**, *52*, 582–594. [CrossRef] [PubMed]
165. Mak, J.W.Y.; Chan, F.K.L.; Ng, S.C. Probiotics and COVID-19: One size does not fit all. *Lancet Gastroenterol. Hepatol.* **2020**, *5*, 644–645. [CrossRef]
166. Guarino, M.P.L.; Altomare, A.; Emerenziani, S.; Di Rosa, C.; Ribolsi, M.; Balestrieri, P.; Iovino, P.; Rocchi, G.; Cicala, M. Mechanisms of Action of Prebiotics and Their Effects on Gastro-Intestinal Disorders in Adults. *Nutrients* **2020**, *12*, 1037. [CrossRef]
167. Peters, V.; Van De Steeg, E.; van Bilsen, J.; Meijerink, M. Mechanisms and immunomodulatory properties of pre- and probiotics. *Benef. Microbes* **2019**, *10*, 225–236. [CrossRef] [PubMed]
168. Shokryazdan, P.; Jahromi, M.F.; Navidshad, B.; Liang, J.B. Effects of prebiotics on immune system and cytokine expression. *Med. Microbiol. Immunol.* **2016**, *206*, 1–9. [CrossRef]
169. Khaled, J.M. Probiotics, prebiotics, and COVID-19 infection: A review article. *Saudi J. Biol. Sci.* **2021**, *28*, 865–869. [CrossRef]
170. Kalantar-Zadeh, K.; Ward, S.A.; Kalantar-Zadeh, K.; El-Omar, E. Considering the Effects of Microbiome and Diet on SARS-CoV-2 Infection: Nanotechnology Roles. *ACS Nano* **2020**, *14*, 5179–5182. [CrossRef]

171. Infusino, F.; Marazzato, M.; Mancone, M.; Fedele, F.; Mastroianni, C.M.; Severino, P.; Ceccarelli, G.; Santinelli, L.; Cavarretta, E.; Marullo, A.G.M.; et al. Diet Supplementation, Probiotics, and Nutraceuticals in SARS-CoV-2 Infection: A Scoping Review. *Nutrients* **2020**, *12*, 1718. [CrossRef]
172. Deschasaux-Tanguy, M.; Srour, B.; Bourhis, L.; Arnault, N.; Druesne-Pecollo, N.; Esseddik, Y.; de Edelenyi, F.S.; Allègre, J.; Allès, B.; Andreeva, V.A.; et al. Nutritional risk factors for SARS-CoV-2 infection: A prospective study within the NutriNet-Santé cohort. *BMC Med.* **2021**, *19*, 290. [CrossRef]
173. Salazar-Robles, E.; Kalantar-Zadeh, K.; Badillo, H.; Calderón-Juárez, M.; García-Bárcenas, C.A.; Ledesma-Pérez, P.D.; Lerma, A.; Lerma, C. Association between severity of COVID-19 symptoms and habitual food intake in adult outpatients. *BMJ Nutr. Prev. Health* **2021**, *4*, 469–478. [CrossRef] [PubMed]

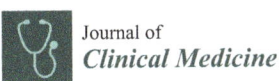

Review

Gut as an Alternative Entry Route for SARS-CoV-2: Current Evidence and Uncertainties of Productive Enteric Infection in COVID-19

Laure-Alix Clerbaux [1,*], Sally A. Mayasich [2], Amalia Muñoz [3], Helena Soares [4], Mauro Petrillo [5], Maria Cristina Albertini [6], Nicolas Lanthier [7], Lucia Grenga [8] and Maria-Joao Amorim [9,10]

1. European Commission, Joint Research Centre (JRC), 21027 Ispra, Italy
2. University of Wisconsin-Madison Aquatic Sciences Center at US EPA, Duluth, MN 55804, USA
3. European Commission, Joint Research Centre (JRC), 2440 Geel, Belgium
4. Laboratory of Human Immunobiology and Pathogenesis, iNOVA4Health, Faculdade de Ciências Médicas—Nova Medical School, Universidade Nova de Lisboa, 1099-085 Lisbon, Portugal
5. Seidor Italy Srl, 20129 Milano, Italy
6. Department of Biomolecular Sciences, University of Urbino Carlo Bo, 61029 Urbino, Italy
7. Laboratoire d'Hépatogastroentérologie, Service d'Hépato-Gastroentérologie, Cliniques Universitaires Saint-Luc, UCLouvain, 1200 Brussels, Belgium
8. Département Médicaments et Technologies pour la Santé, Commissariat à l'Énergie Atomique et aux Énergies Alternatives (CEA), Institut National de Recherche pour l'Agriculture, l'Alimentation et l'Environnement (INRAE), Université Paris-Saclay, 91190 Paris, France
9. Instituto Gulbenkian de Ciência, 2780-156 Lisbon, Portugal
10. Católica Biomedical Research Centre, Católica Medical School, Universidade Católica Portuguesa, 1649-023 Lisbon, Portugal
* Correspondence: laure-alix.clerbaux@ec.europa.eu

Abstract: The gut has been proposed as a potential alternative entry route for SARS-CoV-2. This was mainly based on the high levels of SARS-CoV-2 receptor expressed in the gastrointestinal (GI) tract, the observations of GI disorders (such as diarrhea) in some COVID-19 patients and the detection of SARS-CoV-2 RNA in feces. However, the underlying mechanisms remain poorly understood. It has been proposed that SARS-CoV-2 can productively infect enterocytes, damaging the intestinal barrier and contributing to inflammatory response, which might lead to GI manifestations, including diarrhea. Here, we report a methodological approach to assess the evidence supporting the sequence of events driving SARS-CoV-2 enteric infection up to gut adverse outcomes. Exploring evidence permits to highlight knowledge gaps and current inconsistencies in the literature and to guide further research. Based on the current insights on SARS-CoV-2 intestinal infection and transmission, we then discuss the potential implication on clinical practice, including on long COVID. A better understanding of the GI implication in COVID-19 is still needed to improve disease management and could help identify innovative therapies or preventive actions targeting the GI tract.

Keywords: SARS-CoV-2 infection; COVID-19; gut microbiota; gastrointestinal disorders; enteric infection

1. Introduction

While COVID-19 is mainly considered a respiratory disease, gastrointestinal (GI) symptomatology in COVID-19 has been reported, though the proportion varies depending on the studies, with patients reporting diarrhea, abdominal discomfort, nausea and/or vomiting, with diarrhea being the predominant GI symptom [1–4]. GI disorders, and particularly diarrhea, are proposed to be a direct consequence of SARS-CoV-2 intestinal infection, as many patients have detectable SARS-CoV-2 RNA in feces [5]. In addition, recent studies showed that non-human primates infected with SARS-CoV-2 had transient diarrhea [6]. However, the mechanisms leading to diarrhea in COVID-19 are largely unknown [7]. Studies from other viruses identified different mechanisms-inducing diarrhea

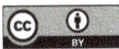

such as malabsorption or inflammation secondary to enterocyte damage and death [8,9], the release of virulent toxins [8] and gut microbiota dysbiosis [10,11]. While SARS-CoV-2 RNA has been found in the stools of many patients, the impact of its presence in the GI tract remains to be clarified; in most cases, infectious particles are not recovered and infection does not always lead to diarrhea. In one study, 50% of the examined COVID-19 patients had a detectable level of virus in their feces, with only half showing diarrhea [12]. In another study the level of fecal viral load was positively associated with diarrhea [5]. Elevated fecal and serum levels of the inflammatory marker calprotectin in COVID-19 were not consistent with GI symptoms [13]. In line, limited intestinal inflammation was observed in patients with acute COVID-19 despite diarrhea, fecal viral RNA and SARS-CoV-2-specific immunoglobulin A (IgA) [14]. Thus, summarizing the current lines of evidence and uncertainties supporting intestinal infection and understanding the impact of intestinal SARS-CoV-2 on the GI system (epithelium damage, inflammation) could improve disease management, help to identify therapies or effective preventive actions targeting the GI tract.

Here, we used a methodological approach well-established in toxicology to evaluate key mechanisms driving SARS-CoV-2 mediated gut pathophysiology: the Adverse Outcome Pathway (AOP) framework which has been developed and is currently used to assess chemical risk for regulatory purposes. Based on existing data and available literature, the AOP approach seeks to pragmatically focus on essential biological key events (KE) at the different biological levels (molecular, cellular, tissue, organ, individual) up to an adverse outcome via a domino effect [15–18]. A KE describes a measurable and essential change in a biological system that can be quantified in experimental or clinical settings [19]. The strength of the relationship between the events is established by demonstrating biological plausibility and causality between pairs of events, called key event relationships (KER) [18,19]. The confidence that each KER occurs within an AOP is postulated by the evaluation of the weight of evidence [20]. Information contained in the KEs, KERs and AOPs are stored in an open access platform (https://aopwiki.org/) where they are identified by assigned unique numbers. Numbers in the text refer to these AOP-wiki pages. There, AOPs can be continuously updated as new information becomes available. This AOP approach highlights important inconsistencies and gaps in the evidence. Interestingly, based on a mechanistic understanding, AOPs help elucidate the pathophysiological mechanisms notably by learning from other inflammatory bowel diseases and other respiratory virus-related diseases (e.g., SARS, MERS, influenza) also presenting GI symptoms. This study was realized under the CIAO project which aims to make sense of the overwhelming flow of publications and data related to COVID-19 pathogenesis by using the AOP framework [21,22]. The project is based on the assumption that such mechanistic organization of the COVID-19 knowledge across the different biological levels will improve the interpretation and efficient application of the scientific understanding of COVID-19 [23]. In addition, we applied this methodology for the first time to map a viral disease of high societal relevance, expanding the AOP scope outside the toxicological field.

We aim to evaluate if the gut can be an alternative route for viral entry, meaning that a productive intestinal infection by SARS-CoV-2 occurs and is responsible for the associated GI disorders (inflammation, permeability, diarrhea). To do so, we explored in the literature the evidence and uncertainties of each event starting with SARS-CoV-2 binding to its cellular receptor towards infection up to intestinal barrier disruption and intestinal inflammation. For this review, we collected evidence reported in tissue cultured cells, human samples and animal models of infection, including mice with human ACE2 (hACE2 mice), hamsters, minks, ferrets and non-human primates.

2. Current Evidence and Uncertainties of an Active SARS-CoV-2 Enteric Infection

Besides GI symptoms experienced by many COVID-19 patients and SARS-CoV-2 RNA detected in feces, the rationale supporting intestinal infection was also based on the high level of expression in the intestines of the main SARS-CoV-2 cellular gateways: angiotensin converting enzyme 2 (ACE2) and transmembrane serine protease 2 (TMPRSS2). Enterocytes in the small intestine express the highest levels of ACE2 in the human body [24] and are one of the few human cell types that co-express TMPRSS2 [24], the main cofactor mediating cellular entry [7,25,26]. To evaluate if SARS-CoV-2 can effectively infect enterocytes, we assessed the evidence from the literature, starting with viable SARS-CoV-2 in the gut lumen binding to ACE2 receptors at the apical surface of the enterocytes, cell entry via TMPRSS2 cleavage and replication while antagonizing the antiviral response in order to release new viral particles (Figure 1).

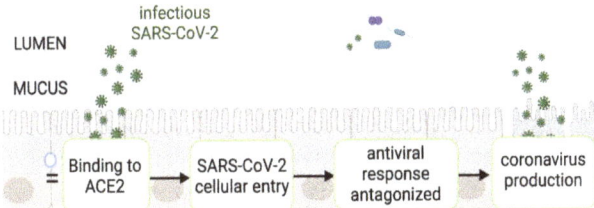

Figure 1. Pathway depicting the proposed sequence of events of a productive SARS-CoV-2 infection in the gut. Virus binding to the ACE2 receptor expressed on enterocytes mediates viral entry inducing an antiviral response that must be antagonized for new virions to be produced. This manuscript will evaluate available published data on the likelihood of their occurrence.

2.1. S Proteins Bind to ACE2 in Enterocytes and Mediates Viral Entry

Biological plausibility. Upon binding of SARS-CoV-2 to ACE2 (KE1739), the spike (S) proteins of the virus need to be activated through proteolytic cleavage to allow fusion between host and viral membranes, a key step in viral entry (KE1738), that releases viral RNA and proteins into host cells. Many proteases were identified as aiding in cell surface entry, such as TMPRSS2. Only three cell types showed co-expression of ACE2 and TMPRSS2, including enterocytes [26,27]. In addition, neuropilin-1 (NRP-1) was proposed to act as ACE2 co-receptor and promote, although to very low levels, SARS-CoV-2 entry even in cells that lack ACE2 and TMPRSS2 [24]. Maximum infection was reported when NRP-1 and ACE2 are co-expressed on the same cell types [28]. NRP-1 is reported to be expressed in the epithelia of the GI tract [29].

Evidence. Regarding ACE2 as the entry receptor for SARS-CoV-2, the level of ACE2 expression did not correlate with infectivity of cells in human intestinal organoids [30]. Both ACE2-positive and ACE2-negative SARS-CoV-2 infected cells in intestinal organoids were observed [31], potentially suggesting the existence of alternative entry receptors, ACE2 downregulation after infection, or reflecting expression levels under the detection limit. However, ACE2-knock-out (KO) intestinal organoids were fully resistant to SARS-CoV-2 infection [31], suggesting that ACE2 is the obligate entry receptor for SARS-CoV-2 in intestinal cells. Accordingly, in human gut-on-chip models composed of intestinal epithelial Caco-2 co-cultured with mucin-secreting HT-29 intestinal cells, the highest levels of ACE2 expression were found in the Caco-2 cells and after viral infection, Spike protein-positive Caco-2 cells were detected [32]. Similarly, higher ACE2 levels correlated with the maturity of enterocytes present in human differentiated enteroids and SARS-CoV-2 was able to infect ACE2+ mature enterocytes [33], therefore mature enterocytes are likely highly susceptible to infection. Further, the entry process was facilitated by TMPRSS2 and TMPRSS4 proteases [33]. However, when using CRISPR-Cas9 to generate different knock-out of key coronavirus host factors in human intestinal organoids, TMPRSS2, and not TMPRSS4, was found to be essential for SARS-CoV-2 entry [31].

As mouse ACE2 has a low affinity for S protein of SARS-CoV-2, different strategies were adopted to circumvent that mice are resistant to SARS-CoV-2 infection [34]. In a transgenic mouse expressing human ACE2 in the lungs, heart, kidneys and intestines (hACE2 mice), viral RNA was detected in the intestines of intranasally inoculated animals [35].

In another stable mouse model generated by CRISPR-Cas9 knock-in technology, hACE2 expression was also detected in the small intestine [36]. Another transgenic mouse model with hACE2 driven by the heterologous promoters (K18-hACE2) showed no viral RNA in the GI tract following nasal inoculation [37], but importantly hACE2 expression was not detected in the gut in these mice [37]. In Syrian golden hamsters, ACE2 protein is highly expressed in surface epithelium of ileum [38] and SARS-CoV-2 nucleocapsid protein was found in the intestine after intranasal infection [39]. In ferrets, ACE2 is expressed in the GI tract [40] and viral RNA was detected in the gut (ileum and colon) of intranasally infected male ferrets [39]. In rhesus monkeys, viral RNA was detectable in GI tissues after intranasal inoculation [41,42].

Uncertainties, inconsistencies and gaps. As previously noted, study in ACE2-KO intestinal organoids indicated ACE2 as the entry receptor of SARS-CoV-2 in enterocytes in vitro facilitated by TMPRSS2 [31]. The authors proposed that the discrepancy with the study considering TMPRSS4 could be explained by the expression in the KO organoids of physiological levels of the proteases rather than overexpression [31]. No studies have specifically investigated the role of NRP-1 in SARS-CoV-2 entry in the gut. However, it is interesting to note that different variants display different affinities for NRP-1, with omicron displaying higher affinity than previous variants. Future studies should elucidate whether this increase in affinity constitutes a functional evolutionary adaptation of SARS-CoV-2 to humans [43], and confer an advantage for viral entry.

2.2. Viral Entry Leads to Antiviral Response

Biological plausibility. Following cellular entry, the primary translation of the SARS-CoV-2 open reading frame (ORF) 1a and ORF1b genomic RNA produces non-structural proteins (NSPs) [44]. The ORF1a produces polypeptide 1a (pp1a) that is cleaved into NSP-1 through NSP11. A -1 ribosomal frameshift occurs immediately upstream of the ORF1a stop codon to allow translation through ORF1b, yielding pp1ab, which is cleaved into 15 NSPs (duplications of NSP1-11 and five additional proteins, NSP12-16). Viral proteases NSP3 and NSP5 cleave the polypeptides through domains functioning as a papain-like protease and a 3C-like protease, respectively [44]. The NSPs, structural proteins, and the accessory proteins are encoded by 10 ORFs in the SARS-CoV-2 RNA genome. They have multiple functions in evasion of the host innate immune response and in viral replication [45].

Evidence. The innate immunity activated by viral infections resulting in quick resolution of disease occurs in many instances of SARS-CoV-2 infection, such as in adults with no or mild symptoms [46], the young [47], and bats that harbor the virus without disease [48]. SARS-CoV-2 infection of human intestinal epithelial cells was associated with a robust innate immune response mediated by type III interferon, which inhibits SARS-CoV-2 replication and de novo virus production [49]. Interestingly, the scRNAseq study by Triana et al. found that SARS-CoV2 induced distinct proinflammatory and interferon-stimulated gene (ISG) expression profiles in infected and bystander cells in organoids. ISG expression was pronounced in bystander cells, while the infected cells showed strong NFkB/TNF-mediated pro-inflammatory response but a limited ISG expression. In intranasally infected hamsters, high levels of viral RNA were detected in the GI tract only in signal transducer and activator of transcription 2 (STAT2) KO animals suggesting that STAT2, the main actor of the interferon (IFN) response, is crucial for preventing intestinal virus replication and production of infectious progeny [50,51].

Uncertainties, inconsistencies and gaps. For SARS-CoV-2 infection, initial transcriptional analyses of infected cells have generated ambiguous results on the induction of type I/III IFNs and the subsequent expression of ISG and many studies associate better prognosis with increased innate immunity activation. However, the effectiveness of IFN treatment is still uncertain due to some studies evaluating IFN and other drugs [52]. There are uncertainties based on differing disease outcomes, mainly associated with the timing of administering IFN; administering late, in the inflammatory stage, led to long-lasting harm and worsened disease outcomes [52]. In the small intestine of infected hamsters, a mild antiviral gene signature was observed coinciding with a low-level inflammatory response and low replication similar to some human cases [53], in contrast to the robust replication seen in human small intestinal organoids [54] and severely ill patients [55].

2.3. Antagonized Antiviral Response Leads to Coronavirus Production

Biological plausibility. The SARS-CoV-2 virus has evolved a repertoire of proteins that bind and block proteins in the IFN cascade so the host antiviral proteins are not expressed, and the virus is free to replicate [56]. Interactions between SARS-CoV-2 proteins and human RNAs have been demonstrated to thwart the IFN response: NSP1 binds to 40S ribosomal RNA in the mRNA entry channel of the ribosome to inhibit host mRNA translation. NSP6 binds TANK binding kinase 1 (TBK1) to suppress interferon regulatory factor 3 (IRF3) phosphorylation, and NSP13 binds and blocks TBK1 phosphorylation [56]. NSP14 induces lysosomal degradation of type 1 IFN-alpha receptor (IFNAR) to prevent STAT activation [57]. ORF6 blocks nuclear import of IRF3 and STAT proteins to silence IFN-I gene expression [58]. ORF7a suppresses STAT2 phosphorylation and ORF7b suppresses STAT1 and STAT2 phosphorylation to block interferon-stimulated gene factor 3 (ISGF 3) complex formation with IRF9 [58]. ORF9b antagonizes IFN-I by targeting multiple components of RIG-I/MDA-5-MAVS, TOMM70, NEMO and cGAS-STING signaling [59–62]. The timely production of type I IFN by host cells is critical for limiting viral replication and promoting antiviral immunity [63]. If the antiviral response is antagonized (KE1901), the viral RNA can be translated, replicated, transcribed and the genomic RNA packaged before the new SARS-CoV-2 virions are assembled and released potentially into feces (KE1847).

Evidence. In human intestinal organoids, following entry, gene expression analysis demonstrated that SARS-CoV-2 replicated with low induction of type I and III IFNs, though increased expression of ISG was observed [27]. Infection of Caco-2 cells leads to a weaker intrinsic immune response, associated with more de novo infectious virus production than T84 cells [49]. In ex vivo human intestinal tissues, SARS-CoV-2 replicated less efficiently (less viral genome copies produced, less infectious particles generated) but induced a more robust innate immune response than SARS-Co-V, including both type I and III IFNs while SARS-Co-V induced only IFNa expression [64]. These findings contrast with data obtained in ex vivo human lung tissues (SARS-CoV-2 replicated more efficiently while triggering an attenuated IFN response) [65]. Studies in human primary nasal epithelial cell cultures have shown that if exogenous IFN-I/III were administered intranasally prior to infection and at sufficient concentration, SARS-CoV-2 infection was inhibited [66]. Furthermore, in a hamster model IFN treatment limited tropism to distal tissues, including the intestine [53]. Also, some people have developed autoimmunity in which they produce autoantibodies that block IFN, resulting in more severe disease [67,68]. Loss of function variants in loci that control TLR3- and IRF7-dependent type I IFN immunity have been identified in a small number of severe adult patients with severe COVID-19 who had not been previously hospitalized for severe illness due to infection with other viruses [69]).

In humans, SARS-CoV-2 could productively replicate in surgically removed intestinal tissue but not in kidney or liver tissues [64]. SARS-CoV-2 RNA has been found in stools of infected individuals consistently, although with different frequencies (ranging from 15.3% to 81.8% of infected people [7]. In a retrospective cohort in China, the median duration of viral RNA in stool was 22 days [70]. In some patients, the viral load in feces reached 10^7 copies/g suggesting an enteric infection not blunted by an interferon response [71]. In addition, SARS-CoV-2 RNA was reported to be detected in untreated wastewater sludge [72]. Viral RNA and intracellular staining of viral nucleocapsid protein were detected in GI epithelium from one patient in China who tested positive for SARS-CoV-2 RNA in feces [73] and duodenal biopsies of 2 out of 5 moderate COVID-19 patients; however, the staining was weak and scattered [74]. In another study, within six patients with GI symptoms subjected to endoscopy, SARS-CoV-2 RNA was detected in stomach, duodenum and rectum specimens of the two patients with severe disease, but only duodenum was positive in one of the four non-severe patients [75]. Another study that tested five COVID-19 patients, presenting with either upper abdominal pain or diarrhea. Early in infection, patients were subjected to a total of four esophagogastroduodenoscopy, and 2 in 5 showed signs of viral replication in the gut and increased numbers of antigen-experienced activated CD8$^+$ T cells were detected within the epithelium [74]. This is in line with another study that found viral nucleocapsid in 5 out of 14 patients at an average of 4 months after initial COVID-19 diagnosis [76].

Uncertainties, inconsistencies and gaps. Contrasting results between ex vivo lung and intestinal tissues prove a line of evidence that SARS-CoV-2 infectivity and antiviral response is different in the gut than in lungs. Studies in lung cells and tissues showed that IFN expression is delayed or reduced by SARS-CoV-2 compared to influenza [66,77–79]. However, one exception to this observation is the response to high multiplicity of infection (MOI) response, where replication was robust with an observed IFN-I and -III signature. At low MOI, the virus might not be a strong inducer of the IFN-I and -III system, as opposed to conditions where the MOI is high [77]. hACE2 mice pre-treated with neutralizing antibodies against IFN-α/β receptors (mimicking pre-existing autoantibodies targeting type I IFNs) were more susceptible to SARS-CoV-2 infection with reduced survival [80]. Autoantibodies against IFN-α have been identified in patients with severe disease and have been shown to contribute to delayed viral clearance in lung cells [80].

While SARS-CoV-2 replication in human enterocytes in vitro is supported by strong evidence, evidence of SARS-CoV-2 infection in the digestive tract of animals showed mixed results. In the intranasally inoculated hACE2 transgenic mice, viral RNA was detected, but no infectious virus was isolated and no viral antigens were detected in the intestines [35]. In another stable mouse model generated by CRISPR-Cas9 knock-in technology [36], robust virus replication were demonstrated in lungs. When infected via the intragastric route, no data were reported on intestinal infection, but interestingly, these mice did exhibit lung infection [36]. K18-hACE2 showed no viral replication in the intestine following nasal inoculation [37]. This is coherent with the fact that hACE2 expression were not observed in the gut of the mice used in that study [37]. No studies in the gut have been reported so far for the HFH4-hACE2 mice developing severe/lethal disease. Thus, multiple strategies for introducing hACE2 into mice have been developed, a comprehensive characterization of the different models as well as of the doses and routes of inoculum used in each case is needed to correctly interpret the results [81]. In golden hamsters, expression of SARS-CoV-2 nucleocapsid protein was found in the intestine after intranasal infection [82]. In ferrets, viral RNA and viral subgenomic mRNA, indicative of a previous or current viral transcription, was detected in the gut but interestingly, in this case did not produce detectable infectious viral particles [39]. Viral RNA but no infectious virus was detected in the ileum of one over three minks inoculated intranasally [83]. In rhesus monkeys, viral RNA was detectable in digestive tissues and in fecal samples after intranasal inoculation and Tissue Culture Infective Dose (TCID50) assays suggested that the virus was infectious [41]. While in rhesus macaques infected via a combination of intranasal, intratracheal and ocular inoculation, viral RNA was and SARS-CoV-2 antigen were detected in the GI tract but not viral mRNA [42]. Thus viral RNA was detected in the intestines after virus inoculation (intranasal or intragastric) in almost all animal models [35,39,41,42,82] providing evidence for SARS-CoV-2 entry into enterocytes. However, evidence that the virus found in the GI tissues was infectious was observed only in rhesus monkeys in one study [41]. As already mentioned, these data calls for precaution of which models are suitable to study SARS-CoV-2 intestinal infection as well as for considering with care the doses and routes of inoculum used in each case [81]. Assessing intestinal infection and IFN response following infection with different dosages in the gut of all types of hACE2 infected mice and non-human infected primates [6] in parallel with ACE2 staining would help provide clear evidence of whether increased coronavirus production occurs in the gut in vivo.

In humans, according to the few endoscopic and histological examinations based on one or two cases [73–76], the GI epithelium is potentially susceptible to infection by SARS-CoV-2 but to date, it remains unclear whether SARS-CoV-2 replicates in the human gut, and for how long it could persist in the gut. Even if difficult to obtain, further staining of COVID-19 patients GI epithelia, as well as omics analysis of intestinal biopsies notably regarding IFN response, are needed to confirm and quantify the proportion of patients with active replication in the gut.

3. Current Evidence and Uncertainties of SARS-CoV-2 Damaging Intestinal Barrier

SARS-CoV-2 infection was reported to be a cytopathic virus in lung cells triggering cell apoptosis in lung epithelial cells and in lungs of infected mice while lung sections of fatal COVID-19 patients revealed cell death markers [84]. Thus, SARS-CoV-2 has been proposed to induce cell death resulting in disruption of the epithelial monolayer integrity or alterations to tight junctions (TJ), the mucus layer and/or the cellular immune system. Disruption of the intestinal barrier layers is associated with increased intestinal permeability, also called "leaky gut", which allows the transfer of commensal or pathogenic bacteria and bacterial components into the lamina propria and later on into the systemic circulation [85] (Figure 2).

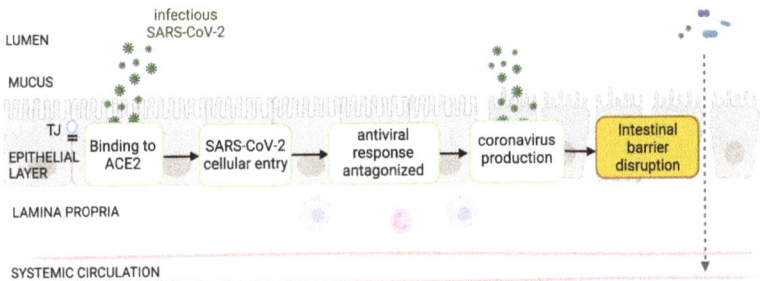

Figure 2. Pathway depicting the sequence of events for SARS-CoV-2 enteric production impairing intestinal barrier (AOP422). Evidence is evaluated in the present work to assess the likelihood of the occurrence.

SARS-CoV-2 Production Impairs Intestinal Barrier

Biological plausibility. Within the host cell, the new virions are assembled (KE1847) and to release viral particles, the virus promotes host lysis, leading to cell death and compromising the integrity of the epithelial monolayer. The intestinal barrier is ensured by the integrity of the monolayer epithelium (via cell integrity and tight junctions/adherens proteins), together with the chemical barrier, the mucosal layer and the cellular immune system located in the lamina propria (KE1931). Alternatively, TJs might be altered following SARS-CoV-2 infection enhancing paracellular permeability. In addition, the mucus layer and/or the cellular immune system might be perturbed.

Evidence. No extensive cell death was observed after SARS-CoV-2 infection in intestinal organoids, compared to MERS-CoV that killed most cells within 48 h of infection [31]. SARS-CoV-2 also replicated less efficiently than SARS-CoV and induced less cytopathology in ex vivo human intestinal epithelium [64]. In contrast, studies in vitro with gut derived organoids report observable organoid disintegration [86] also associated with markers of apoptosis, such as caspase 3 [54,86]. No substantial histopathological changes were observed in the intestines of hACE2 intranasally inoculated mice in which no virus was isolated, nor viral antigens detected [35]. In Syrian hamsters, the histological analysis did not reveal intestinal damage or structural remodeling of the epithelium in hamsters but a trend towards increased blood concentration of intestinal fatty-acid binding protein (FABP), a systemic marker associated with disrupted gut integrity, has been detected [87]. This agrees with other studies [82,88] but contrasts with another study [89] in which severe epithelial cell necrosis and damaged intestinal villi were observed at 4dpi (but not at 2dpi). The reason for this discrepancy is unclear according to the authors, but they proposed differences in the virus preparations and the dose used to inoculate animals, which are well summarized in [81]. In rhesus monkeys, exfoliation of mucosal epithelium in the GI tract was observed after intranasal inoculation of SARS-CoV-2 as well as a reduced number of mucin-containing goblet cells at the earlier stage of infection [41]. In humans, no relation was noted between fecal calprotectin (FC) levels and fecal SARS-CoV-2 RNA in a cohort of 40 hospitalized patients with COVID-19 [1]. In another exploratory study, COVID-19 patients had elevated plasma levels of LPS-binding protein (a gut leakage marker) but not of intestinal FABP (a marker of enterocyte damage) [90]. These data suggest impaired gut barrier function without excessive enterocyte damage and highlight gaps to comprehensively understand under which experimental or clinical conditions, SARS-CoV-2 productively infects and kills enterocytes. However, in a human gut-on-chip model composed of intestinal epithelial Caco-2 co-cultured with intestinal mucin-secreting HT-29 cells, after SARS-CoV-2 infection, S-positive epithelial cells were detected along with damage to the intestinal villus-like structures, disturbance of the mucus layer and reduced expression of TJ (E-cadherin) [32]. Severe COVID-19 was associated with high levels of markers of tight junction permeability and microbial translocation [1,91,92], signaling a loss of the intestinal barrier function.

Uncertainties, inconsistencies and gaps. While the biological plausibility was high, currently, there is not enough evidence to support that enterocyte massive cell death following SARS-CoV-2 infection occurs systematically [93]. Number of cases showing histomorphologic changes due intestinal infection by SARS-CoV-2 is still limited. While not easy to obtain, more (post-mortem) intestinal biopsies of COVID-19 patients showing the presence of replicating SARS-CoV-2 along with cell death markers in epithelial cells of the small intestine would be needed to determine precisely if cell death occurs. A small body of evidence points toward a potential alteration of TJs upon SARS-CoV-2 infection. However, definitive evidence is still limited and warrants further research. The role of Ca/Zn/VitD depletions in COVID-19 patients which weaken physical tissue barrier integrity by interacting with TJ [94] is still unclear. Using biomimetic human intestinal gut-on-chip able to partially mirror intestinal barrier injury and response to viral infection [32] or human intestinal organoids could provide insight into the essentiality of these events in COVID-19. In addition, it would informative to assess the tight junction permeability in infected mice, hamsters or nonhuman primate models described above.

4. Current Evidence and Uncertainties of SARS-CoV-2 Enteric Infection Contributing to the Inflammatory Response

While productive replication still needs further studies, strong evidence supports SARS-CoV-2 entry in intestinal epithelial cells. There it might trigger a coordinated innate immune response due to the recognition of SARS-CoV-2 associated molecular patterns, similar to that reported in the lung cells [49,95], inducing an antiviral response as described above but also releasing proinflammatory mediators which recruit immune cells to the gut, which in turn secrete cytokines leading to gut inflammation (Figure 3).

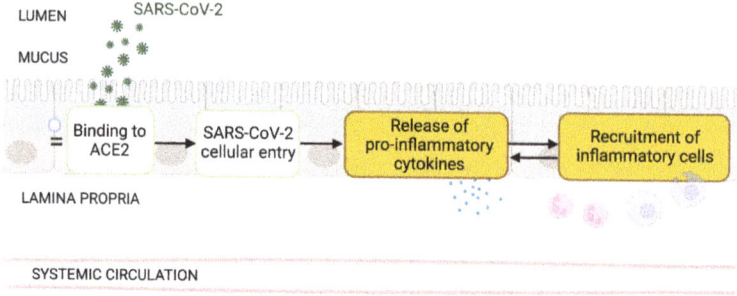

Figure 3. Pathway depicting the sequence of events of SARS-CoV-2 enteric infection contributing to the inflammatory response. This manuscript assesses whether evidence supports these events.

4.1. Viral Entry Induces Pro-Inflammatory Mediators Release

Biological plausibility. Viral infections induce a proinflammatory response including expression of cytokines and chemokines via signal transduction pathways activation, such as NF-kB [96], JAK-STAT [97] and NFAT [98].

Evidence. Infection of human intestinal organoids with SARS-CoV-2 elicited a broad signature of cytokines [54] mediated by NFkB/TNF [30]. Lamers et al. [54] showed that the infection of human intestinal organoids with SARS-CoV-2 can induce Il7 expression. Intestinal viral infections cause IL22 expression in T cells via IFNβ1-mediated IL7 production by epithelial cells and IL6 production in fibroblasts. In non-human primates infected with SARS-CoV-2, increased serum concentrations of interleukin (IL)-8, IL-1RA, C-C motif chemokine ligand (CCL)2, CCL11, and chemokine (C-X-C motif) ligand (CXCL)13 were observed [6,42,99,100]. Higher levels of the pro-inflammatory cytokine IL-8 and lower levels of the anti-inflammatory cytokine IL-10 were detected in the feces of COVID-19 patients when compared to uninfected controls [14]. However, the lack of increase of other cytokines and of calprotectin in this study suggests that the immune response within the gut to this viral infection is limited.

Inconsistencies, uncertainties and gaps. Several components of inflammation exist but we have limited knowledge on the nature of inflammatory pathways triggered in the GI tract by SARS-CoV-2. Additional investigations in COVID-19 patients are still needed, such as analysis of in situ produced cytokines in gut biopsies from COVID-19 patients with distinct disease severity profiles. Of key importance it would be to dissect, if similarly to other enteric viral infections, to what extent does intestinal inflammatory response contribute to the systemic cytokine profile and which are the parallels and differences between in the epithelial response in the gut versus in the lung. In lung samples, a signature of low IFN-I and -III and high pro-inflammatory mediators was consistently observed in vitro, ex vivo, in vivo in longitudinal studies and in COVID-19 patients [77], performing similar analysis in the gut would be informative.

4.2. Pro-Inflammatory Mediators Recruit Inflammatory Cells in the Gut

Biological plausibility. Pro-inflammatory signaling (KE1496) recruits' pro-inflammatory cells, such as neutrophils, macrophages, and T cells to the site of infection (KE1497).

Evidence. When cytokines are released, immune cells, such as neutrophils, macrophages, and lymphocytes, are recruited to the gut environment and facilitates an adaptive immune response [101]. In golden Syrian hamsters intranasally infected with SARS-CoV-2, the viral N protein was detected in the intestine, IL-4, IL-6, TNF-α and IL-12 were upregulated and the lamina propria exhibited mononuclear cell infiltration at 2dpi [102]. Histological examination of human intestinal samples revealed that lymphocytes and inflammatory cells infiltrate the lamina propria [103]. Neutrophils recruitment has been demonstrated by gut calprotein (neutrophil-specific alarmin protein) presence in COVID-19 patients where elevated fecal calprotectin and systemic IL-6 response were identified [1] and associated to intestine inflammation, adding to the evidence that SARS-CoV-2 triggers an inflammatory response in the intestine [104]. Recent studies also described that the cytokine storm may be associated with the expression of calprotectin [105,106] but another preprint study showed that the level of calprotectin was not linked to COVID-19 severity [14].

Uncertainties. Whether direct or indirect modulation in the gut immune activation during SARS-CoV-2 infection is responsible for immune cell recruitment needs to be examined more thoroughly. Direct cell death in intestinal epithelial and goblet cells can cause apoptosis and recruit immune cells or, alternatively, an indirect loss of GI tract integrity caused by viral infection can activate immune cell recruitment. A recent study in ferrets infected with SARS-CoV-2 by gavage compared the immunomodulation of probiotics in the duodenum, however a noninfected placebo group was missing, which would be informative [40]. Recently, in a non-human primate (rhesus monkey) model of SARS-CoV-2 infection, in vivo infection of GI tract increased apoptosis of intestinal epithelial and goblet cells along with intestinal inflammation by macrophages has been reported [41]. However, these results could not explain whe, ther immune modulation in the GI tract was due to direct infection of GI tract cells by the virus or due to changes in the GI tract integrity and microbiota under the influence of systemic cytokines and hypoxic conditions or a combination of all [104]. Certain patient subgroups such as the elderly and patients with type 2 diabetes or obesity have been shown to be associated with more severe disease [107]. Immune defense mechanisms at the digestive level are described as impaired in these populations [108,109]. It is not currently known whether this impaired digestive immunity is a risk factor for infection.

5. Current Insights, Research Needs and Potential Impact on Clinical Practices
5.1. Productive Enteric Infection

An important aspect is that to infect intestinal cells, viable SARS-CoV-2 must reach the gut lumen as an infectious particle, meaning able to actively replicate in the GI tract. In contrast to enteric viruses, enveloped respiratory viruses, such as influenza virus or SARS-CoV-2, are thought to be cleared by the exposure to digestive juices (gastric acid, bile, pancreatic juice) and mucus layer in the GI tract. SARS-CoV-2 was found to be extremely stable over a wide range of pH values (pH 3–10) [110] but rapidly lost infectivity in vitro in the low pH simulated gastric fluid (pH 1.5–3.5, fasting state) [33]. Furthermore, SARS-CoV-2 was rapidly inactivated in the lumen of the colon by enteric fluid [33]. This suggests that, predominantly, noninfectious particles reach the gut lumen [33]. However, while MERS-CoV also rapidly lost infectivity in fasting-state simulated gastric fluid, the infectivity was unaffected in fed-state-simulated gastric fluid (pH 5) [111,112]. Using human coronavirus OC43 (causing mild symptoms and not requiring a biosafety level 3 lab) as a surrogate for the pathogenic SARS-CoV-2, a very recent study showed that, except for fasting-state gastric fluid (pH 1.6), the virus remained infectious in all other GI fluids for 1 h and the presence of food improved viral survival in gastric fluids [112]. A similar strategy should be done for SARS-CoV-2 and investigate infectivity in this fluid simulating stomach acidity after meals. This would allow determining whether SARS-CoV-2 tolerates gastric acid and survives passage to the gut in all settings and whether SARS-CoV-2 ingestion with food could protect the virus against inactivation by the GI fluids [7]. Interestingly, in this regard, it was described that the usage of H pump inhibitors was associated with worse clinical outcomes for COVID-19 patients, despite not being associated with increased susceptibility to SARS-CoV-2 infection. This observation raises the question of whether some medicines permit SARS-CoV-2 replication in the gut [113]. In addition, if other conditions, including for example highly viscous mucus, protect virus particles, allowing the virus to retain its infectivity, as shown for influenza virions, should be evaluated to determine conditions in which SARS-CoV-2 could actively replicate in the gut [114]. In infected hamsters, SARS-CoV-2 intranasal infection was more efficient than oral infection. However, increasing viral dose in the initial inoculum, both intranasal and oral, resulted in higher levels of SARS-CoV-2 RNA in the lungs and in the intestines of these animals, suggesting that the initial dose is an important factor when considering gut infection and mechanisms that protect the virus from the harsh environment of the stomach [88]. Alternatively, other cell types may be able to transport SARS-CoV-2 to the gut, as for example, a small number of lymphocytes has been shown to be infected by SARS-CoV-2 [103] or even bacteria. A recent study showed that SARS-CoV-2 replicates outside the human body in vitro in bacterial growth medium, following bacterial growth and influenced by antibiotics administration, suggesting a bacteriophage-like behavior for SARS-CoV-2 [115] or the activation of other bacteriophages [116]. Electron and fluorescence microscopy images showed the presence of SARS-CoV-2 both outside and inside bacteria [116,117]. Further research is needed as these results could lead to a rethinking of SARS-CoV-2 biology and of effective management of COVID-19 transmission [115]. In addition, it cannot be excluded that both the viscous mucus and the gut microbiome could protect viral RNA and virus particles, allowing the virus to retain its infectivity.

Thus, while the human gut expresses high levels of ACE2, and SARS-CoV-2 infection of human enterocytes in vitro is supported by strong evidence, human healthy gut may not be systematically permeable to viral entry due to the GI fluids, antiviral response and/or the protective multi-layers of the intestinal barrier. However, evidence of intestinal infection of SARS-CoV-2 has been reported, suggesting that there are some conditions that may render people susceptible to SARS-CoV-2 infection in the gut or that may protect the virus from degradation. For example, individuals with altered intestinal barrier prior to infection, or under certain medication or comorbidities, might be more vulnerable to gastrointestinal SARS-CoV-2 infection [118]. An inflammatory environment, as seen in many other conditions such as diabetes, obesity, or resulting from the cytokine storm in severe COVID-19, disrupting the intestinal barrier, may render the GI entry of the SARS-CoV-2 significant [33]. Different experimental models mimicking diseases known to be associated with an altered intestinal barrier exist. Literature describing their use to unravel the mechanisms behind SARS-CoV-2 GI infection is starting to emerge. A mouse preclinical T2DM/obesity co-morbidity model of COVID-19 [119] and a mouse model mimicking obesity-associated COVID-19 comorbidities were established [119]. Such models could accelerate the development of therapeutics for this highly susceptible population. Sex and diet-specific responses partially explaining the effects of obesity and diabetes on COVID-19 disease were observed [119]. The detrimental impact of continuous Western diet on COVID-19 outcome has been reported in Syrian hamsters [120]. The age dependent increase in disease can be observed in Syrian hamsters and nonhuman primates [81]. Thus age, medication, metabolic syndrome, via high fat diet for example, could be incorporated into models to mimic human comorbidities in order to investigate this important question.

In addition, the colonic mucus barrier is shaped by the composition of the gut microbiota [121]. Alteration of the gut microbiota has been associated with severity in COVID-19 [122,123] and might contribute to disrupting the mucus barrier, rendering the gut more permissive to SARS-CoV-2. A body of evidence indicates that gut dysbiosis, prior to infection, represents a risk factor, meaning contributes to more severe outcomes in COVID-19 patients, potentially by modulating intestinal ACE2 expression, intestinal and systemic inflammation and gut barrier integrity [124].

In conclusion, further research is needed to acquire a comprehensive understanding of the conditions under which SARS-CoV-2 productively infects enterocytes in humans in vivo. Notably, it is important to understand if specific conditions, including age, comorbidities or medication are associated with release of infectious particles from feces by tracking and surveillance of several groups in the population. These studies could be complemented by in situ hybridization or staining of human tissues acquired from biopsies or post-mortem samples of gut retried from COVID-19 positive people.

5.2. Infectious Virus in the Feces

If SARS-CoV-2 can establish an intestinal infection, then it remains unknown whether infectious viral particles can tolerate GI fluids and be shed alive through feces with sufficient concentration and infectivity for subsequent transmission. Despite SARS-CoV-2 RNA being detected in stools, and the persistent viral shedding of SARS-CoV-2 in feces, current data from different studies are conflicting regarding the detection of infectious particles in feces. Infectious viral particles may be retrieved from anecdotal cases, although studies indicate that the vast majority of individuals infected with SARS-CoV-2 do not release infectious particles from stools [125]. While high viral RNA concentrations were observed in stools in two different studies (9 and 10 patients, respectively), infectious virus was not recovered in those samples [33,125,126]. In contrast, replicating SARS-CoV-2 virus was detected in feces in [127] and viable SARS-CoV-2 particles in stool samples in [128]. Several aspects could complicate SARS-CoV-2 isolation from fecal material, such as the stability of the virus in the feces [129] and the potential presence of numerous other viruses. These aspects could also make viral activity assays technically challenging. A procedure using filtered diluted specimens without the addition of any potentially toxic antibacterial agents and cell culture medium changing after centrifugation was described as responsible for high virus recovery [130]. Using a similar method Jeong et al. [128] failed to demonstrate the presence of viable virus in stools, but they were able to isolate SARS-CoV-2 from ferrets that were inoculated with stool samples from COVID-19 patients. Other SARS-like viruses have been isolated from animal feces (see [131] as example), coronaviruses related to SARS-CoV-2 were isolated from bat rectal swabs and guano and were tested as able to infect in vitro human cells [132]. Understanding whether and when fecal-oral transmission of SARS-CoV-2 might occur will be of critical importance for health workers since feces from infected hosts could be a transmission source.

In addition, the potential risk of transmission via feces had implications on fecal microbiota transplantation (FMT) highly effective for recurrent *Clostridium difficile* infections. It is speculated that COVID-19 might be transmitted via FMT particularly from asymptomatic donors, specifically those who tested negative for the presence of the virus in their respiratory tract but potentially positive in their fecal samples [133]. No cases of COVID-19 transmission through FMT treatment have been reported, but only FMT products generated from stool donated before December 2019 or before November 2019 can be used according to the FDA recommendations and Hong Kong guidelines, respectively.

Finally, fecal shedding may have important epidemiological implications for community surveillance tools such as wastewater monitoring, which inform public health measures. Detection of SARS-CoV-2 RNA in untreated wastewater has been reported [134]. Detecting SARS-CoV-2 in wastewater might represent a way to better surveille the status of the population and detect peaks of infection and admissions to hospital up to one week ahead development of symptoms or detection in nasopharyngeal swabs [135]. In a recent study [136] fecal viral RNA was observed up to 7 months post infection in patients with mild to moderate COVID-19. Understanding the temporal dynamics of fecal shedding in individuals with mild or even asymptomatic disease is essential for inferring population-prevalence of COVID-19 from wastewater studies [137]. Currently the majority of the longitudinal studies of fecal viral RNA shedding have been limited to hospitalized patients with severe COVID-19 and/or with co-morbidities [138]. As stated by the authors, the continued presence of fecal viral RNA in wastewater may be mistakenly interpreted as evidence of the prevalence of infectious individuals in a community. Since wastewater viral RNA levels are being considered for use in guiding community level policies, it is critical to better understand how aerosol transmissibility of SARS-CoV-2 RNA are temporally related to fecal viral RNA shedding [136].

More evidence is required to demonstrate whether and in which conditions SARS-CoV-2 can establish a fecal–oral transmission route. This requires determining which people are susceptible to GI infection, and from this pool, in what conditions may people shed infectious virus particles in feces. Another important outstanding question to resolve is determining the minimum infectious dose of SARS-CoV-2, which may vary for the different SARS-CoV-2 variants.

5.3. Gut Implication in the Severity of the COVID-19 Outcomes

While a first Asian analysis at the beginning of the pandemic suggested that the presence of GI symptoms in COVID-19 patients was associated with increased clinical deterioration [139], other European or American studies have subsequently found the opposite [140–142]. An initial study showed no significant correlation consistent with GI tract symptomatology and disease severity [143]. Later on, a first meta-analysis did not show a statistically significant difference in mortality between patients with or without GI symptoms [144]. A second recently published (March 2022) large meta-analysis including 53 studies with 55,245 patients also showed no association [144], but two studies including more groups and people associated GI symptoms with worse prognosis of the disease [5,145]. Thus, it is still unclear whether GI symptoms could be predictive of disease severity.

An important body of evidence, however, supports the crucial implication of the gut in the excessive inflammatory response in COVID-19. Under normal conditions, inflammation is a protective process that combats infection. However, prolonged inflammatory response has long been known to play a detrimental role in human diseases, and clinical markers of excessive systemic inflammatory response were associated with severe and fatal COVID-19 [146,147]. Hyperinflammation contributes to broad tissue damage, acute respiratory distress syndrome, multiple-organ failure and ultimately death [148] and has been described as central in inducing severe outcomes in COVID-19 patients [149,150]. Impaired intestinal barrier function enhances the translocation of gut bacteria and of bacterial toxins, such as peptidoglycans and lipopolysaccharides (LPS), from the gut lumen into the blood. Increased levels of LPS in the blood (endotoxemia) activate Toll-Like Receptors, leading to the production of numerous pro-inflammatory cytokines and, hence, low-grade systemic inflammation [151]. In severely ill patients, intestinal barrier disruption and associated bacterial translocation exacerbates systemic inflammation [152,153]. Three studies found higher gut permeability markers in (severe) COVID-19 patients with abnormal presence of gut microbes in their bloodstream [7,91,92]. High levels of zonulin (gut permeability marker) were associated with severe COVID-19 and bacterial products in the blood correlated strongly with higher levels of markers of systemic inflammation and immune activation (such as C-reactive peptide levels) [7,91,92,123]. This does not imply that microbial translocation is the primary trigger of the inflammation, but supports the hypothesis that disrupted intestinal barrier and associated bacterial translocation play an additive or synergistic role in the cytokine storm underlying severe COVID-19 [92,154]. In addition, bacteria translocation from the gut into the systemic circulation might result in secondary infections and aggravate pulmonary symptoms in COVID-19 patients [155,156].

Disruption of the intestinal barrier also induces a local inflammatory response. It remains unclear whether permeability changes are primary events or secondary effects triggered by inflammation. Increased intestinal permeability and chronic intestinal inflammation are hallmarks of inflammatory bowel diseases (IBD), such as Crohn's disease (CD) [157]. Taking advantage of the genetic aspect in CD, several studies reported that increased permeability might precede CD onset as abnormal lactulose-to-mannitol ratios in asymptomatic first-degree relatives of CD patients was associated with a CD diagnosis during the follow up time [158–160]. In line, in the IL-10 gene-deficient IBD mouse model, increased intestinal permeability was observed early in life and then mice spontaneously developed colitis at 12 weeks age [161]. In addition, IL-10 deficient animals treated with AT-1001, a zonulin peptide inhibitor previously shown to reduce small intestinal permeability, developed less colitis later in life. Results from IBD mouse models suggest that investigation of intestinal permeability and inflammation in SARS-CoV-2 infected mice or cells treated with AT-1001 could be informative of the sequential process. Recently, a drug repurposing approach identified AT-1001, currently in phase 3 trials in celiac disease, as a potential therapeutic approach for COVID-19, however still requiring optimization steps [162]. In light of the central role of inflammation in COVID-19, concerns were raised that IBD patients may have an increased risk of worse outcomes. Corticosteroids, commonly used medications for IBD, were associated with adverse outcomes in COVID-19, but overall IBD patients did not have an increased risk of COVID-19 and had largely similar outcomes as the general population [163].

Finally yet importantly, associations between levels of inflammatory markers and gut microbiota composition in COVID-19 patients suggest that the gut microbiota might be involved in the magnitude of COVID-19 severity [122]. Significant alterations in fecal microbiomes of COVID-19 patients were reported at all times of hospitalization [122,164–166]. Recently, animal studies in mice, hamsters and nonhuman primates provided evidence that SARS-CoV-2 infection directly alters the gut microbiome [6,87,166]. However, the underlying mechanisms are still poorly understood. A body of evidence supports that intestinal and systemic inflammation, dysregulation of intestinal ACE2 or infection of intestinal bacteria can be interconnected pathways leading to gut dysbiosis as an adverse outcome following SARS-CoV-2 in the gut, but further laboratory research and large-scale population-based studies are needed to validate these pathways [167]. In addition, changes in the lung microbiome with increase of bacteria normally found in the GI tract were reported in COVID-19 patients [168]. Besides, gut dysbiosis during respiratory viral infection has been shown to worsen lung pathology and to promote secondary infections [156]. Based on the current insights, modulating the gut microbiota with probiotics, prebiotics or diet to improve disease prevention and management might represent easy to implement strategies [169]. Clinical trials in COVID-19 of probiotics with expected anti-inflammatory effects in the gut–lung axis are currently underway [170].

5.4. Gut Implication in Long COVID

Finally, GI disorders described in patients appeared to precede, accompany or follow the respiratory symptoms [5,171,172]. Long-term sequelae of COVID-19, collectively termed the post-acute COVID-19 syndrome (PACS) or long COVID, are rapidly emerging across the globe and many studies following patients who have recovered from the respiratory effects of COVID-19 identified persistent GI sequelae [173–175]. In a study from China, around half of the patients (41 of 74) had fecal samples positive for SARS-CoV-2 RNA, which remained positive for longer than the respiratory samples [173]. A recent study detected fecal RNA in around half of participants (113 patients with mild to moderate COVID-19) within the first week after diagnosis and around 4% of the patients shed up viral RNA up to 7 months after diagnosis while respiratory samples were negative [136]. No association between symptomatology and fecal viral RNA shedding was found in this study in participants with active respiratory infection, but when focusing on participants with extended shedding of fecal viral RNA after respiratory shedding ceased, fecal viral RNA was associated with GI symptoms [136]. Another recent study using a cohort of IBD patients showed that SARS-CoV-2 antigens could persist in the gut up to 7 months after infection. Importantly, only those IBD with detectable viral RNA in the gut were found to display post-acute COVID-19 symptoms [176]. In non-human primates infected with SARS-CoV-2, the viral RNA load decreased less rapidly over time in rectal samples than in nasopharyngeal and tracheal swabs [6]. These studies support the possibility that a prolonged SARS-CoV-2 presence in the GI tract, after the respiratory infection is cleared, might represent long-term viral reservoirs contributing to long COVID. A potential bacteriophage-like behavior of SARS-CoV-2 might also offer a way to explain the intestinal/fecal long-term presence of SARS-CoV-2. While the pathogenesis of long COVID is still under intense investigation, on the four current leading hypotheses [63], it is interestingly to note that two involve the gut: (i) gut dysbiosis [177,178] and (ii) viral reservoir with residual SARS-CoV-2 viral antigens [179] and persistent SARS-CoV-2 nucleic acids [76,177] reported in GI tissues in patients months after diagnosis and proposed to drive chronic inflammation. However, the concept that viral antigen persistence instigates immune perturbation and post-acute COVID-19 still requires validation in controlled clinical trials [176]. Towards that end, the RECOVER initiative (https://recovercovid.org/about) aims to bring together patients, caregivers, clinicians and scientists to understand, prevent and treat Long COVID, notably by collecting biopsies from the lower intestines of some participants [180]. Continuing the unprecedented degree of scientific collaboration, such unified interdisciplinary actions to collect and characterize sufficient PASC cases will enable to identify which factors affects long COVID. In addition, animal models such as humanized mice [181] or Syrian hamsters [182] will help to highlight molecular mechanism of long COVID and to explore future therapeutics.

Finally, currently the definition of long COVID differs depending of the health organizations [183,184]. There is a need for either a universal definition or to stop treating long COVID as a single entity as this umbrella term might represent multiple conditions (203 symptoms reported in 10 organs systems) [185]. Defining long COVID (categories) will help deciphering underlying mechanisms to ultimately improve disease prevention, management and treatment.

6. Conclusions

There are multiple outstanding questions regarding SARS-CoV-2 interaction with the human gut. First, it is not firmly established whether SARS-CoV-2 can actively replicate in human intestine. Evidence from multiple in vitro and in vivo animal studies points towards a direct viral tropism of intestinal cells and a productive enteric infection by SARS-CoV-2, however species, dose, virus preparations and route of inoculum are important factors to consider that can influence the occurrence of productive intestinal infection in animal studies. In addition, it is possible that specific conditions increase susceptibility to SARS-CoV-2 replication in the gut. Further studies are clearly needed to determine the experimental and clinical conditions under the gut represents an alternative entry route for the virus into the body. Such conditions encompass comorbidities, age, medication, inflammatory status, dysbiosis, fasted-fed status or ingestion with food. Secondly, based on the current evidence, it remains unclear whether GI symptoms, and particularly diarrhea, are caused by direct infection of the GI tract by SARS-CoV-2 or whether they are a consequence of a local and systemic immune activation. The wide range in reported rates of diarrhea in clinical studies of SARS-CoV-2 positive patients (from as low as 2% up to 50%) calls for more clinical studies and meta-analysis to elucidate the percentage of COVID-19 patients who develop GI symptoms, and particularly diarrhea, and whether GI disorders depend on active SARS-CoV-2 enteric infection and/or on factors such as those cited above. Answering those questions will be important for deciding the course of medical treatment. Thirdly, at this time, there is a moderate level of evidence to support the idea that the GI tract serves as an alternative route of virus dissemination. Finally, the potential implication of the gut on long COVID possibly by acting as viral reservoir or due to alteration of gut microbiota requires and deserves significant further investment in research, treatment and care of the PACS patients. In conclusion, in addition to calling for further research and large-scale studies, the potential impacts of SARS-CoV-2 productive enteric infection recommends applying appropriate precautions and potential preventive actions.

Author Contributions: This study was performed under the CIAO project (https://www.ciao-covid.net/) aiming at providing a holistic overview of the COVID-19 pathogenesis through the Adverse Outcome Pathway framework, offering to scientists from different fields an international platform to collaborate across disciplines [1]. L.-A.C. conceptualized the manuscript and edited the figures. All authors (L.-A.C., S.A.M., A.M., H.S., M.P., M.C.A., N.L., L.G. and M.-J.A.) contributed to deep reviewing of the literature and to writing of the different parts of the manuscript. All authors have read and agreed to the published version of the manuscript.

Funding: This research was funded by Fundação para a Ciência e Tecnologia through CEECIND/01049/2020 for H.S. and CEECIND/02373/2020 for M.-J.A. For the other authors, this research received no external funding.

Acknowledgments: The authors aim to thank Anna Sjodin and Christopher Schaupp for their careful reading and valuable inputs. The work was performed under the JRC Exploratory Research project CIAO—Modelling COVID-19 pathogenesis using the Adverse Outcome Pathway (AOP).

Conflicts of Interest: The authors declare no conflict of interest.

Disclaimer: This study is solely associated with individual scientist participation and their expressions of interest and opinions; it does not represent the official position of any institution.

References

1. Effenberger, M.; Grabherr, F.; Mayr, L.; Schwaerzler, J.; Nairz, M.; Seifert, M.; Hilbe, R.; Seiwald, S.; Scholl-Buergi, S.; Fritsche, G.; et al. Faecal calprotectin indicates intestinal inflammation in COVID-19. *Gut* **2020**, *69*, 1543–1544. [CrossRef]
2. Hayashi, Y. The characteristics of gastrointestinal symptoms in patients with severe COVID-19: A systematic review and meta-analysis. *J. Gastroenterol.* **2021**, *56*, 409–420. [CrossRef] [PubMed]
3. Jin, X.; Lian, J.S.; Hu, J.H.; Gao, J.; Zheng, L.; Zhang, Y.M.; Hao, S.R.; Jia, H.Y.; Cai, H.; Zhang, X.L.; et al. Epidemiological, clinical and virological characteristics of 74 cases of coronavirus-infected disease 2019 (COVID-19) with gastrointestinal symptoms. *Gut* **2020**, *69*, 1002–1009. [CrossRef] [PubMed]

4. Nobel, Y.R.; Phipps, M.; Zucker, J.; Lebwohl, B.; Wang, T.C.; Sobieszczyk, M.E.; Freedberg, D.E. Gastrointestinal Symptoms and Coronavirus Disease 2019: A Case-Control Study from the United States. *Gastroenterology* **2020**, *159*, 373–375. [CrossRef] [PubMed]
5. Cheung, K.S.; Hung, I.F.N.; Chan, P.P.Y.; Lung, K.C.; Tso, E.; Liu, R.; Ng, Y.Y.; Chu, M.Y.; Chung, T.W.H.; Tam, A.R.; et al. Gastrointestinal Manifestations of SARS-CoV-2 Infection and Virus Load in Fecal Samples from a Hong Kong Cohort: Systematic Review and Meta-analysis. *Gastroenterology* **2020**, *159*, 81–95. [CrossRef] [PubMed]
6. Sokol, H.; Contreras, V.; Maisonnasse, P.; Desmons, A.; Delache, B.; Sencio, V.; Machelart, A.; Brisebarre, A.; Humbert, L.; Deryuter, L.; et al. SARS-CoV-2 infection in nonhuman primates alters the composition and functional activity of the gut microbiota. *Gut Microbes* **2021**, *13*, 1893113. [CrossRef]
7. Guo, M.; Tao, W.; Flavell, R.A.; Zhu, S. Potential intestinal infection and faecal-oral transmission of SARS-CoV-2. *Nat. Rev. Gastroenterol. Hepatol.* **2021**, *18*, 269–283. [CrossRef]
8. Crawford, S.E.; Ramani, S.; Tate, J.E.; Parashar, U.D.; Svensson, L.; Hagbom, M.; Franco, M.A.; Greenberg, H.B.; O'Ryan, M.; Kang, G.; et al. Rotavirus infection. *Nat. Rev. Dis. Primers* **2017**, *3*, 17083. [CrossRef]
9. Glass, R.I.; Parashar, U.D.; Estes, M.K. Norovirus Gastroenteritis. *N. Engl. J. Med.* **2009**, *361*, 1776–1785. [CrossRef]
10. DuPont, H.L. Acute infectious diarrhea in immunocompetent adults. *N. Engl. J. Med.* **2014**, *370*, 1532–1540. [CrossRef]
11. Wang, J.; Li, F.; Wei, H.; Lian, Z.X.; Sun, R.; Tian, Z. Respiratory influenza virus infection induces intestinal immune injury via microbiota-mediated Th17 cell-dependent inflammation. *J. Exp. Med.* **2014**, *211*, 2397–2410. [CrossRef] [PubMed]
12. Young, B.E.; Ong, S.W.X.; Kalimuddin, S.; Low, J.G.; Tan, S.Y.; Loh, J.; Ng, O.T.; Marimuthu, K.; Ang, L.W.; Mak, T.M.; et al. Epidemiologic Features and Clinical Course of Patients Infected with SARS-CoV-2 in Singapore. *JAMA* **2020**, *323*, 1488–1494. [CrossRef] [PubMed]
13. Shokri-Afra, H.; Alikhani, A.; Moradipoodeh, B.; Noorbakhsh, F.; Fakheri, H.; Moradi-Sardareh, H. Elevated fecal and serum calprotectin in COVID-19 are not consistent with gastrointestinal symptoms. *Sci. Rep.* **2021**, *11*, 22001. [CrossRef] [PubMed]
14. Britton, G.J.; Chen-Liaw, A.; Cossarini, F.; Livanos, A.E.; Spindler, M.P.; Plitt, T.; Eggers, J.; Mogno, I.; Gonzalez-Reiche, A.S.; Siu, S.; et al. Limited intestinal inflammation despite diarrhea, fecal viral RNA and SARS-CoV-2-specific IgA in patients with acute COVID-19. *Sci. Rep.* **2021**, *11*, 13308. [CrossRef]
15. Draskau, M.K.; Spiller, C.M.; Boberg, J.; Bowles, J.; Svingen, T. Developmental biology meets toxicology: Contributing reproductive mechanisms to build adverse outcome pathways. *Mol. Hum. Reprod.* **2020**, *26*, 111–116. [CrossRef]
16. Siwicki, A.K.; Terech-Majewska, E.; Grudniewska, J.; Malaczewska, J.; Kazun, K.; Lepa, A. Influence of deltamethrin on nonspecific cellular and humoral defense mechanisms in rainbow trout (*Oncorhynchus mykiss*). *Environ. Toxicol. Chem.* **2010**, *29*, 489–491. [CrossRef]
17. Villeneuve, D.L.; Crump, D.; Garcia-Reyero, N.; Hecker, M.; Hutchinson, T.H.; LaLone, C.A.; Landesmann, B.; Lettieri, T.; Munn, S.; Nepelska, M.; et al. Adverse outcome pathway (AOP) development I: Strategies and principles. *Toxicol. Sci.* **2014**, *142*, 312–320. [CrossRef]
18. Villeneuve, D.L.; Crump, D.; Garcia-Reyero, N.; Hecker, M.; Hutchinson, T.H.; LaLone, C.A.; Landesmann, B.; Lettieri, T.; Munn, S.; Nepelska, M.; et al. Adverse outcome pathway development II: Best practices. *Toxicol. Sci.* **2014**, *142*, 321–330. [CrossRef]
19. *Users' Handbook Supplement to the Guidance Document for Developing and Assessing Adverse Outcome Pathways*; OECD Series on Adverse Outcome Pathways No. 12018; Organisation for Economic Co-operation and Development (OECD): Paris, France, 2018.
20. Svingen, T.; Villeneuve, D.L.; Knapen, D.; Panagiotou, E.M.; Draskau, M.K.; Damdimopoulou, P.; O'Brien, J.M. A Pragmatic Approach to Adverse Outcome Pathway Development and Evaluation. *Toxicol. Sci.* **2021**, *184*, 183–190. [CrossRef]
21. Wittwehr, C.; Amorim, M.J.; Clerbaux, L.A.; Krebs, C.; Landesmann, B.; Macmillan, D.S.; Nymark, P.; Ram, R.; Garcia-Reyero, N.; Sachana, M.; et al. Understanding COVID-19 through adverse outcome pathways—2nd CIAO AOP Design Workshop. *ALTEX* **2021**, *38*, 351–357. [CrossRef] [PubMed]
22. Clerbaux, L.A.; Amigo, N.; Amorim, M.J.; Bal-Price, A.; Batista Leite, S.; Beronius, A.; Bezemer, G.F.G.; Bostroem, A.C.; Carusi, A.; Coecke, S.; et al. COVID-19 through Adverse Outcome Pathways: Building networks to better understand the disease—3rd CIAO AOP Design Workshop. *ALTEX* **2022**, *39*, 322–335. [CrossRef] [PubMed]
23. Nymark, P.; Sachana, M.; Leite, S.B.; Sund, J.; Krebs, C.E.; Sullivan, K.; Edwards, S.; Viviani, L.; Willett, C.; Landesmann, B.; et al. Systematic Organization of COVID-19 Data Supported by the Adverse Outcome Pathway Framework. *Front. Public Health* **2021**, *9*, 638605. [CrossRef] [PubMed]
24. Hamming, I.; Timens, W.; Bulthuis, M.L.; Lely, A.T.; Navis, G.; van Goor, H. Tissue distribution of ACE2 protein, the functional receptor for SARS coronavirus. A first step in understanding SARS pathogenesis. *J. Pathol.* **2004**, *203*, 631–637. [CrossRef]
25. Lee, J.J.; Kopetz, S.; Vilar, E.; Shen, J.P.; Chen, K.; Maitra, A. Relative Abundance of SARS-CoV-2 Entry Genes in the Enterocytes of the Lower Gastrointestinal Tract. *Genes* **2020**, *11*, 645. [CrossRef]
26. Ziegler, C.G.K.; Allon, S.J.; Nyquist, S.K.; Mbano, I.M.; Miao, V.N.; Tzouanas, C.N.; Cao, Y.; Yousif, A.S.; Bals, J.; Hauser, B.M.; et al. SARS-CoV-2 Receptor ACE2 Is an Interferon-Stimulated Gene in Human Airway Epithelial Cells and Is Detected in Specific Cell Subsets across Tissues. *Cell* **2020**, *181*, 1016–1035.e19. [CrossRef]
27. Zhang, H.; Kang, Z.; Gong, H.; Xu, D.; Wang, J.; Li, Z.; Li, Z.; Cui, X.; Xiao, J.; Zhan, J.; et al. Digestive system is a potential route of COVID-19: An analysis of single-cell coexpression pattern of key proteins in viral entry process. *Gut* **2020**, *69*, 1010–1018. [CrossRef]

28. Daly, J.L.; Simonetti, B.; Klein, K.; Chen, K.E.; Williamson, M.K.; Anton-Plagaro, C.; Shoemark, D.K.; Simon-Gracia, L.; Bauer, M.; Hollandi, R.; et al. Neuropilin-1 is a host factor for SARS-CoV-2 infection. *Science* **2020**, *370*, 861–865. [CrossRef]
29. Thul, P.J.; Akesson, L.; Wiking, M.; Mahdessian, D.; Geladaki, A.; Ait Blal, H.; Alm, T.; Asplund, A.; Bjork, L.; Breckels, L.M.; et al. A subcellular map of the human proteome. *Science* **2017**, *356*, 3321. [CrossRef]
30. Triana, S.; Metz-Zumaran, C.; Ramirez, C.; Kee, C.; Doldan, P.; Shahraz, M.; Schraivogel, D.; Gschwind, A.R.; Sharma, A.K.; Steinmetz, L.M.; et al. Single-cell analyses reveal SARS-CoV-2 interference with intrinsic immune response in the human gut. *Mol. Syst. Biol.* **2021**, *17*, e10232. [CrossRef]
31. Beumer, J.; Geurts, M.H.; Lamers, M.M.; Puschhof, J.; Zhang, J.; van der Vaart, J.; Mykytyn, A.Z.; Breugem, T.I.; Riesebosch, S.; Schipper, D.; et al. A CRISPR/Cas9 genetically engineered organoid biobank reveals essential host factors for coronaviruses. *Nat. Commun.* **2021**, *12*, 5498. [CrossRef] [PubMed]
32. Guo, Y.; Luo, R.; Wang, Y.; Deng, P.; Song, T.; Zhang, M.; Wang, P.; Zhang, X.; Cui, K.; Tao, T.; et al. SARS-CoV-2 induced intestinal responses with a biomimetic human gut-on-chip. *Sci. Bull.* **2021**, *66*, 783–793. [CrossRef] [PubMed]
33. Zang, R.; Gomez Castro, M.F.; McCune, B.T.; Zeng, Q.; Rothlauf, P.W.; Sonnek, N.M.; Liu, Z.; Brulois, K.F.; Wang, X.; Greenberg, H.B.; et al. TMPRSS2 and TMPRSS4 promote SARS-CoV-2 infection of human small intestinal enterocytes. *Sci. Immunol.* **2020**, *5*, 3582. [CrossRef] [PubMed]
34. Parolin, C.; Virtuoso, S.; Giovanetti, M.; Angeletti, S.; Ciccozzi, M.; Borsetti, A. Animal Hosts and Experimental Models of SARS-CoV-2 Infection. *Chemotherapy* **2021**, *66*, 8–16. [CrossRef] [PubMed]
35. Bao, L.; Deng, W.; Huang, B.; Gao, H.; Liu, J.; Ren, L.; Wei, Q.; Yu, P.; Xu, Y.; Qi, F.; et al. The pathogenicity of SARS-CoV-2 in hACE2 transgenic mice. *Nature* **2020**, *583*, 830–833. [CrossRef] [PubMed]
36. Sun, S.H.; Chen, Q.; Gu, H.J.; Yang, G.; Wang, Y.X.; Huang, X.Y.; Liu, S.S.; Zhang, N.N.; Li, X.F.; Xiong, R.; et al. A Mouse Model of SARS-CoV-2 Infection and Pathogenesis. *Cell Host Microbe* **2020**, *28*, 124–133.e4. [CrossRef]
37. Winkler, E.S.; Bailey, A.L.; Kafai, N.M.; Nair, S.; McCune, B.T.; Yu, J.; Fox, J.M.; Chen, R.E.; Earnest, J.T.; Keeler, S.P.; et al. SARS-CoV-2 infection of human ACE2-transgenic mice causes severe lung inflammation and impaired function. *Nat. Immunol.* **2020**, *21*, 1327–1335. [CrossRef] [PubMed]
38. Suresh, V.; Parida, D.; Minz, A.P.; Sethi, M.; Sahoo, B.S.; Senapati, S. Tissue Distribution of ACE2 Protein in Syrian Golden Hamster (Mesocricetus auratus) and Its Possible Implications in SARS-CoV-2 Related Studies. *Front Pharmacol.* **2020**, *11*, 579330. [CrossRef]
39. van de Ven, K.; van Dijken, H.; Wijsman, L.; Gomersbach, A.; Schouten, T.; Kool, J.; Lenz, S.; Roholl, P.; Meijer, A.; van Kasteren, P.B.; et al. Pathology and Immunity After SARS-CoV-2 Infection in Male Ferrets Is Affected by Age and Inoculation Route. *Front Immunol.* **2021**, *12*, 750229. [CrossRef]
40. Lehtinen, M.J.; Kumar, R.; Zabel, B.; Makela, S.M.; Nedveck, D.; Tang, P.; Latvala, S.; Guery, S.; Budinoff, C.R. The effect of the probiotic consortia on SARS-CoV-2 infection in ferrets and on human immune cell response in vitro. *iScience* **2022**, *25*, 104445. [CrossRef]
41. Jiao, L.; Li, H.; Xu, J.; Yang, M.; Ma, C.; Li, J.; Zhao, S.; Wang, H.; Yang, Y.; Yu, W.; et al. The Gastrointestinal Tract Is an Alternative Route for SARS-CoV-2 Infection in a Nonhuman Primate Model. *Gastroenterology* **2021**, *160*, 1647–1661. [CrossRef] [PubMed]
42. Munster, V.J.; Feldmann, F.; Williamson, B.N.; van Doremalen, N.; Perez-Perez, L.; Schulz, J.; Meade-White, K.; Okumura, A.; Callison, J.; Brumbaugh, B.; et al. Respiratory disease in rhesus macaques inoculated with SARS-CoV-2. *Nature* **2020**, *585*, 268–272. [CrossRef] [PubMed]
43. Baindara, P.; Roy, D.; Mandal, S.M.; Schrum, A.G. Conservation and Enhanced Binding of SARS-CoV-2 Omicron Spike Protein to Coreceptor Neuropilin-1 Predicted by Docking Analysis. *Infect. Dis. Rep.* **2022**, *14*, 243–249. [CrossRef] [PubMed]
44. Kim, D.; Lee, J.Y.; Yang, J.S.; Kim, J.W.; Kim, V.N.; Chang, H. The Architecture of SARS-CoV-2 Transcriptome. *Cell* **2020**, *181*, 914–921.e10. [CrossRef] [PubMed]
45. Amor, S.; Fernandez Blanco, L.; Baker, D. Innate immunity during SARS-CoV-2: Evasion strategies and activation trigger hypoxia and vascular damage. *Clin. Exp. Immunol.* **2020**, *202*, 193–209. [CrossRef] [PubMed]
46. Chandran, A.; Rosenheim, J.; Nageswaran, G.; Swadling, L.; Pollara, G.; Gupta, R.K.; Burton, A.R.; Guerra-Assuncao, J.A.; Woolston, A.; Ronel, T.; et al. Rapid synchronous type 1 IFN and virus-specific T cell responses characterize first wave non-severe SARS-CoV-2 infections. *Cell. Rep. Med.* **2022**, *3*, 100557. [CrossRef]
47. Chou, J.; Thomas, P.G.; Randolph, A.G. Immunology of SARS-CoV-2 infection in children. *Nat. Immunol.* **2022**, *23*, 177–185. [CrossRef]
48. Christie, M.J.; Irving, A.T.; Forster, S.C.; Marsland, B.J.; Hansbro, P.M.; Hertzog, P.J.; Nold-Petry, C.A.; Nold, M.F. Of bats and men: Immunomodulatory treatment options for COVID-19 guided by the immunopathology of SARS-CoV-2 infection. *Sci. Immunol.* **2021**, *6*, eabd0205. [CrossRef]
49. Stanifer, M.L.; Kee, C.; Cortese, M.; Zumaran, C.M.; Triana, S.; Mukenhirn, M.; Kraeusslich, H.G.; Alexandrov, T.; Bartenschlager, R.; Boulant, S. Critical Role of Type III Interferon in Controlling SARS-CoV-2 Infection in Human Intestinal Epithelial Cells. *Cell Rep.* **2020**, *32*, 107863. [CrossRef]
50. Boudewijns, R.; Thibaut, H.J.; Kaptein, S.J.F.; Li, R.; Vergote, V.; Seldeslachts, L.; Van Weyenbergh, J.; De Keyzer, C.; Bervoets, L.; Sharma, S.; et al. STAT2 signaling restricts viral dissemination but drives severe pneumonia in SARS-CoV-2 infected hamsters. *Nat. Commun.* **2020**, *11*, 5838. [CrossRef]

51. Imai, M.; Iwatsuki-Horimoto, K.; Hatta, M.; Loeber, S.; Halfmann, P.J.; Nakajima, N.; Watanabe, T.; Ujie, M.; Takahashi, K.; Ito, M.; et al. Syrian hamsters as a small animal model for SARS-CoV-2 infection and countermeasure development. *Proc. Natl. Acad. Sci. USA* **2020**, *117*, 16587–16595. [CrossRef] [PubMed]
52. Sodeifian, F.; Nikfarjam, M.; Kian, N.; Mohamed, K.; Rezaei, N. The role of type I interferon in the treatment of COVID-19. *J. Med. Virol.* **2022**, *94*, 63–81. [CrossRef] [PubMed]
53. Hoagland, D.A.; Moller, R.; Uhl, S.A.; Oishi, K.; Frere, J.; Golynker, I.; Horiuchi, S.; Panis, M.; Blanco-Melo, D.; Sachs, D.; et al. Leveraging the antiviral type I interferon system as a first line of defense against SARS-CoV-2 pathogenicity. *Immunity* **2021**, *54*, 557–570. [CrossRef] [PubMed]
54. Lamers, M.M.; Beumer, J.; van der Vaart, J.; Knoops, K.; Puschhof, J.; Breugem, T.I.; Ravelli, R.B.G.; Paul van Schayck, J.; Mykytyn, A.Z.; Duimel, H.Q.; et al. SARS-CoV-2 productively infects human gut enterocytes. *Science* **2020**, *369*, 50–54. [CrossRef] [PubMed]
55. Cholankeril, G.; Podboy, A.; Aivaliotis, V.I.; Tarlow, B.; Pham, E.A.; Spencer, S.P.; Kim, D.; Hsing, A.; Ahmed, A. High Prevalence of Concurrent Gastrointestinal Manifestations in Patients with Severe Acute Respiratory Syndrome Coronavirus 2: Early Experience from California. *Gastroenterology* **2020**, *159*, 775–777. [CrossRef]
56. Xia, H.; Cao, Z.; Xie, X.; Zhang, X.; Chen, J.Y.; Wang, H.; Menachery, V.D.; Rajsbaum, R.; Shi, P.Y. Evasion of Type I Interferon by SARS-CoV-2. *Cell Rep.* **2020**, *33*, 108234. [CrossRef]
57. Hayn, M.; Hirschenberger, M.; Koepke, L.; Nchioua, R.; Straub, J.H.; Klute, S.; Hunszinger, V.; Zech, F.; Prelli Bozzo, C.; Aftab, W.; et al. Systematic functional analysis of SARS-CoV-2 proteins uncovers viral innate immune antagonists and remaining vulnerabilities. *Cell Rep.* **2021**, *35*, 109126. [CrossRef]
58. Xia, H.; Shi, P.Y. Antagonism of Type I Interferon by Severe Acute Respiratory Syndrome Coronavirus 2. *J. Interferon Cytokine Res.* **2020**, *40*, 543–548. [CrossRef]
59. Han, L.; Zhuang, M.W.; Deng, J.; Zheng, Y.; Zhang, J.; Nan, M.L.; Zhang, X.J.; Gao, C.; Wang, P.H. SARS-CoV-2 ORF9b antagonizes type I and III interferons by targeting multiple components of the RIG-I/MDA-5-MAVS, TLR3-TRIF, and cGAS-STING signaling pathways. *J. Med. Virol.* **2021**, *93*, 5376–5389. [CrossRef]
60. Jiang, H.W.; Zhang, H.N.; Meng, Q.F.; Xie, J.; Li, Y.; Chen, H.; Zheng, Y.X.; Wang, X.N.; Qi, H.; Zhang, J.; et al. SARS-CoV-2 Orf9b suppresses type I interferon responses by targeting TOM70. *Cell. Mol. Immunol.* **2020**, *17*, 998–1000. [CrossRef]
61. Wu, J.; Shi, Y.; Pan, X.; Wu, S.; Hou, R.; Zhang, Y.; Zhong, T.; Tang, H.; Du, W.; Wang, L.; et al. SARS-CoV-2 ORF9b inhibits RIG-I-MAVS antiviral signaling by interrupting K63-linked ubiquitination of NEMO. *Cell Rep.* **2021**, *34*, 108761. [CrossRef] [PubMed]
62. Gordon, D.E.; Jang, G.M.; Bouhaddou, M.; Xu, J.; Obernier, K.; White, K.M.; O'Meara, M.J.; Rezelj, V.V.; Guo, J.Z.; Swaney, D.L.; et al. A SARS-CoV-2 protein interaction map reveals targets for drug repurposing. *Nature* **2020**, *583*, 459–468. [CrossRef] [PubMed]
63. Merad, M.; Blish, C.A.; Sallusto, F.; Iwasaki, A. The immunology and immunopathology of COVID-19. *Science* **2022**, *375*, 1122–1127. [CrossRef]
64. Chu, H.; Chan, J.F.; Wang, Y.; Yuen, T.T.; Chai, Y.; Shuai, H.; Yang, D.; Hu, B.; Huang, X.; Zhang, X.; et al. SARS-CoV-2 Induces a More Robust Innate Immune Response and Replicates Less Efficiently Than SARS-CoV in the Human Intestines: An Ex Vivo Study with Implications on Pathogenesis of COVID-19. *Cell Mol. Gastroenterol. Hepatol.* **2021**, *11*, 771–781. [CrossRef] [PubMed]
65. Chu, H.; Chan, J.F.; Wang, Y.; Yuen, T.T.; Chai, Y.; Hou, Y.; Shuai, H.; Yang, D.; Hu, B.; Huang, X.; et al. Comparative Replication and Immune Activation Profiles of SARS-CoV-2 and SARS-CoV in Human Lungs: An Ex Vivo Study with Implications for the Pathogenesis of COVID-19. *Clin. Infect. Dis.* **2020**, *71*, 1400–1409. [CrossRef]
66. Hatton, C.F.; Botting, R.A.; Duenas, M.E.; Haq, I.J.; Verdon, B.; Thompson, B.J.; Spegarova, J.S.; Gothe, F.; Stephenson, E.; Gardner, A.I.; et al. Delayed induction of type I and III interferons mediates nasal epithelial cell permissiveness to SARS-CoV-2. *Nat. Commun.* **2021**, *12*, 7092. [CrossRef]
67. Bastard, P.; Gervais, A.; Le Voyer, T.; Rosain, J.; Philippot, Q.; Manry, J.; Michailidis, E.; Hoffmann, H.H.; Eto, S.; Garcia-Prat, M.; et al. Autoantibodies neutralizing type I IFNs are present in ~4% of uninfected individuals over 70 years old and account for ~20% of COVID-19 deaths. *Sci. Immunol.* **2021**, *6*, abl4340. [CrossRef]
68. Lopez, J.; Mommert, M.; Mouton, W.; Pizzorno, A.; Brengel-Pesce, K.; Mezidi, M.; Villard, M.; Lina, B.; Richard, J.C.; Fassier, J.B.; et al. Early nasal type I IFN immunity against SARS-CoV-2 is compromised in patients with autoantibodies against type I IFNs. *J. Exp. Med.* **2021**, *218*, 20211211. [CrossRef]
69. Zhang, Q.; Bastard, P.; Liu, Z.; Le Pen, J.; Moncada-Velez, M.; Chen, J.; Ogishi, M.; Sabli, I.K.D.; Hodeib, S.; Korol, C.; et al. Inborn errors of type I IFN immunity in patients with life-threatening COVID-19. *Science* **2020**, *370*, abd4570. [CrossRef]
70. Zheng, S.; Fan, J.; Yu, F.; Feng, B.; Lou, B.; Zou, Q.; Xie, G.; Lin, S.; Wang, R.; Yang, X.; et al. Viral load dynamics and disease severity in patients infected with SARS-CoV-2 in Zhejiang province, China, January-March 2020: Retrospective cohort study. *BMJ* **2020**, *369*, m1443. [CrossRef]
71. Wang, X.; Zheng, J.; Guo, L.; Yao, H.; Wang, L.; Xia, X.; Zhang, W. Fecal viral shedding in COVID-19 patients: Clinical significance, viral load dynamics and survival analysis. *Virus Res.* **2020**, *289*, 198147. [CrossRef] [PubMed]
72. Peccia, J.; Zulli, A.; Brackney, D.E.; Grubaugh, N.D.; Kaplan, E.H.; Casanovas-Massana, A.; Ko, A.I.; Malik, A.A.; Wang, D.; Wang, M.; et al. Measurement of SARS-CoV-2 RNA in wastewater tracks community infection dynamics. *Nat. Biotechnol.* **2020**, *38*, 1164–1167. [CrossRef] [PubMed]

73. Xiao, F.; Tang, M.; Zheng, X.; Liu, Y.; Li, X.; Shan, H. Evidence for Gastrointestinal Infection of SARS-CoV-2. *Gastroenterology* **2020**, *158*, 1831–1833. [CrossRef] [PubMed]
74. Lehmann, M.; Allers, K.; Heldt, C.; Meinhardt, J.; Schmidt, F.; Rodriguez-Sillke, Y.; Kunkel, D.; Schumann, M.; Bottcher, C.; Stahl-Hennig, C.; et al. Human small intestinal infection by SARS-CoV-2 is characterized by a mucosal infiltration with activated CD8+ T cells. *Mucosal. Immunol.* **2021**, *14*, 1381–1392. [CrossRef]
75. Lin, L.; Jiang, X.; Zhang, Z.; Huang, S.; Zhang, Z.; Fang, Z.; Gu, Z.; Gao, L.; Shi, H.; Mai, L.; et al. Gastrointestinal symptoms of 95 cases with SARS-CoV-2 infection. *Gut* **2020**, *69*, 997–1001. [CrossRef]
76. Gaebler, C.; Wang, Z.; Lorenzi, J.C.C.; Muecksch, F.; Finkin, S.; Tokuyama, M.; Cho, A.; Jankovic, M.; Schaefer-Babajew, D.; Oliveira, T.Y.; et al. Evolution of antibody immunity to SARS-CoV-2. *Nature* **2021**, *591*, 639–644. [CrossRef]
77. Blanco-Melo, D.; Nilsson-Payant, B.E.; Liu, W.C.; Uhl, S.; Hoagland, D.; Moller, R.; Jordan, T.X.; Oishi, K.; Panis, M.; Sachs, D.; et al. Imbalanced Host Response to SARS-CoV-2 Drives Development of COVID-19. *Cell* **2020**, *181*, 1036–1045. [CrossRef]
78. Galani, I.E.; Rovina, N.; Lampropoulou, V.; Triantafyllia, V.; Manioudaki, M.; Pavlos, E.; Koukaki, E.; Fragkou, P.C.; Panou, V.; Rapti, V.; et al. Untuned antiviral immunity in COVID-19 revealed by temporal type I/III interferon patterns and flu comparison. *Nat. Immunol.* **2021**, *22*, 32–40. [CrossRef]
79. Rouchka, E.C.; Chariker, J.H.; Alejandro, B.; Adcock, R.S.; Singhal, R.; Ramirez, J.; Palmer, K.E.; Lasnik, A.B.; Carrico, R.; Arnold, F.W.; et al. Induction of interferon response by high viral loads at early stage infection may protect against severe outcomes in COVID-19 patients. *Sci. Rep.* **2021**, *11*, 15715. [CrossRef]
80. Wang, E.Y.; Mao, T.; Klein, J.; Dai, Y.; Huck, J.D.; Jaycox, J.R.; Liu, F.; Zhou, T.; Israelow, B.; Wong, P.; et al. Diverse functional autoantibodies in patients with COVID-19. *Nature* **2021**, *595*, 283–288. [CrossRef]
81. Shou, S.; Liu, M.; Yang, Y.; Kang, N.; Song, Y.; Tan, D.; Liu, N.; Wang, F.; Liu, J.; Xie, Y. Animal Models for COVID-19: Hamsters, Mouse, Ferret, Mink, Tree Shrew, and Non-human Primates. *Front Microbiol.* **2021**, *12*, 626553. [CrossRef] [PubMed]
82. Sia, S.F.; Yan, L.M.; Chin, A.W.H.; Fung, K.; Choy, K.T.; Wong, A.Y.L.; Kaewpreedee, P.; Perera, R.; Poon, L.L.M.; Nicholls, J.M.; et al. Pathogenesis and transmission of SARS-CoV-2 in golden hamsters. *Nature* **2020**, *583*, 834–838. [CrossRef] [PubMed]
83. Shuai, L.; Zhong, G.; Yuan, Q.; Wen, Z.; Wang, C.; He, X.; Liu, R.; Wang, J.; Zhao, Q.; Liu, Y.; et al. Replication, pathogenicity, and transmission of SARS-CoV-2 in minks. *Natl. Sci. Rev.* **2021**, *8*, nwaa291. [CrossRef] [PubMed]
84. Li, S.; Zhang, Y.; Guan, Z.; Li, H.; Ye, M.; Chen, X.; Shen, J.; Zhou, Y.; Shi, Z.L.; Zhou, P.; et al. SARS-CoV-2 triggers inflammatory responses and cell death through caspase-8 activation. *Signal Transduct. Target Ther.* **2020**, *5*, 235. [CrossRef] [PubMed]
85. Vanuytsel, T.; Tack, J.; Farre, R. The Role of Intestinal Permeability in Gastrointestinal Disorders and Current Methods of Evaluation. *Front Nutr.* **2021**, *8*, 717925. [CrossRef]
86. Heuberger, J.; Trimpert, J.; Vladimirova, D.; Goosmann, C.; Lin, M.; Schmuck, R.; Mollenkopf, H.J.; Brinkmann, V.; Tacke, F.; Osterrieder, N.; et al. Epithelial response to IFN-gamma promotes SARS-CoV-2 infection. *EMBO Mol. Med.* **2021**, *13*, e13191. [CrossRef]
87. Sencio, V.; Machelart, A.; Robil, C.; Benech, N.; Hoffmann, E.; Galbert, C.; Deryuter, L.; Heumel, S.; Hantute-Ghesquier, A.; Flourens, A.; et al. Alteration of the gut microbiota following SARS-CoV-2 infection correlates with disease severity in hamsters. *Gut Microbes* **2022**, *14*, 2018900. [CrossRef]
88. Lee, A.C.; Zhang, A.J.; Chan, J.F.; Li, C.; Fan, Z.; Liu, F.; Chen, Y.; Liang, R.; Sridhar, S.; Cai, J.P.; et al. Oral SARS-CoV-2 Inoculation Establishes Subclinical Respiratory Infection with Virus Shedding in Golden Syrian Hamsters. *Cell Rep. Med.* **2020**, *1*, 100121. [CrossRef]
89. Chan, J.F.; Yuan, S.; Zhang, A.J.; Poon, V.K.; Chan, C.C.; Lee, A.C.; Fan, Z.; Li, C.; Liang, R.; Cao, J.; et al. Surgical Mask Partition Reduces the Risk of Noncontact Transmission in a Golden Syrian Hamster Model for Coronavirus Disease 2019 (COVID-19). *Clin. Infect. Dis.* **2020**, *71*, 2139–2149. [CrossRef]
90. Hoel, H.; Heggelund, L.; Reikvam, D.H.; Stiksrud, B.; Ueland, T.; Michelsen, A.E.; Otterdal, K.; Muller, K.E.; Lind, A.; Muller, F.; et al. Elevated markers of gut leakage and inflammasome activation in COVID-19 patients with cardiac involvement. *J. Intern. Med.* **2021**, *289*, 523–531. [CrossRef]
91. Prasad, R.; Patton, M.J.; Floyd, J.L.; Vieira, C.P.; Fortmann, S.; DuPont, M.; Harbour, A.; Jeremy, C.S.; Wright, J.; Lamendella, R.; et al. Plasma microbiome in COVID-19 subjects: An indicator of gut barrier defects and dysbiosis. *bioRxiv* **2021**. [CrossRef] [PubMed]
92. Giron, L.B.; Dweep, H.; Yin, X.; Wang, H.; Damra, M.; Goldman, A.R.; Gorman, N.; Palmer, C.S.; Tang, H.Y.; Shaikh, M.W.; et al. Plasma Markers of Disrupted Gut Permeability in Severe COVID-19 Patients. *Front Immunol.* **2021**, *12*, 686240. [CrossRef] [PubMed]
93. Mitsuyama, K.; Tsuruta, K.; Takedatsu, H.; Yoshioka, S.; Morita, M.; Niwa, M.; Matsumoto, S. Clinical Features and Pathogenic Mechanisms of Gastrointestinal Injury in COVID-19. *J. Clin. Med.* **2020**, *9*, 3630. [CrossRef]
94. Name, J.J.; Souza, A.C.R.; Vasconcelos, A.R.; Prado, P.S.; Pereira, C.P.M. Zinc, Vitamin D and Vitamin C: Perspectives for COVID-19 with a Focus on Physical Tissue Barrier Integrity. *Front Nutr.* **2020**, *7*, 606398. [CrossRef] [PubMed]
95. Scaldaferri, F.; Ianiro, G.; Privitera, G.; Lopetuso, L.R.; Vetrone, L.M.; Petito, V.; Pugliese, D.; Neri, M.; Cammarota, G.; Ringel, Y.; et al. The Thrilling Journey of SARS-CoV-2 into the Intestine: From Pathogenesis to Future Clinical Implications. *Inflamm. Bowel. Dis.* **2020**, *26*, 1306–1314. [CrossRef] [PubMed]
96. Mogensen, T.H.; Paludan, S.R. Molecular pathways in virus-induced cytokine production. *Microbiol. Mol. Biol. Rev.* **2001**, *65*, 131–150. [CrossRef] [PubMed]

97. Ezeonwumelu, I.J.; Garcia-Vidal, E.; Ballana, E. JAK-STAT Pathway: A Novel Target to Tackle Viral Infections. *Viruses* **2021**, *13*, 2379. [CrossRef]
98. Fric, J.; Zelante, T.; Wong, A.Y.; Mertes, A.; Yu, H.B.; Ricciardi-Castagnoli, P. NFAT control of innate immunity. *Blood* **2012**, *120*, 1380–1389. [CrossRef]
99. Rockx, B.; Kuiken, T.; Herfst, S.; Bestebroer, T.; Lamers, M.M.; Oude Munnink, B.B.; de Meulder, D.; van Amerongen, G.; van den Brand, J.; Okba, N.M.A.; et al. Comparative pathogenesis of COVID-19, MERS, and SARS in a nonhuman primate model. *Science* **2020**, *368*, 1012–1015. [CrossRef]
100. Nelson, C.E.; Namasivayam, S.; Foreman, T.W.; Kauffman, K.D.; Sakai, S.; Dorosky, D.E.; Lora, N.E.; NIAID/DIR Tuberculosis Imaging Program; Brooks, K.; Potter, E.L.; et al. Mild SARS-CoV-2 infection in rhesus macaques is associated with viral control prior to antigen-specific T cell responses in tissues. *Sci. Immunol.* **2022**, *2022*, eabo0535. [CrossRef]
101. Zohar, T.; Loos, C.; Fischinger, S.; Atyeo, C.; Wang, C.; Slein, M.D.; Burke, J.; Yu, J.; Feldman, J.; Hauser, B.M.; et al. Compromised Humoral Functional Evolution Tracks with SARS-CoV-2 Mortality. *Cell* **2020**, *183*, 1508–1519. [CrossRef] [PubMed]
102. Chan, J.F.; Zhang, A.J.; Yuan, S.; Poon, V.K.; Chan, C.C.; Lee, A.C.; Chan, W.M.; Fan, Z.; Tsoi, H.W.; Wen, L.; et al. Simulation of the Clinical and Pathological Manifestations of Coronavirus Disease 2019 (COVID-19) in a Golden Syrian Hamster Model: Implications for Disease Pathogenesis and Transmissibility. *Clin. Infect. Dis.* **2020**, *71*, 2428–2446. [CrossRef]
103. Qian, Q.; Fan, L.; Liu, W.; Li, J.; Yue, J.; Wang, M.; Ke, X.; Yin, Y.; Chen, Q.; Jiang, C. Direct Evidence of Active SARS-CoV-2 Replication in the Intestine. *Clin. Infect. Dis.* **2021**, *73*, 361–366. [CrossRef]
104. Roy, K.; Agarwal, S.; Banerjee, R.; Paul, M.K.; Purbey, P.K. COVID-19 and gut immunomodulation. *World J. Gastroenterol.* **2021**, *27*, 7925–7942. [CrossRef] [PubMed]
105. Zhou, F.; Yu, T.; Du, R.; Fan, G.; Liu, Y.; Liu, Z.; Xiang, J.; Wang, Y.; Song, B.; Gu, X.; et al. Clinical course and risk factors for mortality of adult inpatients with COVID-19 in Wuhan, China: A retrospective cohort study. *Lancet* **2020**, *395*, 1054–1062. [CrossRef]
106. Chen, L.; Long, X.; Xu, Q.; Tan, J.; Wang, G.; Cao, Y.; Wei, J.; Luo, H.; Zhu, H.; Huang, L.; et al. Elevated serum levels of S100A8/A9 and HMGB1 at hospital admission are correlated with inferior clinical outcomes in COVID-19 patients. *Cell Mol. Immunol.* **2020**, *17*, 992–994. [CrossRef]
107. Stefan, N.; Sippel, K.; Heni, M.; Fritsche, A.; Wagner, R.; Jakob, C.E.M.; Preissl, H.; von Werder, A.; Khodamoradi, Y.; Borgmann, S.; et al. Obesity and Impaired Metabolic Health Increase Risk of COVID-19-Related Mortality in Young and Middle-Aged Adults to the Level Observed in Older People: The LEOSS Registry. *Front Med.* **2022**, *9*, 875430. [CrossRef]
108. Winer, D.A.; Luck, H.; Tsai, S.; Winer, S. The Intestinal Immune System in Obesity and Insulin Resistance. *Cell Metab.* **2016**, *23*, 413–426. [CrossRef] [PubMed]
109. Bosco, N.; Noti, M. The aging gut microbiome and its impact on host immunity. *Genes Immun.* **2021**, *22*, 289–303. [CrossRef]
110. Chin, A.W.H.; Chu, J.T.S.; Perera, M.R.A.; Hui, K.P.Y.; Yen, H.-L.; Chan, M.C.W.; Peiris, M.; Poon, L.L.M. Stability of SARS-CoV-2 in different environmental conditions. *Lancet Microbe* **2020**, *1*, e10. [CrossRef]
111. Zhou, J.; Li, C.; Zhao, G.; Chu, H.; Wang, D.; Yan, H.H.; Poon, V.K.; Wen, L.; Wong, B.H.; Zhao, X.; et al. Human intestinal tract serves as an alternative infection route for Middle East respiratory syndrome coronavirus. *Sci. Adv.* **2017**, *3*, eaao4966. [CrossRef]
112. Harlow, J.; Dallner, M.; Nasheri, N. Protective Effect of Food Against Inactivation of Human Coronavirus OC43 by Gastrointestinal Fluids. *Food Environ. Virol.* **2022**, *14*, 212–216. [CrossRef] [PubMed]
113. Lee, S.W.; Ha, E.K.; Yeniova, A.O.; Moon, S.Y.; Kim, S.Y.; Koh, H.Y.; Yang, J.M.; Jeong, S.J.; Moon, S.J.; Cho, J.Y.; et al. Severe clinical outcomes of COVID-19 associated with proton pump inhibitors: A nationwide cohort study with propensity score matching. *Gut* **2021**, *70*, 76–84. [CrossRef]
114. Hirose, R.; Nakaya, T.; Naito, Y.; Daidoji, T.; Watanabe, Y.; Yasuda, H.; Konishi, H.; Itoh, Y. Mechanism of Human Influenza Virus RNA Persistence and Virion Survival in Feces: Mucus Protects Virions from Acid and Digestive Juices. *J. Infect. Dis.* **2017**, *216*, 105–109. [CrossRef]
115. Petrillo, M.; Brogna, C.; Cristoni, S.; Querci, M.; Piazza, O.; Van den Eede, G. Increase of SARS-CoV-2 RNA load in faecal samples prompts for rethinking of SARS-CoV-2 biology and COVID-19 epidemiology. *F1000Research* **2021**, *10*, 370. [CrossRef]
116. Brogna, C.; Brogna, B.; Bisaccia, D.R.; Lauritano, F.; Marino, G.; Montano, L.; Cristoni, S.; Prisco, M.; Piscopo, M. Could SARS-CoV-2 Have Bacteriophage Behavior or Induce the Activity of Other Bacteriophages? *Vaccines* **2022**, *10*, 708. [CrossRef] [PubMed]
117. Petrillo, M.; Querci, M.; Brogna, C.; Ponti, J.; Cristoni, S.; Markov, P.V.; Valsesia, A.; Leoni, G.; Benedetti, A.; Wiss, T.; et al. Evidence of SARS-CoV-2 bacteriophage potential in human gut microbiota. *F1000Research* **2022**, *11*, 292. [CrossRef]
118. Liu, R.; Hong, J.; Xu, X.; Feng, Q.; Zhang, D.; Gu, Y.; Shi, J.; Zhao, S.; Liu, W.; Wang, X.; et al. Gut microbiome and serum metabolome alterations in obesity and after weight-loss intervention. *Nat. Med.* **2017**, *23*, 859–868. [CrossRef]
119. Caldera-Crespo, L.A.; Paidas, M.J.; Roy, S.; Schulman, C.I.; Kenyon, N.S.; Daunert, S.; Jayakumar, A.R. Experimental Models of COVID-19. *Front Cell Infect. Microbiol.* **2021**, *11*, 792584. [CrossRef]
120. Port, J.R.; Adney, D.R.; Schwarz, B.; Schulz, J.E.; Sturdevant, D.E.; Smith, B.J.; Avanzato, V.A.; Holbrook, M.G.; Purushotham, J.N.; Stromberg, K.A.; et al. Western diet increases COVID-19 disease severity in the Syrian hamster. *bioRxiv* **2021**. [CrossRef]
121. Jakobsson, H.E.; Rodriguez-Pineiro, A.M.; Schutte, A.; Ermund, A.; Boysen, P.; Bemark, M.; Sommer, F.; Backhed, F.; Hansson, G.C.; Johansson, M.E. The composition of the gut microbiota shapes the colon mucus barrier. *EMBO Rep.* **2015**, *16*, 164–177. [CrossRef] [PubMed]

122. Yeoh, Y.K.; Zuo, T.; Lui, G.C.; Zhang, F.; Liu, Q.; Li, A.Y.; Chung, A.C.; Cheung, C.P.; Tso, E.Y.; Fung, K.S.; et al. Gut microbiota composition reflects disease severity and dysfunctional immune responses in patients with COVID-19. *Gut* **2021**, *70*, 698–706. [CrossRef] [PubMed]
123. Moreira-Rosario, A.; Marques, C.; Pinheiro, H.; Araujo, J.R.; Ribeiro, P.; Rocha, R.; Mota, I.; Pestana, D.; Ribeiro, R.; Pereira, A.; et al. Gut Microbiota Diversity and C-Reactive Protein Are Predictors of Disease Severity in COVID-19 Patients. *Front Microbiol.* **2021**, *12*, 705020. [CrossRef]
124. Clerbaux, L.A.; Albertini, M.C.; Amigo, N.; Beronius, A.; Bezemer, G.F.G.; Coecke, S.; Daskalopoulos, E.P.; Del Giudice, G.; Greco, D.; Grenga, L.; et al. Factors Modulating COVID-19: A Mechanistic Understanding Based on the Adverse Outcome Pathway Framework. *J. Clin. Med.* **2022**, *11*, 4464. [CrossRef] [PubMed]
125. Cerrada-Romero, C.; Berastegui-Cabrera, J.; Camacho-Martinez, P.; Goikoetxea-Aguirre, J.; Perez-Palacios, P.; Santibanez, S.; Jose Blanco-Vidal, M.; Valiente, A.; Alba, J.; Rodriguez-Alvarez, R.; et al. Excretion and viability of SARS-CoV-2 in feces and its association with the clinical outcome of COVID-19. *Sci. Rep.* **2022**, *12*, 7397. [CrossRef] [PubMed]
126. Wolfel, R.; Corman, V.M.; Guggemos, W.; Seilmaier, M.; Zange, S.; Muller, M.A.; Niemeyer, D.; Jones, T.C.; Vollmar, P.; Rothe, C.; et al. Virological assessment of hospitalized patients with COVID-2019. *Nature* **2020**, *581*, 465–469. [CrossRef]
127. Wang, D.; Hu, B.; Hu, C.; Zhu, F.; Liu, X.; Zhang, J.; Wang, B.; Xiang, H.; Cheng, Z.; Xiong, Y.; et al. Clinical Characteristics of 138 Hospitalized Patients with 2019 Novel Coronavirus-Infected Pneumonia in Wuhan, China. *JAMA* **2020**, *323*, 1061–1069.
128. Jeong, H.W.; Kim, S.M.; Kim, H.S.; Kim, Y.I.; Kim, J.H.; Cho, J.Y.; Kim, S.H.; Kang, H.; Kim, S.G.; Park, S.J.; et al. Viable SARS-CoV-2 in various specimens from COVID-19 patients. *Clin. Microbiol. Infect.* **2020**, *26*, 1520–1524. [CrossRef]
129. Liu, Y.; Li, T.; Deng, Y.; Liu, S.; Zhang, D.; Li, H.; Wang, X.; Jia, L.; Han, J.; Bei, Z.; et al. Stability of SARS-CoV-2 on environmental surfaces and in human excreta. *J. Hosp. Infect.* **2021**, *107*, 105–107. [CrossRef]
130. Dergham, J.; Delerce, J.; Bedotto, M.; La Scola, B.; Moal, V. Isolation of Viable SARS-CoV-2 Virus from Feces of an Immunocompromised Patient Suggesting a Possible Fecal Mode of Transmission. *J. Clin. Med.* **2021**, *10*, 2696. [CrossRef]
131. Mendenhall, I.H.; Kerimbayev, A.A.; Strochkov, V.M.; Sultankulova, K.T.; Kopeyev, S.K.; Su, Y.C.F.; Smith, G.J.D.; Orynbayev, M.B. Discovery and Characterization of Novel Bat Coronavirus Lineages from Kazakhstan. *Viruses* **2019**, *11*, 356. [CrossRef] [PubMed]
132. Temmam, S.; Vongphayloth, K.; Baquero, E.; Munier, S.; Bonomi, M.; Regnault, B.; Douangboubpha, B.; Karami, Y.; Chretien, D.; Sanamxay, D.; et al. Bat coronaviruses related to SARS-CoV-2 and infectious for human cells. *Nature* **2022**, *604*, 330–336. [CrossRef] [PubMed]
133. Kazemian, N.; Kao, D.; Pakpour, S. Fecal Microbiota Transplantation during and Post-COVID-19 Pandemic. *Int. J. Mol. Sci.* **2021**, *22*, 4. [CrossRef] [PubMed]
134. Ahmed, W.; Angel, N.; Edson, J.; Bibby, K.; Bivins, A.; O'Brien, J.W.; Choi, P.M.; Kitajima, M.; Simpson, S.L.; Li, J.; et al. First confirmed detection of SARS-CoV-2 in untreated wastewater in Australia: A proof of concept for the wastewater surveillance of COVID-19 in the community. *Sci. Total Environ.* **2020**, *728*, 138764. [CrossRef] [PubMed]
135. Gawlik, B.; Tavazzi, S.; Mariani, G.; Skejo, H.; Sponar, M.; Higgins, T.; Medema, G.; Wintgens, T. *SARS-CoV-2 Surveillance Employing Sewage: Towards a Sentinel System*; Publications Office of the European Union: Luxembourg, 2021.
136. Natarajan, A.; Zlitni, S.; Brooks, E.F.; Vance, S.E.; Dahlen, A.; Hedlin, H.; Park, R.M.; Han, A.; Schmidtke, D.T.; Verma, R.; et al. Gastrointestinal symptoms and fecal shedding of SARS-CoV-2 RNA suggest prolonged gastrointestinal infection. *Med* **2022**, *3*, 371–387.e9. [CrossRef] [PubMed]
137. Miura, F.; Kitajima, M.; Omori, R. Duration of SARS-CoV-2 viral shedding in faeces as a parameter for wastewater-based epidemiology: Re-analysis of patient data using a shedding dynamics model. *Sci. Total. Environ.* **2021**, *769*, 144549. [CrossRef]
138. Zhang, S.; Zhu, H.; Ye, H.; Hu, Y.; Zheng, N.; Huang, Z.; Xiong, Z.; Fu, L.; Cai, T. Risk factors for prolonged virus shedding of respiratory tract and fecal in adults with severe acute respiratory syndrome coronavirus-2 infection. *J. Clin. Lab. Anal.* **2021**, *35*, e23923. [CrossRef]
139. Zheng, T.; Yang, C.; Wang, H.Y.; Chen, X.; Yu, L.; Wu, Z.L.; Sun, H. Clinical characteristics and outcomes of COVID-19 patients with gastrointestinal symptoms admitted to Jianghan Fangcang Shelter Hospital in Wuhan, China. *J. Med. Virol.* **2020**, *92*, 2735–2741. [CrossRef]
140. Schettino, M.; Pellegrini, L.; Picascia, D.; Saibeni, S.; Bezzio, C.; Bini, F.; Omazzi, B.F.; Devani, M.; Arena, I.; Bongiovanni, M.; et al. Clinical Characteristics of COVID-19 Patients with Gastrointestinal Symptoms in Northern Italy: A Single-Center Cohort Study. *Am. J. Gastroenterol.* **2021**, *116*, 306–310. [CrossRef]
141. Lanthier, N.; Mahiat, C.; Henrard, S.; Starkel, P.; Gilard, I.; De Brauwer, I.; Cornette, P.; Boland, B. Gastro-intestinal symptoms are associated with a lower in-hospital mortality rate in frail older patients hospitalized for COVID-19. *Acta Gastroenterol. Belg.* **2021**, *84*, 135–136. [CrossRef]
142. Soares, R.C.M.; Mattos, L.R.; Raposo, L.M. Risk Factors for Hospitalization and Mortality due to COVID-19 in Espirito Santo State, Brazil. *Am. J. Trop. Med. Hyg.* **2020**, *103*, 1184–1190. [CrossRef]
143. Liu, J.; Cui, M.; Yang, T.; Yao, P. Correlation between gastrointestinal symptoms and disease severity in patients with COVID-19: A systematic review and meta-analysis. *BMJ Open Gastroenterol.* **2020**, *7*, e000437. [CrossRef]
144. Mao, R.; Qiu, Y.; He, J.S.; Tan, J.Y.; Li, X.H.; Liang, J.; Shen, J.; Zhu, L.R.; Chen, Y.; Iacucci, M.; et al. Manifestations and prognosis of gastrointestinal and liver involvement in patients with COVID-19: A systematic review and meta-analysis. *Lancet Gastroenterol. Hepatol.* **2020**, *5*, 667–678, Correction to *Lancet Gastroenterol. Hepatol.* **2020**, *5*, 625–710.e6. [CrossRef]

145. Wan, Y.; Li, J.; Shen, L.; Zou, Y.; Hou, L.; Zhu, L.; Faden, H.S.; Tang, Z.; Shi, M.; Jiao, N.; et al. Enteric involvement in hospitalised patients with COVID-19 outside Wuhan. *Lancet Gastroenterol. Hepatol.* **2020**, *5*, 534–535. [CrossRef]
146. Chidambaram, V.; Tun, N.L.; Haque, W.Z.; Majella, M.G.; Sivakumar, R.K.; Kumar, A.; Hsu, A.T.; Ishak, I.A.; Nur, A.A.; Ayeh, S.K.; et al. Factors associated with disease severity and mortality among patients with COVID-19: A systematic review and meta-analysis. *PLoS ONE* **2020**, *15*, e0241541. [CrossRef] [PubMed]
147. Mudatsir, M.; Fajar, J.K.; Wulandari, L.; Soegiarto, G.; Ilmawan, M.; Purnamasari, Y.; Mahdi, B.A.; Jayanto, G.D.; Suhendra, S.; Setianingsih, Y.A.; et al. Predictors of COVID-19 severity: A systematic review and meta-analysis. *F1000Research* **2020**, *9*, 1107. [CrossRef]
148. Doig, C.J.; Sutherland, L.R.; Sandham, J.D.; Fick, G.H.; Verhoef, M.; Meddings, J.B. Increased intestinal permeability is associated with the development of multiple organ dysfunction syndrome in critically ill ICU patients. *Am. J. Respir. Crit. Care Med.* **1998**, *158*, 444–451. [CrossRef]
149. Fajgenbaum, D.C.; June, C.H. Cytokine Storm. *N. Engl. J. Med.* **2020**, *383*, 2255–2273. [CrossRef]
150. Mulchandani, R.; Lyngdoh, T.; Kakkar, A.K. Deciphering the COVID-19 cytokine storm: Systematic review and meta-analysis. *Eur. J. Clin. Investig.* **2021**, *51*, e13429. [CrossRef]
151. Rhee, S.H. Lipopolysaccharide: Basic biochemistry, intracellular signaling, and physiological impacts in the gut. *Intest. Res.* **2014**, *12*, 90–95. [CrossRef]
152. Openshaw, P.J. Crossing barriers: Infections of the lung and the gut. *Mucosal. Immunol.* **2009**, *2*, 100–102. [CrossRef] [PubMed]
153. Cardinale, V.; Capurso, G.; Ianiro, G.; Gasbarrini, A.; Arcidiacono, P.G.; Alvaro, D. Intestinal permeability changes with bacterial translocation as key events modulating systemic host immune response to SARS-CoV-2: A working hypothesis. *Dig. Liver. Dis.* **2020**, *52*, 1383–1389. [CrossRef]
154. Vignesh, R.; Swathirajan, C.R.; Tun, Z.H.; Rameshkumar, M.R.; Solomon, S.S.; Balakrishnan, P. Could Perturbation of Gut Microbiota Possibly Exacerbate the Severity of COVID-19 via Cytokine Storm? *Front Immunol.* **2020**, *11*, 607734. [CrossRef]
155. Venzon, M.; Bernard-Raichon, L.; Klein, J.; Axelrad, J.E.; Zhang, C.; Hussey, G.A.; Sullivan, A.P.; Casanovas-Massana, A.; Noval, M.G.; Valero-Jimenez, A.M.; et al. Gut microbiome dysbiosis during COVID-19 is associated with increased risk for bacteremia and microbial translocation. *bioRxiv* **2022**. [CrossRef]
156. Manna, S.; Baindara, P.; Mandal, S.M. Molecular pathogenesis of secondary bacterial infection associated to viral infections including SARS-CoV-2. *J. Infect. Public Health* **2020**, *13*, 1397–1404. [CrossRef] [PubMed]
157. Antoni, L.; Nuding, S.; Wehkamp, J.; Stange, E.F. Intestinal barrier in inflammatory bowel disease. *World J. Gastroenterol.* **2014**, *20*, 1165–1179. [CrossRef] [PubMed]
158. Turpin, W.; Lee, S.H.; Raygoza Garay, J.A.; Madsen, K.L.; Meddings, J.B.; Bedrani, L.; Power, N.; Espin-Garcia, O.; Xu, W.; Smith, M.I.; et al. Increased Intestinal Permeability Is Associated with Later Development of Crohn's Disease. *Gastroenterology* **2020**, *159*, 2092–2100. [CrossRef] [PubMed]
159. Hollander, D.; Vadheim, C.M.; Brettholz, E.; Petersen, G.M.; Delahunty, T.; Rotter, J.I. Increased intestinal permeability in patients with Crohn's disease and their relatives. A possible etiologic factor. *Ann. Intern. Med.* **1986**, *105*, 883–885. [CrossRef]
160. May, G.R.; Sutherland, L.R.; Meddings, J.B. Is small intestinal permeability really increased in relatives of patients with Crohn's disease? *Gastroenterology* **1993**, *104*, 1627–1632. [CrossRef]
161. Arrieta, M.C.; Madsen, K.; Doyle, J.; Meddings, J. Reducing small intestinal permeability attenuates colitis in the IL10 gene-deficient mouse. *Gut* **2009**, *58*, 41–48. [CrossRef] [PubMed]
162. Di Micco, S.; Musella, S.; Sala, M.; Scala, M.C.; Andrei, G.; Snoeck, R.; Bifulco, G.; Campiglia, P.; Fasano, A. Peptide Derivatives of the Zonulin Inhibitor Larazotide (AT1001) as Potential Anti SARS-CoV-2: Molecular Modelling, Synthesis and Bioactivity Evaluation. *Int. J. Mol. Sci.* **2021**, *22*, 9367. [CrossRef] [PubMed]
163. Lin, S.; Lau, L.H.; Chanchlani, N.; Kennedy, N.A.; Ng, S.C. Recent advances in clinical practice: Management of inflammatory bowel disease during the COVID-19 pandemic. *Gut* **2022**, *71*, 1426–1439. [CrossRef] [PubMed]
164. Gu, S.; Chen, Y.; Wu, Z.; Chen, Y.; Gao, H.; Lv, L.; Guo, F.; Zhang, X.; Luo, R.; Huang, C.; et al. Alterations of the Gut Microbiota in Patients with Coronavirus Disease 2019 or H1N1 Influenza. *Clin. Infect. Dis.* **2020**, *71*, 2669–2678. [CrossRef]
165. Zuo, T.; Zhang, F.; Lui, G.C.Y.; Yeoh, Y.K.; Li, A.Y.L.; Zhan, H.; Wan, Y.; Chung, A.C.K.; Cheung, C.P.; Chen, N.; et al. Alterations in Gut Microbiota of Patients with COVID-19 During Time of Hospitalization. *Gastroenterology* **2020**, *159*, 944–955. [CrossRef] [PubMed]
166. Venzon, M.; Bernard-Raichon, L.; Klein, J.; Axelrad, J.; Hussey, G.; Sullivan, A.; Casanovas-Massana, A.; Noval, M.; Valero-Jimenez, A.; Gago, J.; et al. Gut microbiome dysbiosis during COVID-19 is associated with increased risk for bacteremia and microbial translocation. *Res. Sq.* **2021**. [CrossRef]
167. Clerbaux, L.-A.; Fillipovska, J.; Muñoz, A.; Petrillo, M.; Coecke, S.; Amorim, M.-J.; Grenga, L. Mechanisms leading to gut dysbiosis in COVID-19: Current evidence and uncertainties based on putative adverse outcome pathways. *J. Clin. Med.* **2022**, Submitted. [CrossRef]
168. He, Y.; Wang, J.; Li, F.; Shi, Y. Main Clinical Features of COVID-19 and Potential Prognostic and Therapeutic Value of the Microbiota in SARS-CoV-2 Infections. *Front Microbiol.* **2020**, *11*, 1302. [CrossRef] [PubMed]
169. Toussaint, B.; Raffael, B.; Petrillo, M.; Puertas Gallardo, A.; Munoz-Pineiro, A.; Patak Dennstedt, A.; Querci, M. *Relationship between the Gut Microbiome and Diseases, Including COVID-19*; JRC125924; Publications Office of the European Union: Luxembourg, 2021. [CrossRef]

170. Baindara, P.; Chakraborty, R.; Holliday, Z.M.; Mandal, S.M.; Schrum, A.G. Oral probiotics in coronavirus disease 2019: Connecting the gut-lung axis to viral pathogenesis, inflammation, secondary infection and clinical trials. *New Microbes New Infect.* **2021**, *40*, 100837. [CrossRef]
171. Sultan, S.; Altayar, O.; Siddique, S.M.; Davitkov, P.; Feuerstein, J.D.; Lim, J.K.; Falck-Ytter, Y.; El-Serag, H.B.; AGA Institute. AGA Institute Rapid Review of the Gastrointestinal and Liver Manifestations of COVID-19, Meta-Analysis of International Data, and Recommendations for the Consultative Management of Patients with COVID-19. *Gastroenterology* **2020**, *159*, 320–334.e27. [CrossRef]
172. El Ouali, S.; Achkar, J.P.; Lashner, B.; Regueiro, M. Gastrointestinal manifestations of COVID-19. *Cleve Clin. J. Med.* **2021**. [CrossRef]
173. Wu, Y.; Guo, C.; Tang, L.; Hong, Z.; Zhou, J.; Dong, X.; Yin, H.; Xiao, Q.; Tang, Y.; Qu, X.; et al. Prolonged presence of SARS-CoV-2 viral RNA in faecal samples. *Lancet Gastroenterol. Hepatol.* **2020**, *5*, 434–435. [CrossRef]
174. Carfi, A.; Bernabei, R.; Landi, F.; Gemelli Against, C.-P.-A.C.S.G. Persistent Symptoms in Patients After Acute COVID-19. *JAMA* **2020**, *324*, 603–605. [CrossRef]
175. Al-Aly, Z.; Xie, Y.; Bowe, B. High-dimensional characterization of post-acute sequelae of COVID-19. *Nature* **2021**, *594*, 259–264. [CrossRef]
176. Zollner, A.; Koch, R.; Jukic, A.; Pfister, A.; Meyer, M.; Rossler, A.; Kimpel, J.; Adolph, T.E.; Tilg, H. Postacute COVID-19 is Characterized by Gut Viral Antigen Persistence in Inflammatory Bowel Diseases. *Gastroenterology* **2022**, *163*, 495–506.e8. [CrossRef] [PubMed]
177. Arostegui, D.; Castro, K.; Schwarz, S.; Vaidy, K.; Rabinowitz, S.; Wallach, T. Persistent SARS-CoV-2 Nucleocapsid Protein Presence in the Intestinal Epithelium of a Pediatric Patient 3 Months After Acute Infection. *JPGN Rep.* **2022**, *3*, e152. [CrossRef]
178. Liu, Q.; Mak, J.W.Y.; Su, Q.; Yeoh, Y.K.; Lui, G.C.; Ng, S.S.S.; Zhang, F.; Li, A.Y.L.; Lu, W.; Hui, D.S.; et al. Gut microbiota dynamics in a prospective cohort of patients with post-acute COVID-19 syndrome. *Gut* **2022**, *71*, 544–552. [CrossRef]
179. Cheung, C.C.L.; Goh, D.; Lim, X.; Tien, T.Z.; Lim, J.C.T.; Lee, J.N.; Tan, B.; Tay, Z.E.A.; Wan, W.Y.; Chen, E.X.; et al. Residual SARS-CoV-2 viral antigens detected in GI and hepatic tissues from five recovered patients with COVID-19. *Gut* **2022**, *71*, 226–229. [CrossRef] [PubMed]
180. Ledford, H. Coronavirus 'ghosts' found lingering in the gut. *Nature* **2022**, *605*, 408–409. [CrossRef] [PubMed]
181. Sefik, E.; Israelow, B.; Mirza, H.; Zhao, J.; Qu, R.; Kaffe, E.; Song, E.; Halene, S.; Meffre, E.; Kluger, Y.; et al. A humanized mouse model of chronic COVID-19. *Nat. Biotechnol.* **2022**, *40*, 906–920. [CrossRef]
182. Frere, J.J.; Serafini, R.A.; Pryce, K.D.; Zazhytska, M.; Oishi, K.; Golynker, I.; Panis, M.; Zimering, J.; Horiuchi, S.; Hoagland, D.A.; et al. SARS-CoV-2 infection in hamsters and humans results in lasting and unique systemic perturbations post recovery. *Sci. Transl. Med.* **2022**, *2022*, eabq3059. [CrossRef] [PubMed]
183. WHO. Coronavirus Disease (COVID-19): Post COVID-19 Condition. Available online: https://www.who.int/news-room/questions-and-answers/item/coronavirus-disease-(covid-19)-post-covid-19-condition (accessed on 15 June 2022).
184. Centers for Disease Control and Prevention (CDC). Long COVID or Post-COVID Conditions. Available online: https://www.cdc.gov/coronavirus/2019-ncov/long-term-effects/index.html (accessed on 15 June 2022).
185. Davis, H.E.; Assaf, G.S.; McCorkell, L.; Wei, H.; Low, R.J.; Re'em, Y.; Redfield, S.; Austin, J.P.; Akrami, A. Characterizing long COVID in an international cohort: 7 months of symptoms and their impact. *EClinicalMedicine* **2021**, *38*, 101019. [CrossRef] [PubMed]

MDPI
St. Alban-Anlage 66
4052 Basel
Switzerland
Tel. +41 61 683 77 34
Fax +41 61 302 89 18
www.mdpi.com

Journal of Clinical Medicine Editorial Office
E-mail: jcm@mdpi.com
www.mdpi.com/journal/jcm

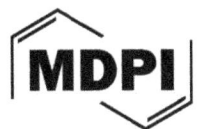

www.ingramcontent.com/pod-product-compliance
Lightning Source LLC
LaVergne TN
LVHW070654100526
838202LV00013B/961